BASIC AUDIOLOGIC EVALUATION

BASIC AUDIOLOGIC EVALUATION

William R. Hodgson, Ph.D.
Professor, Department of Speech and Hearing Sciences
University of Arizona
Tucson, Arizona

WILLIAMS & WILKINS
Baltimore/London

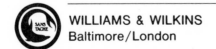

Made in the United States of America

Library of Congress Cataloging in Publication Data

Hodgson, William R
Basic audiologic evaluation.
Bibliography: p.
Includes indexes.
1. Audiometry. I. Title [DNLM: 1. Hearing tests. WV272 H691b]
RF294.H63 617.8 80-12883
ISBN 0-683-04091-X

Composed and printed at the
Waverly Press, Inc.
Mt. Royal and Guilford Aves.
Baltimore, MD 21202, U.S.A.

Preface

I feel too little attention is given to preparing students for administration of the basic audiologic evaluation. Students coming into our graduate program routinely tell me they have had a course which covered the basic audiologic evaluation. Frequently, it develops that the course to which they referred was a survey in which they did not study the basic test battery in depth. Therefore, students may begin clinical practice in audiology without having come to grips with problems of masking, valid bone conduction testing, patient control, or assessment of the validity and meaning of auditory test results.

The basic audiologic evaluation involves concepts as difficult as any area of clinical audiology. The difficulty of obtaining consistently valid pure tone thresholds is often underestimated. Air conduction threshold testing of a cooperative adult is simple. Obtaining valid thresholds from an uncooperative, very young, old, or ill person with a complex hearing loss can be most difficult. Knowledge, skill, and the ability to understand and control behavior are required.

The purpose of this book is a thorough study of the administration of the basic audiologic evaluation as well as validation and interpretation of test results. The major tests discussed are pure tone air and bone conduction threshold audiometry, speech threshold and discrimination assessment, and basic impedance measurement. I hope that students, before reading this text, will have had a course in hearing science to verse them in the structure and function of the ear, the physical aspects of sound, and the measurement units used in auditory testing.

I am indebted to Ron Leavitt for reading the manuscript and for his many helpful suggestions. I would like to thank LeAnn Marin, Lorin Wilde, and Leslie Peterson for their help in preparing the manuscript. I am grateful to my wife and children for their assistance and support.

William R. Hodgson, Ph.D.

Contents

CHAPTER 1 The Audiologic Evaluation

With some overlap and exclusions, auditory tests can be divided into four areas: (1) the basic test battery, (2) pediatric assessment, (3) site-of-lesion testing, and (4) hearing aid evaluation. The basic battery establishes the magnitude and configuration of hearing loss, assesses ability to differentiate sounds, and provides some insight into the type of loss and possible etiology. Pediatric assessment involves special techniques appropriate for testing children. In addition to hearing testing, pediatric assessment may require measurement of other functions affected by impaired hearing, such as language development. Site-of-lesion testing involves special auditory tests which help to locate the source of the problem in the auditory system. Some site-of-lesion testing is routinely included in the basic battery. Hearing aid evaluation provides an estimate of how much a person needs and may benefit from amplification. Ordinarily the basic test battery is an important preliminary to both site-of-lesion testing and hearing aid evaluation.

This text covers only the basic test battery. Pediatric assessment, site-of-lesion testing beyond that routinely included in the basic battery, and hearing aid evaluation are not discussed in detail. For more information about pediatric assessment, see Northern and Downs (1978). Site-of-lesion testing is covered by Katz (1978). Hodgson and Skinner (1977) give details of hearing aid evaluation and use. Although this text covers only the basic battery, you should be aware that many of the concepts and skills associated with the basic battery are also requisites for administration of "more advanced" auditory tests. For example, appropriate use of masking, control of patients behavior, and assessment of validity of test results are essential to all auditory tests.

THE BASIC TEST BATTERY

The objective of this book is to help you achieve competence in the administration and interpretation of the basic audiologic test battery.

Depending on philosophy and circumstances, this battery usually is made up of the tests described below.

Pure tone air conduction thresholds provide a measure of hearing sensitivity as a function of frequency. When a hearing loss is present, the pure tone air conduction test indicates reduced hearing sensitivity.

Pure tone bone conduction thresholds are obtained when air conduction testing indicates reduced hearing sensitivity. Bone conduction evaluation is intended to be a direct measure of inner ear sensitivity. Comparison of air and bone conduction thresholds establishes the location in the peripheral auditory system of the problem causing the hearing loss. In other words, the type of hearing loss can be established.

Speech thresholds, through agreement with pure tone threshold averages, corroborate pure tone test results and constitute a direct measure of hearing sensitivity for speech. Disagreement between speech threshold and pure tone threshold averages suggests invalid results and the need for additional testing to establish actual thresholds.

Speech discrimination testing measures the patient's ability to differentiate speech sounds. Discrimination ability is an important auditory function which may be affected in varying amounts, depending on the type, etiology, and magnitude of hearing loss. Auditory discrimination scores contribute to estimates of the amount of handicap to be expected from the hearing loss and the prognosis for rehabilitation.

Impedance measures assess the status of the middle ear (the sound conducting mechanism) as well as confirm and extend information gained in the other tests of the basic battery. Impedance measures tell us about the functioning of the Eustachian tube and the ossicular chain and the probability of fluid in the middle ear space. Additionally, impedance measures support or refute information about type of loss obtained from other tests.

These are the major tests of the basic battery. In some cases, not all are administered. In other instances, the basic battery suggests the need for additional testing.

The difficulty of obtaining consistently valid pure tone test results is often underestimated. Obtaining air conduction thresholds from a cooperative adult with normal hearing is simple. Obtaining valid thresholds from an uncooperative, very young, old, or ill person with a complex hearing loss can be quite difficult. Knowledge, skill, and the ability to understand and control behavior are required.

The basic audiologic evaluation involves concepts as difficult as those found in any phase of clinical audiology. Jerger (1974) states:

> The assumption that comparatively low-level technicians can be quickly trained to carry out basic audiometry is one of the great myths of our time. It should not go unchallenged. One of the first lessons the observant clinical

> supervisor learns is that obtaining a seemingly simple pure tone audiogram often requires a considerable degree of prior training and insight. . . . People who trust the audiograms of minimally trained personnel have not yet learned how terribly wrong they can be in all but mild to moderate, bilaterally symmetrical loss.

Good audiometry requires more than simply knowing audiometric techniques and being skillful in manipulation of audiometric controls. Price (1978) states:

> The pure tone audiometer is commonly used improperly by those who have no basic understanding of the correct underlying concepts and, as a result, improper medical diagnosis and educational placement are not an uncommon occurrence.

Mistakes made by inadequately trained individuals may include giving visual clues to which the patient may respond, incorrect instrument settings, establishing an invalid response criterion, incorrect masking procedures, and erroneous recordings of results. All of these problems emphasize the difficulty of obtaining valid test results and the importance of thorough training in administering and interpreting audiometric test results.

Accurate administration of the basic test battery should establish the presence and the characteristics of the hearing loss. Through observation of the patient's behavior and analysis of the test results the audiologist should also be able to answer the following questions:

1. Are test results valid? Should limitation be placed on interpretation of test results because of test conditions?
2. Is the loss as measured sufficient to explain the behavior observed, or is it likely that problems in addition to hearing loss are present?
3. What additional audiologic tests are indicated?
4. Do the results suggest a medical problem and the need for examination by a physician?
5. Is evaluation by other professionals indicated?
6. What are the social, educational, and vocational implications of the loss?
7. What corrective procedures are feasible?

Explanation of results to the patient or to parents of children being evaluated is an important part of the basic audiologic evaluation. Results must be explained in a way that is comprehensible and acceptable. Recommendations must be made clearly and in a fashion which will lead the patient to follow the recommendations. These topics—administration, interpretation, and explanation of the basic test battery—are discussed in the following chapters.

Before reading this book I hope you will have studied the structure and function of the auditory system. Some knowledge about the causes of hearing loss will also be helpful. It will help you to know something about the physical nature of sound—a very brief review is presented below. If you have difficulty understanding the following sections, or otherwise feel the need for more background, refer to the suggested readings at the end of this chapter.

STRUCTURE AND FUNCTION OF THE EAR

You must know something of how the ear is constructed and how it works to understand how disorders in various parts of the auditory system cause characteristic audiometric tests results. This knowledge is vital to understanding difficult audiometric procedures, such as obtaining valid bone conduction results, the proper use of masking to prevent participation of the nontest ear, and the accurate interpretation of test results.

The outer ear and the middle ear are the sound conducting parts of the peripheral auditory system. They deliver sound energy to the deeper parts of the ear and perform additional functions described below. As shown in Figure 1.1, the outer ear consists of the pinna and the external auditory canal.

The pinna is the visible part of the ear which protrudes from the head, and is not very functional in humans. The dimensions of the external auditory canal vary, about an inch in length and ¼ inch in diameter. The outer (lateral) part of the canal has cartilaginous walls while the inner (medial) part passes through the bone of the skull. In some individuals the cartilaginous part may collapse under pressure from earphones, causing difficulty in auditory testing. This problem is discussed in Chapter 3. A bend in the canal necessitates pulling the pinna upward and backward in order to see the eardrum at the end of the canal. Ear wax (cerumen) secreted into the canal may occasionally accumulate to cause a small hearing loss or difficulty in impedance testing. Resonance in the canal enhances energy of sound waves between 2000 and 4000 Hz by about 15 dB, including the small effect contributed by the pinna (Wiener and Ross, 1946).

The middle ear is a small (1–2 cm^3) air filled cavity in the temporal bone. Much of its outer (lateral) wall is made up of the eardrum, or tympanic membrane (Fig. 1.2). Through this membrane can be seen part of the outermost of three small bones which form the ossicular chain. These auditory ossicles consist of the malleus (hammer), incus (anvil), and stapes (stirrup). They are suspended within the middle ear cavity by small ligaments. The ossicular chain acts as an impedance matching system, promoting an efficient transfer between air borne energy of sound waves and fluid borne energy within the inner ear.

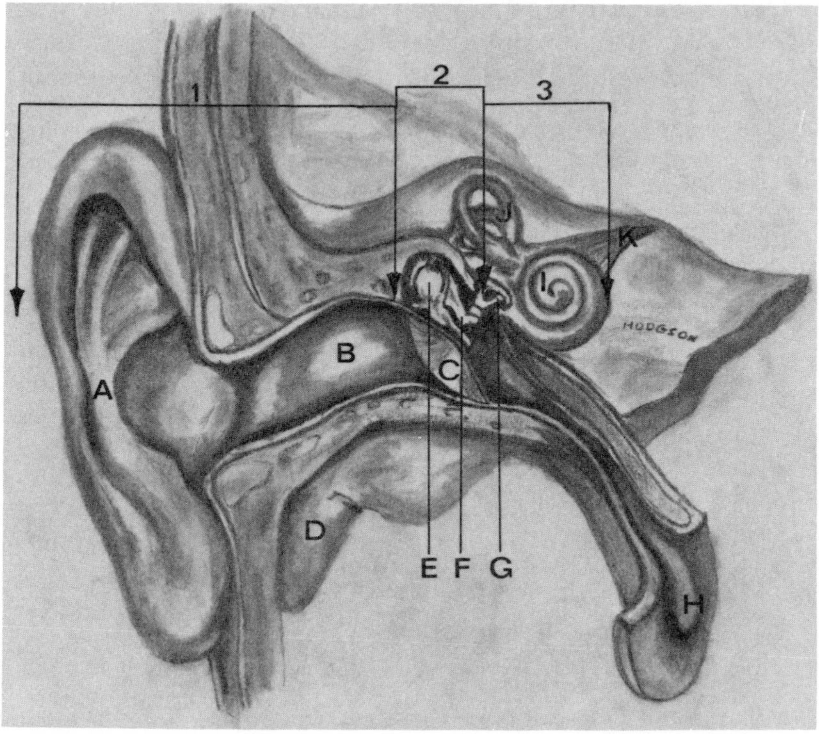

Fig. 1.1. The ear. *1*, outer ear; *2*, middle ear; *3*, inner ear (labyrinth); *A*, pinna; *B*, external ear canal; *C*, eardrum (tympanic membrane); *D*, mastoid process; *E*, malleus (hammer); *F*, incus (anvil); *G*, stapes (stirrup); *H*, Eustachian tube; *I*, cochlea; *J*, semicircular canal; *K*, VIIIth nerve.

On the front (anterior) wall of the middle ear cavity is the opening of the Eustachian tube. This tube passes to the back (posterior) wall of the nasopharynx. The part of the tube adjacent to the middle ear is bony, but that part near the nasopharynx is cartilaginous and normally closed. The tube in the region of the nasopharynx usually opens on swallowing, through the action of the tensor palatini muscle.

The roof of the middle ear cavity is a thin shelf of bone, above which is the middle cranial fossa area of the brain case. On the back (posterior) wall of the middle ear space is an opening into the large air cells of the mastoid bone. The inner (medial) wall of the middle ear space bulges outward because of the basal turn of the inner ear. This bulge is called the promontory. On the upper back (superior-posterior) edge of the promontory is the oval window, an opening between the middle and inner ear. The opening is covered with a membrane and the footplate of the stapes. On the bottom front (inferior-anterior) part of the promontory is the round window, another opening between the middle and

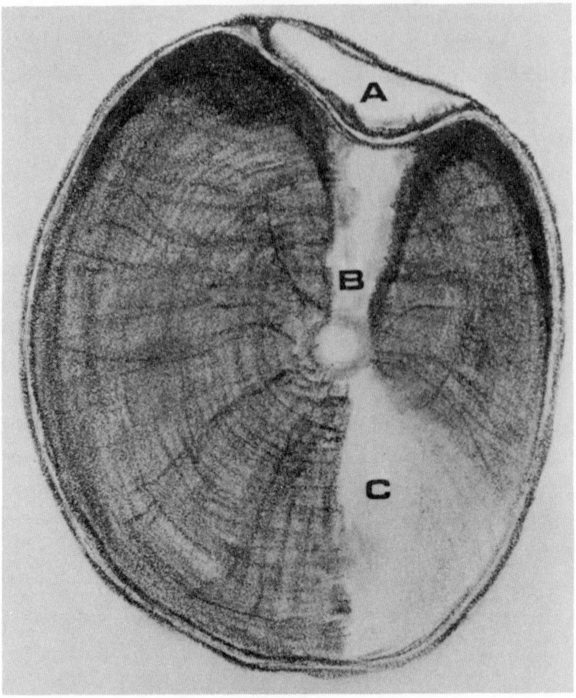

Fig. 1.2. The eardrum (tympanic membrane). *A*, *pars flaccida*, with fewer fibers, is less stiff than the rest of the eardrum; *B*, manubrium (handle) of the malleus, visible through the eardrum; *C*, cone of light reflected from examining illumination in the normal eardrum.

inner ear. This window is also covered by a membrane. The membrane permits displacement of inner ear fluid when the footplate of the stapes moves inward.

Two small muscles are associated with the middle ear. The tensor tympani muscle lies in a bony channel above the Eustachian tube. It enters the middle ear space and attaches by a tendon to the malleus. The stapedius muscle emerges from a bony cavity and attaches to the innermost bone of the ossicular chain, the stapes. When these muscles contract they increase the stiffness of the middle ear mechanism. The stapedius, innervated by the VIIth cranial (facial) nerve, contracts reflexively when an individual hears a sound of sufficient loudness. Measuring certain aspects of this acoustic reflex is an important part of impedance measures, as discussed in Chapter 7.

The walls and contents of the middle ear space are covered with mucous membrane. This lining is continuous with that of the mastoid cells behind the middle ear space and with the Eustachian tube.

The inner ear, or labyrinth, contains sections important to balance and to hearing. The bony labyrinth is a series of channels in the temporal bone and contains a fluid, perilymph. The membraneous labyrinth, inside the bony labyrinth, contains a different fluid, endolymph. Blood is supplied to the inner ear by a single artery, the internal auditory artery.

The part of the labyrinth which contributes to balance is called the vestibular system. It consists of three semicircular canals and the vestibule. Sensory cells within these structures respond to gravitational and accelerative forces. Clinically, vestibular function can be measured by insertion of cool and warm water into the ear canal. Eye movement (nystagmus) resulting from this caloric stimulation provides a measure of vestibular function.

The cochlea is the part of the inner ear concerned with hearing. It is a snail-shaped space in the temporal bone with a bony core, the modiolus. Through the internal auditory canal and the modiolus enters the cochlear part of the VIIIth cranial (auditory) nerve. The fibers are distributed throughout the cochlea.

In cross-section you can see (Fig. 1.3) that the cochlear channel is divided by membranes into three parts. The upper part is called the scala vestibuli because it opens into the vestibule. The lower part is called the scala tympani because it terminates at the round window, sometimes called the tympanic window. The triangular middle part is

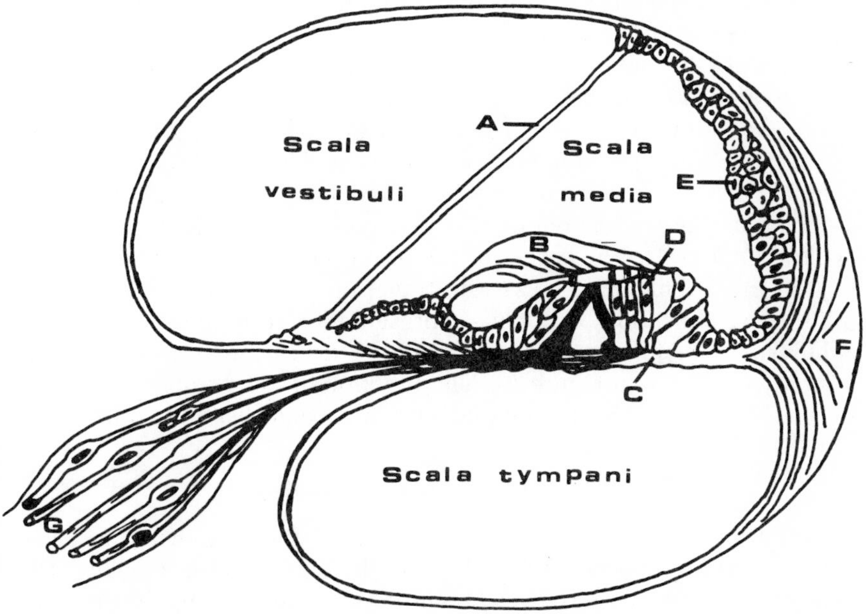

Fig. 1.3. Cross-section of the cochlea. *A*, Reissner's membrane; *B*, tectorial membrane; *C*, basilar membrane; *D*, sensory cells; *E*, stria vascularis; *F*, spiral ligament; *G*, spiral ganglion (VIIIth nerve).

called the scala media or cochlear duct. The scala media terminates just short of the apex of the bony cochlea, permitting interchange of fluid (perilymph) between scalae vestibuli and tympani. As mentioned previously, the fluid in the scala media and in the membraneous vestibular areas is endolymph.

Situated on the basilar membrane, one of the membranes which forms the scala media, is the organ of Corti. This structure, which traverses the entire length of the membraneous cochlea, contains thousands of sensory and supporting cells. The sensory cells function to convert the physical energy of sound waves into the electrical energy of nerve impulses. Fibers of the cochlear portion of the auditory nerve are distributed to these sensory cells in a complex fashion. Sound waves displace the cochlear fluid, causing distortion of the sensory cells and resultant initiation of nerve impulses. Cilia (hairs) extending from the sensory cells contact the overlying tectorial membrane. Relative movement in the scala media subjects the sensory cells to a shearing force with the tectorial membrane, which appears to be an important prelude to the generation of a nerve impulse. Mechanical properties of the basilar membrane and neural tuning of the cochlear nerve fibers implement frequency and intensity analysis. Different frequencies elicit response along different areas of the basilar membrane. The area near the base of the cochlea is important for high frequency sounds and that at the apex for low frequency sounds.

Fibers of the cochlear nerve travel from the organ of Corti into the modiolus where the cell bodies (spiral ganglion) are located. These fibers then join the vestibular branch of the nerve and travel with the facial nerve through the internal auditory canal into the brain stem. The cochlear nerve fibers terminate in the cochlear nucleus in the brain stem. From there two major pathways depart, one to travel in a complex synaptic pattern to the cortex of the brain on the same side of the ear of the origin. The other crosses to travel upward to the cortex on the other side. Thus, both ears have representation in both cerebral hemispheres. The major ascending pathways of the central auditory nervous system are shown in Figure 1.4. The function of this complex system is to integrate and reform neural impulses into a code useful to other parts of the brain.

TYPES OF HEARING LOSS

From the brief review of the structure and function of the ear, you can see that hearing loss is divisible into the types discussed below. The type of loss is based on the location of the disorder causing the problem.

Conductive Hearing Loss

Conductive disorders arise from problems in the outer or middle ear, which reduce their sound conducting ability. Examples are a buildup of

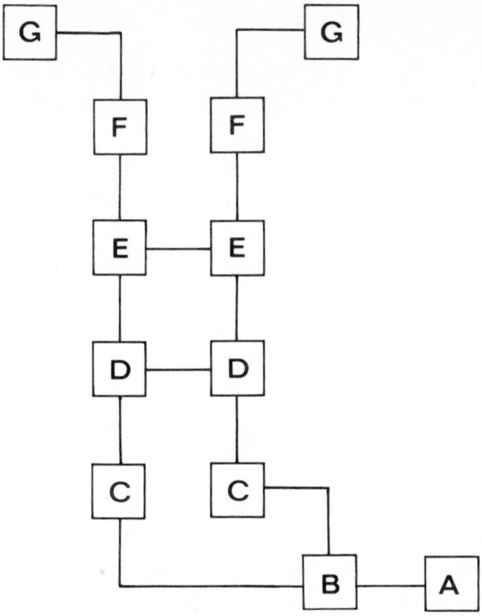

Fig. 1.4. Diagram of the ascending (afferent) pathways of the central auditory nervous system. *A*, cochlea; *B*, cochlear nucleus; *C*, superior olivary complex; *D*, lateral lemniscus; *E*, inferior colliculus; *F*, medial geniculate; *G*, auditory cortex.

wax that blocks the ear canal or fluid in the middle ear. In a purely conductive loss the inner ear remains normal but a hearing loss is present because of the reduction of sound energy reaching the inner ear.

Sensorineural Hearing Loss

Sensorineural disorders are caused by problems in the cochlea (sensory) or in the cochlear nerve (neural). The disorders are called sensorineural, rather than sensory or neural, because the basic audiologic battery does not differentiate sensory and neural pathology. An example of a sensorineural loss that is cochlear in origin is reduced sensory cell function from long exposure to high noise levels. A tumor growing on the auditory nerve can cause a neural loss. Older terms for sensorineural loss are "nerve" hearing loss and "perceptive" hearing loss.

Mixed Hearing Loss

Mixed loss consists of a conductive and a sensorineural loss coexisting in the same ear. Conductive loss is often remediable. Therefore, if the conductive disorder is successfully treated, hearing will improve, leaving only the sensorineural component. Sensorineural loss is usually permanent and irreversible.

Central Auditory Disorders

Because of the proliferation of auditory pathways in the brain, it is unlikely that damage to these pathways will cause a loss of auditory sensitivity. Rather, more subtle manifestations may occur. For example, individuals with known lesions in the central auditory nervous system have shown reduced auditory discrimination scores for distorted speech on the ear contralateral to the lesion (Snow *et al.*, 1977). More difficult to measure defects may be associated with a diffuse central auditory nervous system disorder, such as that associated with auditory processing problems (Beasley and Rintelmann, 1979). Ordinarily, the tests of the basic battery are not sensitive to the presence of a central auditory disorder.

THE DECIBEL

A brief review of the unit used to express magnitude of hearing loss may be helpful. The basic unit for reporting sound level values, the Bel, was named to honor Alexander Graham Bell. For more precise reporting the decibel (dB, 1/10 Bel) is used. The decibel is suitable for sound measurement because the values involved are usually so small and because the ranges involved are often so large. Take, for example, the difference between sounds that measure 0 and 140 dB sound pressure level (SPL). These two values approximate the level necessary for audibility and that which causes pain, respectively. On the decibel scale, a change of 140 dB is represented, but on a linear pressure scale, there is an increase of 10,000,000.

The decibel is defined as a logarithmic, dimensionless unit which expresses the ratio of two values. Let us take this rather formidable definition apart to see what it means. A logarithmic, rather than linear, scale is used to obviate the large numbers which would otherwise result because of the great range which must be covered when measuring sound values. Logarithms are exponents which tell how many times a number is to be multiplied by itself. For example, $10^2 = 10 \times 10$, or 100. The number 10 is called the base. The number 2 is the logarithm (to the base 10) of 100.

The decibel is dimensionless in the sense that it has no fixed absolute value. It is a ratio, telling the proportion by which one value is greater or less than another. Therefore, an expressed dB value must have a specified or understood reference value. Because this reference value can be changed to suit particular needs, the absolute value of the decibel is unknown unless the reference value is known.

A number of reference values are used in sound measurement. Sound power has as its usual reference value 10^{-12} W and represents the total acoustic power output of a sound source. Sound intensity, which is power per unit area, has the usual reference of 10^{-16} W/cm^2 and is the basis for measuring the sound power which flows through a square centimeter.

The dyne (or Newton) is a unit of force, and sound force is a value commonly used to express the output of bone conduction vibrators. Pressure is force per unit area, and constitutes the most common sound measurement reference, 0.0002 dyne/cm^2. The value equivalent to 0.0002 dyne/cm^2 is sometimes expressed in different fashions, all of which are equal: 0.0002 microbar or 2×10^{-5} Newtons/m^2. More recently the term 20 micro Pascals has been used. The Pascal is a pressure unit and the value equivalent to 0.0002 dyne/cm^2 is written 20 μ Pa.

Use of the word "level" means that a value is expressed in decibels. Without "level," sound values are expressed in Watts, Pascals, etc. The result of all this is a scale which can conveniently express values across a wide range without using extremely large numbers and which can be very flexible through use of different reference values. There are a few differences which separate use of the decibel from our more commonly used linear measures. Zero dB does not mean an absence of sound but rather that the sound value observed or measured is the same as the reference value. Positive dB values mean that the sound value observed is greater than the reference value, and negative dB values mean that the sound value observed is less than the reference value. Furthermore, because of the logarithmic scale, doubling pressure of a sound does not double the number of decibels. In fact, doubling sound pressure increases SPL by 6 dB. Additional relationships are shown in Table 1.1.

The sound pressure levels (dB re: 20 μ Pa) necessary for audibility of tones by a normal human ear have been established. Because sensitivity of the ear varies for different frequencies, the SPLs representing threshold vary according to the frequency of the tone in question. To simplify measurement, audiometers (instruments for measurement of auditory sensitivity) are designed so that an intensity control (hearing loss dial)

Table 1.1
Relationships Between Sound Pressure and Sound Pressure Level

Sound Pressure	Ratio	Sound Pressure Level
0.0002 dyne/cm^2 (0.000020 Pa)[a]	1:1	0 dB
0.002 dyne/cm^2 (0.00020 Pa)	10:1	20 dB
0.02 dyne/cm^2 (0.0020 Pa)	100:1	40 dB
0.2 dyne/cm^2 (0.020 Pa)	1,000:1	60 dB
2.0 dynes/cm^2 (0.20 Pa)	10,000:1	80 dB
20.0 dynes/cm^2 (2.0 Pa)	100,000:1	100 dB
200.0 dynes/cm^2 (20.0 Pa)	1,000,000:1	120 dB
2000.0 dynes/cm^2 (200.0 Pa)	10,000,000:1	140 dB

[a] 20 μPa.

setting of 0 dB for each audiometric frequency generates the SPL necessary to just reach audibility for a normal ear. Therefore, 0 dB hearing level (HL, or dB re: the audiometer hearing loss dial) represents a different SPL for each audiometric frequency, depending on the sensitivity of the normal ear for that frequency. This convention permits us to represent normal hearing by a straight line across a graph at 0 dB rather than the curved line which would result if 0 dB on the audiometer utilized 20 μ Pa as a reference value. The actual SPLs which represent 0 dB HL at each audiometer frequency are given in the next chapter.

To reiterate, the physical reference for SPL is dB re: 20 μ Pa. Audiometers, however, are calibrated so that when the hearing loss dial is set at zero they generate, at each audiometric frequency, the SPL necessary to reach threshold of audibility for a normal hearing person. Thus, dB HL means dB re: audiometer zero. The actual SPL required for 0 dB HL varies from frequency to frequency, according to the sensitivity of the normal ear.

Another convention is to refer to dB sensation level (SL). Decibels SL refers to decibels above or below the auditory threshold of a particular individual. That is, 0 dB SL refers to the threshold of the individual, 10 dB SL describes a signal 10 dB above the person's threshold, −10 dB is 10 dB below the person's threshold, and so on. Such usage simplifies terminology when discussing the presentation level of suprathreshold tests. As an example, for a test to be delivered at 40 dB SL means that the test should be presented at a level 40 dB above the threshold of any person taking the test.

SUMMARY

Auditory tests can be divided into four groups: the basic test battery, pediatric assessment, site-of-lesion testing, and hearing aid evaluation. This text is concerned with the basic test battery, which consists of pure tone air and bone conduction thresholds, speech thresholds, speech discrimination testing, and basic impedance measures. Although "advanced" tests are not discussed, you should remember that many of the concepts and skills that apply when administering and interpreting the basic battery are also vital for use of the advanced tests.

The basic audiologic battery establishes the magnitude and configuration of hearing loss. Through measurements of sensitivity and discrimination ability it contributes to estimation of probable handicap, to determination of rehabilitative needs, and to prognosis for a rehabilitative program. Comparison of air and bone conduction thresholds establishes the type of hearing loss. Conductive loss results from disorders in the outer or middle ear. Sensorineural loss is associated with cochlear or VIIIth nerve disorders. Mixed hearing loss consists of a conductive and a sensorineural component in the same ear.

The unit of intensity commonly used in hearing evaluation is the decibel (dB). It is a logarithmic unit expressing the ratio between two values. A common reference value for sound pressure level (SPL) is 20 μ Pa, a pressure equivalent to 0.0002 dyne/cm^2. Audiometers are calibrated so that when their hearing loss dial is set at 0, they generate the SPL just necessary for audibility for a normal ear. For each audiometric frequency, this SPL is designated 0 dB hearing level (HL). Thus, 10 dB HL means 10 dB re: the audiometer dial, or 10 dB above the threshold of normal human auditory sensitivity. Decibels sensation level (SL) refers to the amount a sound is above or below the threshold of a particular individual. Ten dB SL means 10 dB above the threshold of that individual and −10 dB SL means a signal which is 10 dB below that particular person's threshold.

Suggested Readings

If you need more background on the material covered in this chapter, the following sources are suggested:

Anatomy and Physiology of the Ear

Glattke, T.: Anatomy and physiology of the auditory system. In *Audiological Assessment* (Rev. Ed.), edited by D. Rose, Ch 2., Englewood Cliffs, N.J.: Prentice-Hall, Inc., 1978.

Yost, W., and Nielsen, D.: *Fundamentals of Hearing*, New York: Holt, Rinehart and Winston, 1977.

The Decibel and the Physical Nature of Sound

Danaloff, R., Schuckers, G., and Feth, L.: Acoustics, the science of sound. In *The Physiology of Speech and Hearing*, Ch. 4, Englewood Cliffs, N.J.: Prentice-Hall, Inc., 1980.

Small, A.: *Elements of Hearing Science: A Programmed Text*, New York: John Wiley & Sons, Inc., 1978.

STUDY QUESTIONS

1. List the tests constituting the basic battery which you would administer to a hearing impaired patient. What is the purpose of each test?
2. What knowledge and skills should you have before administering the basic audiologic test battery? What are some common mistakes?
3. After reviewing the structure and function of the ear, answer these questions: Which areas of the ear are involved in (a) conductive loss? (b) sensorineural loss? (c) mixed loss?
4. Why is it convenient to use a logarithmic unit to express sound levels?
5. What is the meaning of the statement that the decibel is "dimensionless"?
6. What are some common reference values used in sound measurement?
7. What is the difference between sound pressure and sound pressure level?

CHAPTER 2 Facilities and Equipment

Sound treated facilities and calibrated equipment are a prerequisite to valid audiometry. An environment is needed which will not invalidate testing because of unwanted sound originating either from inside or outside the test room. Frequent calibration (checking) of the audiometric equipment is necessary.

Failure to calibrate at appropriate intervals is probably a major cause of invalid test results. Cozad (1966) surveyed calibration practices in a hearing conservation program. The most common answer to the question, "When do you calibrate your audiometer?" was, "When it doesn't work anymore". In other words, the majority of the respondents reported giving no attention to the functioning of their equipment until it was not working at all. To ensure accurate signals, audiometers must be checked when first purchased and regularly thereafter. It is the audiologist's responsibility to ascertain the proper functioning of all test equipment. This task includes caring for equipment, detecting malfunctions, making minor repairs, appropriate calibration, and monitoring adequacy of test conditions. These topics are the subject of this chapter.

SOUND ROOMS

To minimize the noise level within the test room, thought should be given to placement of the facility during the planning stage. In addition to noise generated within the room itself, noise from outside the room will determine suitability for testing. Finding a good place to set up a sound room is a particular problem in industry, where noise levels may be high throughout the facility.

Permissible noise levels for audiometric test environments are shown in Table 2.1. The higher levels permitted for air conduction testing assume noise attenuation (reduction) by the earphone-cushion combination covering the ears. Bienvenue and Michael (1978) reported significant differences in noise attenuation, depending on headband tension. They pointed out that earphone calibration can also be affected by leakage and recommended appropriate care to ensure adequate headset tension. Measurement of noise levels in the sound room should be made with a sound level meter with octave band measuring capacity.

Commercially available prefabricated sound rooms are in common use. An efficient testing arrangement consists of a sound suite made up of a control room and an examination room as shown in Figure 2.1. The control room contains the audiometer and related test equipment which will be described later. Test signals are sent electrically from the

Table 2.1
Maximum Permissible Noise Levels in dB SPL for Pure Tone Threshold Testing[a]

	Frequency in Hz[b]										
	125	250	500	750	1000	1500	2000	3000	4000	6000	8000
Under earphones[c]	34.5	23.0	21.5	22.5	29.5	29.0	34.5	39.0	42.0	41.0	45.0
Bone conduction	28.0	18.5	14.5	12.5	14.0	10.5	8.5	8.5	9.0	14.0	20.5

[a] ANSI (1977).
[b] Hz (Hertz), cycles per second.
[c] Mounted in MX 41/AR cushions.

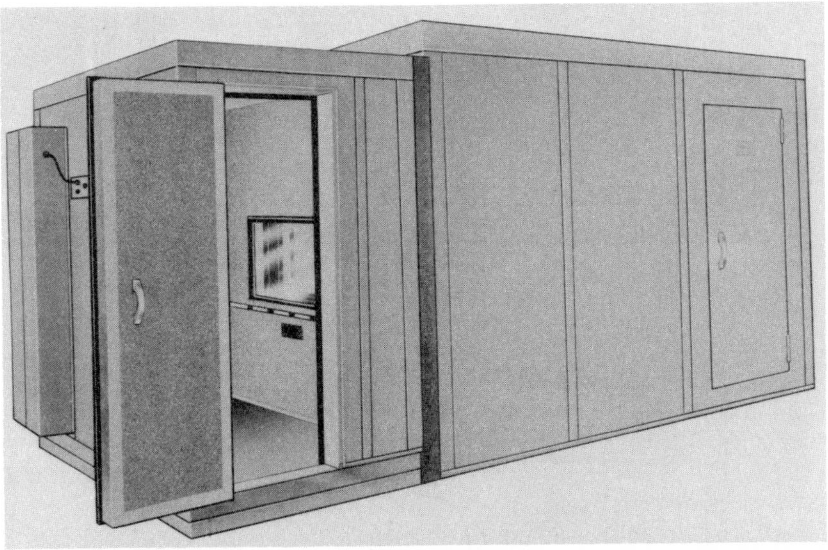

Fig. 2.1. A commercially available prefabricated sound suite. There is a single wall control room and a double wall examination room. The double walls of the examination room, where the patient is seated, give additional attenuation of outside noise. (Courtesy of Industrial Acoustics Co.)

audiometer into the examination room where the earphones and loudspeakers are located. During the audiologic evaluation, the audiologist is seated in front of the audiometer and the patient either listens through earphones or a bone vibrator or is placed at a designated position near the loudspeakers. A common arrangement is shown in Figure 2.2.

Because of the need for additional noise attenuation, the examination room often has double walls. This arrangement generally assures a sufficiently quiet test situation, although the adequacy of such a room should never be taken for granted. Double wall rooms also permit live voice testing at high levels through loudspeakers without feedback produced by sound leaking through the examination room back into the

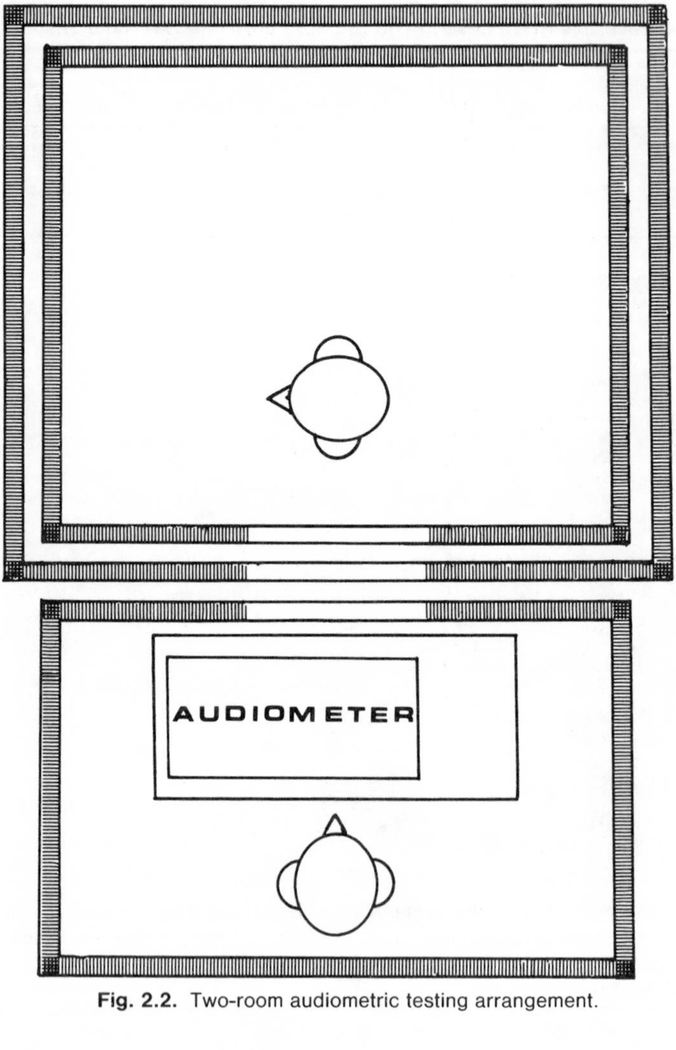

Fig. 2.2. Two-room audiometric testing arrangement.

test microphone. In addition, the possibility is eliminated that the patient with good hearing may hear test words delivered by live voice directly through the wall of the sound room rather than via the audiometer circuit.

The size of the examination room depends on its uses. Sound field testing, via loudspeakers, is not routinely a part of the basic test battery and is not covered in this text. However, hearing clinics should be equipped for sound field testing and the room should be large enough to seat the patient at least 1 m from the loudspeaker (Sivian and White, 1933). Testing of children is facilitated by a larger room to permit the presence of an assistant. Patients in wheelchairs necessitate several modifications. Sound rooms, doors, and hallways must accomodate the wheelchair, and entrance ramps are necessary.

The inner door on many double wall sound rooms opens inward and may reduce usable space. It is possible to mount both doors on the same hinges so that both open outward. Unfortunately, this arrangement sometimes creates problems because of the increased weight on the hinges.

In addition to space for the sound room, an adequately equipped clinic needs (1) a waiting room; (2) a quiet and private area for case history taking, interpreting test results, and counseling; and (3) an area for impedance measurement. In clinics where more than the basic audiometric battery is administered, additional space and facilities are needed, but these are not considered in this text.

AUDIOMETRIC EQUIPMENT FOR THE BASIC BATTERY

A pure tone and speech audiometer and an impedance meter are required to administer the basic battery. A diagram of a pure tone speech audometer's controls is shown in Figure 2.3. The pure tone audiometer should have two channels so that two independent signals may be generated and controlled separately. It is not strictly necessary that all signals be duplicated on each channel. For example, it is fairly common to have a speech input on only one channel and a noise input on only the second channel. In this case, however, there should be a switch in the audiometer circuitry which allows the speech input to be sent to both channels with separate intensity controls for each channel. These controls are called attenuators, or hearing loss dials. While not required for tests described in this book, the audiometer should have separate pure tone generating capacity for each channel to do the site-of-lesion testing that is common in most hearing clinics. For testing children and for hearing aid evaluation, capacity to generate warble (frequency modulated) tones is useful. These signals, used in sound field, will also require booster amplifiers and loudspeakers.

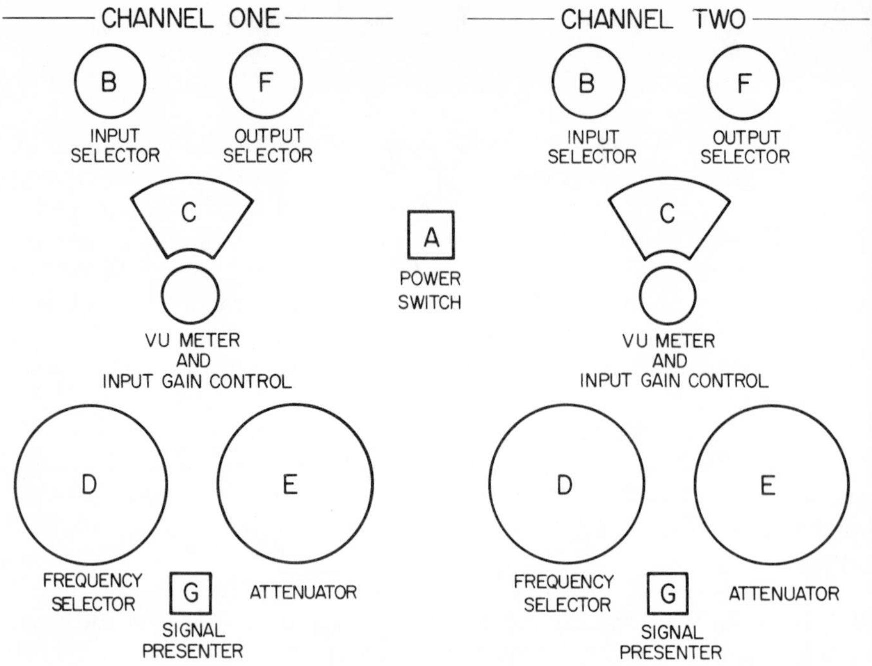

Fig.2.3. Controls of a two-channel pure tone and speech audiometer. *A*, off-on power switch; *B*, input selectors for microphone, phonograph, tape recorder, pure tone, or broad band or narrow band masking signals; *C*, input gain controls and VU meters for calibration of input signals; *D*, frequency selectors for determination of pure tone or narrow band noise frequencies; *E*, attenuators, or hearing loss dials, to control output levels; *F*, output selector to direct signals to desired transducer (earphones, bone vibrator, loudspeakers); *G*, signal presenters to control presentation of signal.

The audiometer should have a white noise generator and provisions for narrow bands of noise. These signals are used as needed to prevent participation of the nontest ear during speech and pure tone testing. The audiometer should generate the tones shown in Table 2.2.

The speech circuit may be combined with the pure tone audiometer, as described above, or it may be housed separately. Either arrangement should provide for masking, live voice testing, and audio tape or phonograph inputs. There must be an input gain control and a VU meter which meets the specifications of the American National Standards Institute (ANSI, 1961). A combined pure tone and speech audiometer is shown in Figure 2.4.

In two-room test arrangements, there should be a talkback circuit permitting the audiologist to listen to the patient's responses. It is helpful to have both earphones and a loudspeaker in the talkback circuit, with a switch to permit monitoring by either. There should be a talk forward

Table 2.2
Minimum Requirements for Test Frequencies and Maximum Outputs for Wide Range Pure Tone Audiometers[a]

Frequency in Hz	Minimum Operating Range (db HL)
125[b]	0–70[b]
250	0–90
500	0–100
750[b]	0–100[b]
1000	0–100
1500	0–100
2000	0–100
3000	0–100
4000	0–100
6000	0–90
8000	0–80

[a] ANSI (1969).
[b] 125 and 750 Hz are not required but are usually included. Most pure tone audiometers have maximum outputs exceeding the minimum requirements: 110 dB HL from 500 to 6000 Hz, and 90 dB at 8000 Hz.

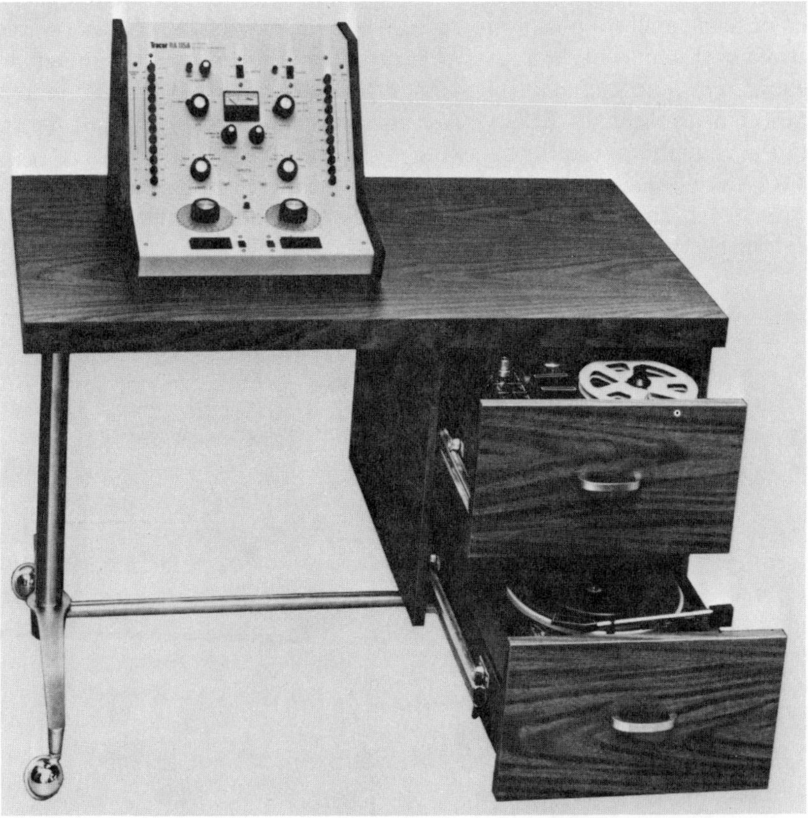

Fig. 2.4. A two-channel audiometer. (Courtesy of Tracor Instruments)

circuit independent of the speech audiometric circuit, permitting conversation with the patient without changing the controls of the test circuit. If young children are to be tested in a two-room setup there should be another talk forward circuit for the assistant in the examining room, to permit conversation between the audiologist and the assistant and to inform the assistant when signals are delivered.

A portable pure tone audiometer should be available for the option of testing young or difficult to test patients. Testing of such individuals in a one-room setup permits simpler and more direct instructions and reinforcement. An appropriate audiometer is shown in Figure 2.5. This audiometer, as well as the other equipment discussed above, should meet ANSI (1969) specifications. These standards are currently being reconsidered, and a revision is pending.

An impedance meter is necessary for obtaining the tympanograms and acoustic reflex thresholds discussed in Chapter 7. One such unit is shown in Figure 2.6. Most impedance units incorporate a pure tone audiometer for elicitation of acoustic reflexes. However, if this is not the case, a separate pure tone audiometer will be needed. A compatible strip chart recorder is a useful addition to the impedance meter, to record tympanograms and acoustic reflexes. All audiometer earphones should be housed in MX 41/AR cushions to permit coupling to the standard artificial ear for checking calibration.

A two-channel, two-or four-track tape recorder is needed for delivery of recorded speech tests to the audiometer. Alternatively, a turntable may be used. Speech tests on audio tape are probably more flexible and

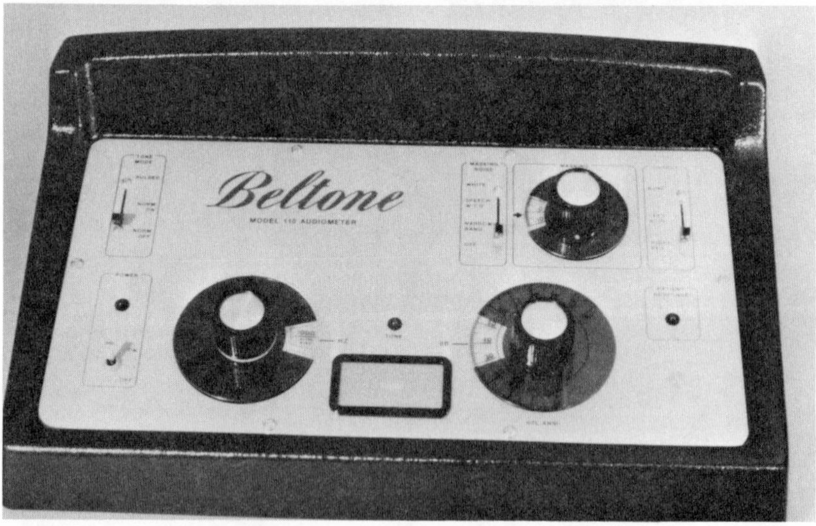

Fig. 2.5. A portable pure tone audiometer. (Courtesy of Beltone Electronics Corp.)

otoscope and impedance tips. Appropriate forms and test materials should be readily available. This material, and its use, is discussed in the following chapters.

AUDIOMETER NORMS

Audiometer frequency, intensity, and time characteristics must be carefully controlled. Several procedures will be discussed for measuring test signal characteristics. These measurements are collectively referred to as calibration procedures.

According to Davis (1978), the calibration of the first commercially available pure tone audiometer was based on the hearing sensitivity of 85 young adults who worked at the Bell Telephone Laboratories, where this instrument was developed in the early 1920s. Davis mentions that the basic decision occurred at that time to make 0 dB on the audiometer intensity dial correspond to normal human threshold for each frequency to be tested. Thus, the physical output, or SPL, for audiometric zero varies from frequency to frequency, depending on the sensitivity norm for the given frequency.

Beasley (1938) reported the SPLs necessary for pure tone thresholds in a survey of normal listeners conducted by the U. S. Public Health Service in 1935-1936. These SPLs were adopted by the American Standards Association (1951) to represent audiometric zero. The standards, known as the ASA 1951 norms, were in general use in the United States until 1964. There was concern that the American standards were not in very good agreement with audiometric norms of other countries. The International Standards Organization (1964) published a new recommended standard based on 15 published studies of hearing sensitivity in normal individuals. After a period of transition, these ISO 1964 norms were in general use. The American National Standards Institute (previously the American Standards Association) adopted a slightly revised version of the ISO norms in 1969. Today, essentially all pure tone audiometers in use in this country will indicate on the face of the audiometer that they are calibrated to the ISO 1964 or the ANSI 1969 norms.

One additional factor complicates the situation slightly. The type of earphone that is used in all standardized measurements changes from time to time and a transfer of norms from the old to the new earphone type is necessary. This process results in slightly different sound pressures representing audiometer zero, or normal human thresholds, depending on the earphone in question. Table 2.3 shows sound pressure levels representing normal thresholds re: the 1951 ASA norms, the 1964 ISO norms, and the 1969 ANSI norms for the TDH 39 earphone, the earphone in standard use throughout much of the period these norms

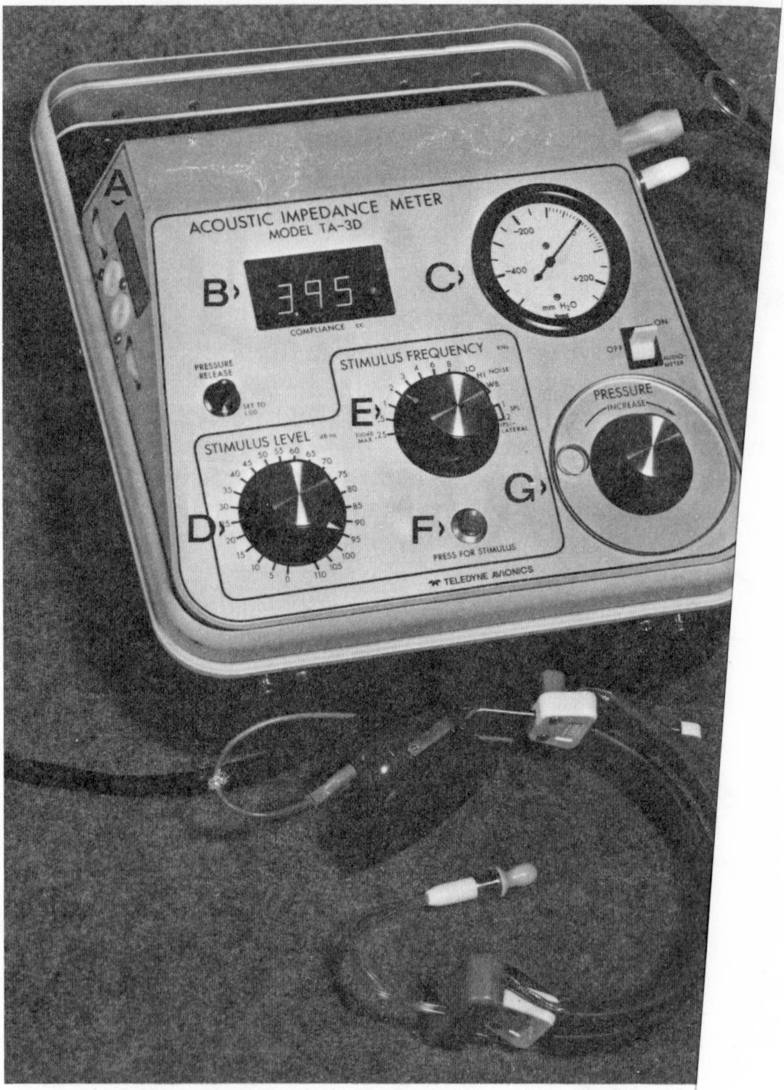

Fig. 2.6. An impedance meter. *A*, calibration cavities; *B*, compliance meter; *D*, audiometer hearing loss dial; *E*, audiometer frequency selector; *F*, a presentation button; *G*, air pressure pump control.

economical than those on phonograph discs. Either unit sho to ANSI (1969) standards.

A self-illuminating otoscope should be available for ob ear canals prior to evaluation. A germicidal fluid such chloride and containers should be available for cleaning

Table 2.3
SPLs in NBS 9 A Coupler Corresponding to Threshold (dB Re: 20 μ Pa); TDH 39 or TDH 49 Earphone in MX 41/AR Cushion

Frequency in Hz	Norm			
	ASA, 1951 TDH 39[a]	ISO, 1964 TDH 39[b]	ANSI, 1969 TDH 39[c]	ANSI, 1969 TDH 49[d]
125	51.8	42.8	45.0	47.5
250	39.5	24.5	25.5	26.5
500	24.1	10.1	11.5	13.5
750		6.5	8.0	8.5
1000	17.2	7.2	7.0	7.5
1500		8.0	6.5	7.5
2000	18.0	9.5	9.0	11.0
3000	15.6	7.1	10.0	9.5
4000	14.3	8.3	9.5	10.5
6000	19.5	10.0	15.5	13.5
8000	26.8	15.3	13.0	13.0

[a] Receiver values proposed by Cox and Bilger (1960). *ASA*, American Standards Association.
[b] WE 705A norms (Davis and Kranz, 1964) corrected to TDH 39 values. *ISO*, International Standards Organization.
[c] ANSI (1969). *ANSI*, American National Standards Institute.
[d] Proposed ANSI values for TDH 49 earphone (Wilber, 1978).

have been available. Additionally, proposed ANSI norms are given for the TDH 49 earphone which is also currently in use. In all cases measurements are made via an NBS 9 A coupler with the earphone housed in the MX 41/AR cushion, as described below and shown in Figure 2.8.

ANSI SPECIFICATIONS FOR AUDIOMETERS

In addition to specifying the sound pressure levels required for threshold, the American National Standards Institute has other standards which audiometers should meet (ANSI, 1969). These standards specify permitted tolerances for accuracy of frequency and time factors of the signal. The specifications are shown in Table 2.4. These values, along with the SPLs shown in Table 2.3, should be used for audiometer calibration, as detailed below.

The tolerances shown in Table 2.4 indicate the deviation permitted in intensity and frequency output. Harmonic distortion tolerances are also specified. Harmonic distortion results when overtones (harmonics) are generated. If these overtones are too strong, the patient may respond to the overtone rather than to the actual test tone, with invalid results. This danger is greatest in patients who have greater loss for lower frequencies. The possibility is increased that, because of their better sensitivity for higher frequencies, they may hear and respond to an overtone if the signal has high harmonic content.

Table 2.4
Specifications for Pure Tone Audiometers[a]

Accuracy of SPL	Earphone SPL shall not vary from the indicated value by more than 3 dB (250–3000 Hz), 4 dB at 4000 Hz, or 5 dB elsewhere.
Frequency	Required frequencies shall be within 3% of the indicated frequency.
Purity of tones	SPL of any harmonic of the fundamental shall be at least 30 dB below the SPL of the fundamental.
Attenuator linearity	Measured difference between each hearing loss dial setting shall not differ from the dial indicated difference by more than (1) 3/10 of the dial interval measured in dB, or (2) 1 dB, whichever is larger.
Rise-decay time	The time required for the SPL to rise from −20 dB to −1 dB re the final steady value shall not be less than 0.02 sec and not more than 0.1 sec. Time required for the SPL to decay by 20 dB shall not be less than 0.005 sec and not more than 0.1 sec.
Sound from second earphone	Any sound not used for testing shall have SPL at least 10 dB below the hearing threshold reference level, except it need not be more than 70 dB below the signal from the "on" earphone.
Other unwanted sound	Any sound due to operation of audiometer controls during the actual test shall be inaudible to a normal hearing person at each hearing loss dial setting up to and including 50 dB.
Freedom from shock hazard	No exposed part shall have an open circuit potential to ground or another exposed part of more than 30 V rms and the current through a 1500 ohm resistor shall not be more than 5 mA. The power cord should be of the 3-wire type if used with other electric devices or in an operating room.

[a] ANSI (1969).

Requirements for attenuator linearity are specified in Table 2.4. An attenuator is linear if the actual change in output corresponds with each equal change in the hearing loss dial. That is, each change in the hearing loss dial of 5 dB should result in a change of 5 dB in output. It is possible for the attenuator's resistor network to change over time, resulting in nonlinearity, especially at low output levels where the resistor network must routinely handle a large current flow. For example, at dial settings less than 20 dB, a 5 dB change in the dial setting may result in less than a 5 dB reduction in output, or no reduction at all. In the latter case, hearing thresholds less than 20 dB could never be measured. Even though a patient had a 20 dB threshold the tone would continue to be audible as the hearing loss dial is turned to 0, since the attenuator actually did not reduce the signal below 20 dB.

Rise time of the signal relates to how fast the signal grows to a specified part of its steady-state level once the tone presenter is depressed. If the rise time is too fast, a click may be generated. The click, a signal of abrupt onset with energy present across a wide band of frequencies, may be audible to the patient with good hearing sensitivity in some part of that frequency band. The patient may respond to the click, rather than to the test tone, and an invalid threshold measurement may result. On the other hand, a signal with rise time too slow may fail to elicit the on-effect, considered important in threshold determination. The result may be somewhat poorer than a threshold obtained by a signal with the proper rise time. A slow rise time may have yet another effect on the manner in which the subject responds. Since the tone takes a longer time to reach its steady state value, the patient will not respond as soon as the tone presentation control is depressed. The patient's immediate response to the tone is a good check of the validity of the response. Without this check, false responses may go undetected. Tolerances for these signal time factors are shown in Table 2.4.

TYPES OF CALIBRATION

To accredit hearing clinics, the Professional Services Board representing the American Speech and Hearing Association (ASHA, 1978c) recommended the following calibration schedule. A *daily* listening check should be done in which the audiologist listens to and looks at the audiometer to detect gross deficiencies. A *monthly* detailed listening check adds examination for crosstalk in the earphones, signal distortion, and abnormal noise. A *quarterly* electroacoustic calibration of solid-state (transitorized) audiometers should be accomplished. The same calibration should be performed monthly on nonsolid-state audiometers. It consists of measuring the sound pressure levels for pure tones, masking noises, and speech signals in both earphones and sound field loudspeakers. *Annual* electroacoustic evaluation requires, in addition to the quarterly check: (1) measurement of output levels for pure tones in the bone vibrator; (2) frequency calibration for pure tones; (3) rise-decay time measures for pure tones; (4) measurement of harmonic distortion for pure tones; (5) measurement of signal-to-noise ratio for all outputs; (6) determination of attenuator linearity; (7) evaluation of special test equipment, including the impedance meter; and (8) determination of freedom from shock hazard.

Calibration should be performed on a regular schedule, as indicated. Needless to say, if the audiometer appears to be malfunctioning, the appropriate check should be instituted immediately rather than waiting until the regularly scheduled date.

Daily Listening Check

To ensure representative performance, ANSI (1969) recommends an initial warm up time of 30 min. You should check the audiometer as it will be used. In a two-room test setting, do not bring the earphones in from the test room and plug them directly into the audiometer. To do so would prevent detection of defects in patch cords or in the panel transferring the signal through the sound room walls. *Look* and *listen* as indicated below.

Visual Inspection. Look at the face of the audiometer. Be sure all controls are in their usual and necessary positions. Incidentally, do not booby trap an audiometer by leaving some seldom used control turned on. For example, some audiometers have a switch for reducing the output by a fixed amount, such as 20 dB, relative to the hearing loss dial setting. This provision permits testing unusually sensitive hearing. If the audiometer is left in that mode, and unnoticed by the next operator, the result will be a 20 dB error in obtained thresholds. Of course, if subsequent operators do *their* listening check carefully, the problem will be prevented.

Check for loose dials, knobs, or switches which can alert you to the possibility of erroneous output signals. Inspect the earphone and bone vibrator cords and earphone cushions. Signs of cord wear suggest the possibility of a broken electrical circuit. Cushions with cracks or missing pieces may cause excess leakage of the acoustic signal. Check the air and bone conduction headsets. Is tension sufficient to maintain adequate pressure? Will the air conduction headset retain the phones as you set them, without slipping? If you are not sure, try the headset on your own head.

Listening Check. Listen to all test signals through each transducer which will be used. Set the output at a moderate level, such as 40 dB, and determine that all signals are present at about the same loudness.

Listen to a continuous signal while wearing the earphones. Gently twist each cord where it attaches to the earphone. An intermittent signal indicates a loose or broken cord which must be repaired before testing. Repeat the check for the bone conduction cord.

Selecting one earphone and one frequency, rotate the hearing loss dial from minimum to maximum setting. Be sure a change in loudness accompanies each 5 dB change. This general check indicates that the attenuator is operating across its entire range and is grossly linear.

A listening check is no substitute for electroacoustic calibration. However, completion of a thorough listening check ensures that the properly calibrated audiometer is ready for use. The daily listening check is often the only safeguard against invalid test results caused by an improperly functioning audiometer. It is important that the steps of the listening check be carefully followed.

Monthly Listening Check

This biologic calibration calls for, in addition to the procedures of the daily listening check, evaluation for abnormal noise, signal distortion, and crosstalk in the earphones. If older, nonsolid-state audiometers are still in use, the quarterly electroacoustic calibration described in the next section should be done on a monthly basis.

With the attenuator turned to maximum output, turn the signal off and listen for hum or other amplifier noise. Excessive noise of this sort may be distracting to patients with high frequency losses. Their good low frequency hearing may permit them to hear this noise at the high output level used to check their defective high frequency sensitivity.

Still at maximum output level, turn the signal on and off, using the tone interrupter. Be sure clicks are not generated which, because of their frequency or intensity characteristics, may be audible to the patient even when the legitimate test signal is not. Be sure the tonal quality sounds free of distortion.

Check for the presence of an unwanted test signal in the nontest earphone. This defect is referred to as crosstalk, or sound from second earphone (ANSI, 1969). It may produce invalid audiograms when testing people with unilateral losses. Although such patients may be unaware of the signal in the impaired test ear, they may hear and respond to the signal leaking into the normal nontest ear. This check must be done at each audiometric frequency, since crosstalk may be audible at some frequencies and not at others. The clinician should always be alerted to the possibility of crosstalk whenever a patient with a large unilateral loss shows normal sensitivity at one or two frequencies. To check for crosstalk, turn the signal to at least 60 dB. Unplug the phone to which the signal is directed or place it well away from the head and listen to the nontest phone. An audible tone in the nontest phone will create invalid results. Crosstalk can originate from two possible sources. The first is a short in the jack panel which carries the signal between the examination and control room. The second source results from a problem in the audiometer circuitry. The first problem is simple to identify and repair. The second is an indicator that the audiometer is functioning very poorly and may require a trip to the manufacturer.

The listening check is a real ear calibration to ensure that the test tone is present in each earphone, that the attenuator is functioning adequately, and that no unwanted noise is present. In addition, the mechanical integrity of the audiometer is evaluated. Table 2.5 provides a checklist which may be helpful.

Quarterly Electroacoustic Calibration

The quarterly calibration should evaluate the SPL output from both earphones, the linearity of the attenuator, and the functioning of the bone conduction vibrator. Because of the different equipment required for bone vibrator calibration, that subject is treated separately in a later section.

Table 2.5
Checklist for Listening Check

Item	Enter Date of Listening Check				
Cushions OK					
Headband OK					
No noise in phones					
No crosstalk					
Earphone cords OK					
Plugs seated					
Jack panel OK					
Dials not loose					
Tones clear					
Attenuator OK					
No clicks					

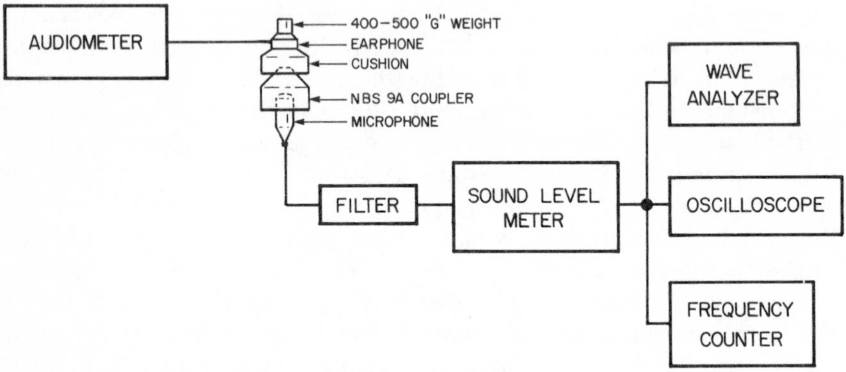

Fig. 2.7. Instrumentation for audiometer calibration.

An audiometer calibration system is shown in Figure 2.7. The most advanced systems permit almost automated calibration. To use these, you need only refer to the manual which is supplied along with the instrument. Less specialized units permit audiometer calibration along with use of the components (the sound level meter, for example) for other purposes. Use of such units is described below.

SPL Check. For earphone calibration, the earphone, housed in its MX 41/AR cushion is coupled to the measuring microphone via the NBS 9 A (6 cm^3) coupler, or its equivalent. This "artificial ear" simulates some of the characteristics occurring when the earphone and its cushion are mounted on a real ear. There are some differences between artificial and real ear coupling, but the NBS 9 A coupler remains the standard for earphone calibration.

The artificial ear couples the earphone-cushion combination to a condensor microphone (Western Electric 640 AA or equivalent). The cushion should be held against the coupler by a 400–500 g wt (ANSI, 1969). This force may be provided by an actual weight which rests on the earphone or by a spring loaded device incorporated into the artificial ear assembly. The arrangement is shown in Figure 2.8. The signal from the microphone system is sent to a preamplifier and then to a volt meter or a sound level meter, permitting a readout of the signal from the earphone.

After the instrumentation is assembled, the earphone-cushion combination is placed on the coupler. A 250 Hz tone of 70 dB HL is turned

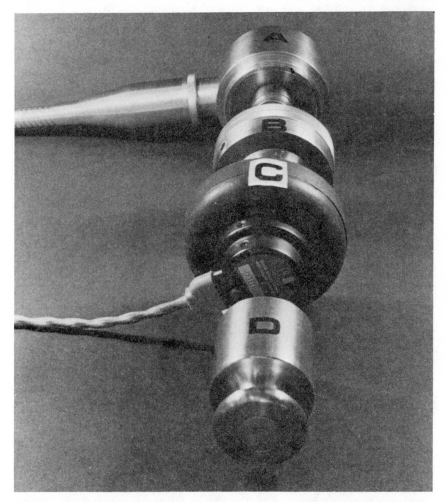

Fig. 2.8. Exploded view of artificial ear arrangement. *A*, microphone assembly (Western Electric 640 AA or equivalent); *B*, coupler (NBS 9 A or equivalent); *C*, earphone mounted in MX 41/AR cushion; *D*, 400–500 g wt.

on. Correct positioning of the earphone is important. It should be well centered and level on the coupler and positioned so that the maximum output, repeatable when the earphone is removed and replaced, is achieved.

It is conventional to set the audiometer hearing loss dial at 70 dB for calibration. This setting is high enough for easy reading of the output without exceeding audiometer output limits. It is helpful to send the signal through octave or third-octave filters to reduce extraneous noise which might interfere with measurement. The filter must be set to pass the signal being tested. The output is read on the sound level meter and recorded. Deviations from the expected results should be noted. The readout if the audiometer is in exact calibration will be the hearing loss dial setting (70) plus the SPL required for threshold at the given frequency. An efficient form for recording results is shown in Table 2.6. The output of each frequency for both phones should be checked.

There are two simple procedures for correcting errors in output. Many audiometers have "trim pots," auxiliary potentiometers which can be adjusted while the earphone is still on the artificial ear, until the output is correct. That is, if the output reads 1 dB stronger than it should, the trim pot can be turned until the output is exactly correct. Figure 2.9 shows how this correction is made on one audiometer.

Alternatively, correction charts can be made to indicate how much the audiometer output is in error and the amount by which thresholds should be corrected. When correction charts are used, it is conventional to make no correction if the error is 2.5 dB or less, to correct the obtained results by 5 dB if the error is between 2.6 and 7.5 dB, and to correct the

Table 2.6
Record Sheet for Audiometer Calibration Check

Audiometer ________ Date ________ By ________

ANSI 1969 Norms

Channel ________ Earphone ________

	Frequency in Hz									
	125	250	500	1000	1500	2000	3000	4000	6000	8000
Norm[a]	45	25.5	11.5	7.0	6.5	9.0	10.0	9.5	15.5	13.0
Attenuator setting	70	70	70	70	70	70	70	70	70	70
Expected result	115.0	95.5	81.5	77.0	76.5	79.0	80.0	79.5	85.5	83.0
Observed result	___	___	___	___	___	___	___	___	___	___
Difference	___	___	___	___	___	___	___	___	___	___
Correction	___	___	___	___	___	___	___	___	___	___

[a] SPLs in NBS 9 A coupler corresponding to threshold in dB re: 20 μ Pa for the TDH 39 earphone.

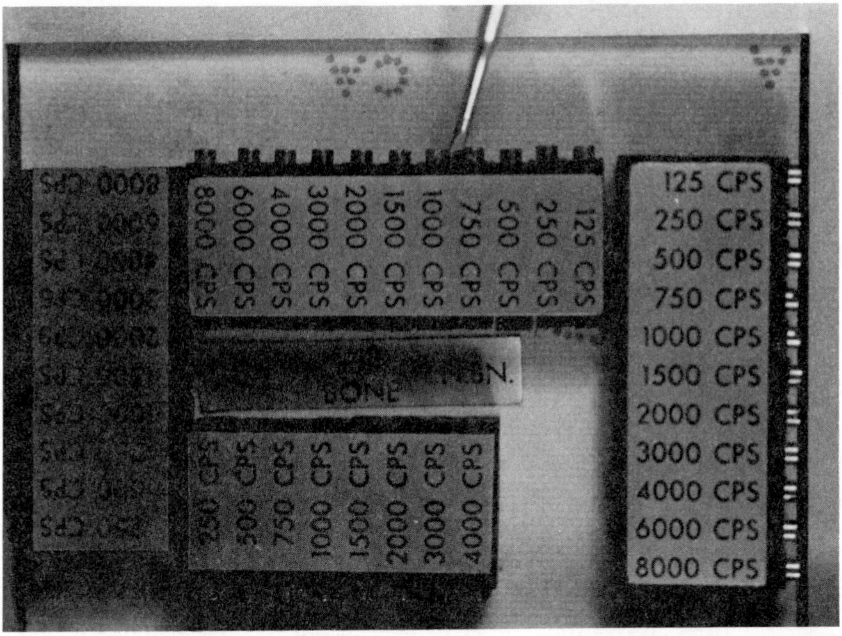

Fig. 2.9. Adjusting audiometer trim pots to correct the output during calibration.

results by 10 dB if the error is between 7.6 and 12.5 dB. Greater deviations indicate that the audiometer is seriously malfunctioning and should not be used. The direction of the correction depends on whether the output is weak or strong. When testing with weak output, the hearing loss dial will be turned to a higher setting than the actual output required to achieve an audible signal. Consequently, the recorded threshold should be made better than the hearing loss dial indicates, by the amount of the error. When testing with strong output, the tone will become audible at a lower hearing loss dial setting than the actual output. As a result, it is necessary to make the recorded thresholds poorer than the hearing loss dial setting indicates. A convenient correction chart is shown in Table 2.7. This chart, posted on the audiometer, indicates the corrections which should be made before recording results on the audiogram.

Attenuator Linearity. This check should be made electrically (ANSI, 1969) with leads from a volt meter attached to the earphone cords. For proper loading, the earphone should be placed on the coupler during the measurement. The hearing loss dial should be set at maximum output and a reading obtained. Next, the hearing loss dial should be reduced 5 dB and a new reading obtained. The output should, of course, drop 5 dB. The process should be continued across the entire range. Permitted tolerances are given in Table 2.4.

Table 2.7
Correction Chart

Date 2-2-80 Examiner Hodgson

Values preceded by (−) mean the output is weak. Make thresholds *better* by the indicated amount.

Values preceded by (+) mean the output is strong. Make threshold *poorer* by the indicated amount.

Ear	Frequency in Hz										
	125	250	500	750	1000	1500	2000	3000	4000	6000	8000
RE	+5	0	0	0	0	0	0	0	0	−5	−10
LE	+5	0	0	0	0	0	0	0	0	−5	−10

Annual Electroacoustic Calibration

The annual evaluation calls for an exhaustive calibration, which includes the following, in addition to the values measured in the quarterly check.

Frequency Check. The frequency of test tones is measured with an electronic frequency counter. Frequency can be measured either by inserting the counter into the electrical circuit of the earphone system or by measuring the output picked up by the artificial ear. The frequency of each test tone should be measured. It is not necessary to repeat the measure for each earphone when one oscillator serves both earphones. On a two-channel audiometer, however, both oscillators should be checked when both are used for pure tone testing.

Rise Time Check. Rise time of the signal is best measured with an oscilloscope which has a storage capacity. This instrument will hold an image of the signal onset so that the characteristics of the rise time can be determined. It also permits visual observation of clicks generated from rise-fall times which are too abrupt. Permitted tolerances are shown in Table 2.4

Harmonic Distortion Check. Measurement should be made of energy in individual harmonics of each test tone (ANSI, 1969). This measurement requires a distortion wave analyzer. Such an instrument passes on to the measuring apparatus only the energy in the individual harmonic of interest. Tolerances for harmonic content are shown in Table 2.4.

CALIBRATION OF THE SPEECH CIRCUIT

The speech circuit, or the speech audiometer, should be checked routinely. It makes sense to evaluate this equipment at the same intervals recommended for pure tone functions.

Testing the speech circuit under earphones is as simple as the pure tone calibration check, and the same instrumentation is used. The speech signal fluctuates rapidly, making precise reading of the sound level meter difficult. Therefore, it is recommended that a 1000 Hz pure tone signal be used for calibration (ANSI, 1969). This signal can be fed into the phono or tape input of the speech circuit. The source can be a pure tone generator or a recorded pure tone. The calibration tone recorded on most phonographic or audio tape speech tests will serve.

With the calibration tone on, the input gain control should be adjusted until the needle of the VU meter reads zero. The pending revision of the ANSI (1969) standard specifies that the norm for speech threshold is 12.5 dB above the SPL required for threshold of a 1000 Hz tone. Thus, the speech threshold norm is 19.5 dB SPL for the TDH 39 earphone or 20 dB SPL for the TDH 49 earphone. ANSI (1969) indicates that a hearing loss dial setting of 60 should be used for calibration. Therefore, the output SPL of a correctly calibrated speech circuit should be 79.5 dB or 80 dB for the TDH 39 or TDH 49 earphone, respectively. Error should be corrected with speech trim pot if the audiometer is equipped with one. If not, the error can be corrected by adjusting the input gain control, while reading the output on the sound level meter, until the output signal is accurate. The reading on the speech audiometer's VU meter should then be noted. A correction factor can then be posted on the audiometer, indicating the VU meter reading which should be used during testing. For example, if accurate output is achieved during calibration with a VU meter reading of −2, then testing should be done with the meter peaking at that level as test words are delivered.

BONE CONDUCTION CALIBRATION

Signals from an earphone can be measured by means of an artificial ear which simulates some of the characteristics of the human ear. To measure signals from a bone vibrator, a system is needed which simulates some of the characteristics of the bone conduction system; an artificial mastoid. Efforts to develop an artificial mastoid were hampered by lack of knowledge about the mechanical impedance of the human mastoid and by difficulty in simulating this impedance in an artificial mastoid. There were also problems finding material that would maintain the characteristics with aging.

Before the development of artificial mastoids, clinicians relied on biologic calibration of bone conduction systems. The American Medical Association (1951) specified a procedure for using 6 to 10 normal ears. There were some problems with this procedure. It was difficult to be sure that both the air and bone conduction thresholds of all subjects were entirely normal, a requirement for calibration of the bone conduction system through comparison with the subjects' air conduction thresholds. Furthermore, the lowest output on the audiometer is not always low enough to establish actual thresholds of normals, and this problem may introduce some error.

Roach and Carhart (1956) proposed using individuals with sensorineural loss and no history or symptoms of conductive disorder as subjects for biologic bone conduction calibration. It is not always possible to ensure that a small conductive component is not present in an individual with sensorineural loss. However, if impedance studies are normal, the presence of a pure sensorineural loss can be inferred. Hearing impaired individuals with normal impedance measures permit the clinician to monitor the bone conduction system during clinical evaluation. If air-bone disagreements are common when testing such patients, more thorough calibration is indicated. Of course, the error may be in the air conduction system instead of, or in addition to, the bone conduction system.

The problems mentioned above with biologic calibration make use of an artificial mastoid preferable although problems remain in reliability of mastoid measures (Dirks *et al.*, 1979). Two commercially available units are the Beltone 5A (Weiss, 1960), and the Bruel and Kjaer 4930 (Stisen and Dahm, 1969). An artificial mastoid is shown in Figure 2.10.

The specific calibration procedure used with a particular artificial mastoid can be found in the unit's instruction manual. In general terms the procedure is as follows: (1) assemble the unit, following the manufacturer's instructions; (2) adjust the sound level meter to be compatible with the mastoid in use; (3) center the bone vibrator on the artificial mastoid and exert a 550-g force; (4) set the audiometer hearing loss dial at the levels recommended by the mastoid manufacturer and turn on the tone; (5) read the output on the sound level meter for each test frequency, 250–4000 Hz; (6) compare the actual and expected values and make corrections where appropriate, using the same tolerances previously recommended in air conduction calibration.

Lybarger (1966) reported values widely used as interim norms for the Beltone artificial mastoid. Wilber (1972) related these values to the Bruel and Kjaer mastoid. These norms are shown in Table 2.8. Corrections specific to the artificial mastoid in use may also be necessary. These corrections are supplied by the manufacturer. Lybarger specified that his norms are applicable to the Sonotone B-9 and Radioear B70A bone vibrators. Radioear B71 and B72 vibrators are now in use as well. Dirks and Kamm (1975) reported only small differences between thresholds obtained with these vibrators and those obtained with the B70A vibrator. More definitive bone conduction standards await the forthcoming revision of ANSI (1969) specifications.

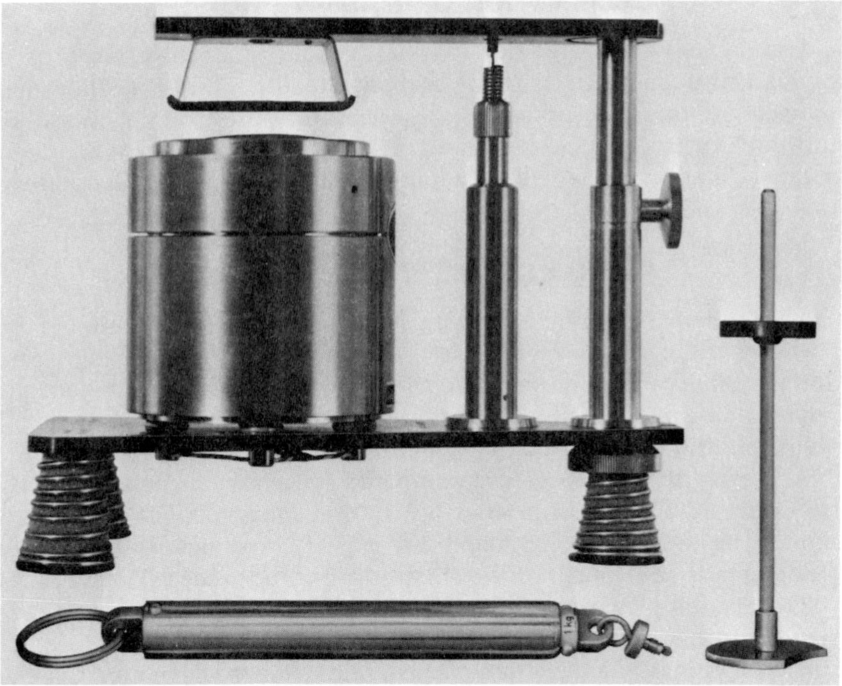

Fig. 2.10 An artificial mastoid. (Courtesy of B & K Instruments, Inc.)

Table 2.8
Mastoid RMS Force Levels in dB Re: 1 Dyne

Frequency in Hz	Beltone M5A Artificial Mastoid[a]	B & K 4930 Artificial Mastoid[b]
250	43	41.4
500	37.5	30.7
750	29	19.3
1000	23	16.9
1500	20.5	15.4
2000	20	8.1
3000	10.5	6.6
4000	15	11.2

[a] Lybarger (1966).
[b] Wilber (1972).

The harmonic content of the signal from the bone vibrator should also be measured. High harmonic distortion is often a problem with bone conduction systems, particularly at 250 Hz. The source may be in the audiometer but is more likely to be in the vibrator. It may be necessary to replace the vibrator to achieve an acceptable level of harmonic distortion.

CALIBRATION OF MASKING NOISE

Stability of noise used for masking should be checked with each biologic and electroacoustic calibration. Broad band noise calibration may follow the same procedure described for pure tone checks. More information is given in Chapter 4 about calibration of narrow band masking noise and the determination of effective masking characteristics.

IMPEDANCE METER CALIBRATION

The audiometer circuit used to elicit acoustic reflexes should be checked in the same way as described above for earphone calibration, and the same calibration schedule should be observed. Some impedance meters do not use Telephonics earphones, and in these cases the manual gives sound pressure levels representing threshold values.

Accuracy of the air pressure pump and gauge may be determined by connecting the air pressure tube to a water manometer. The system can then be tested at +200, 0, and −200 mm H_2O settings. Wilber (1978) recommends adjustment of the apparatus if error exceeds 25 mm H_2O.

The accuracy of the probe tone can be determined by directing that signal into an appropriate coupler attached to an audiometer calibration system. Ordinarily a 2 cm^3 coupler is used. Refer to the manual for the coupler type and the expected level of the probe tone for a particular model. If the probe tone is in error, there are internal adjustments, explained in the manual, which will permit appropriate corrections.

SUMMARY

Correctly calibrated and well maintained audiometers and adequate facilities are necessary for valid audiologic evaluation. Equipment and facilities should meet appropriate standards. The equipment for the basic audiometric battery includes a two-channel pure tone audiometer with masking noise, a bone conduction circuit, and a speech circuit. Provisions for recorded speech tests, via tape recorder or phonograph, should be made. A portable audiometer should be available for more direct contact with difficult to test patients.

A listening check and visual inspection should be made daily, or each time the equipment is used. More extensive monthly listening checks should be conducted. Evaluation of SPL output and attenuator linearity should be made at least quarterly. The speech and bone conduction circuits should be checked, as well as the earphones. Yearly, an exhaustive calibration should evaluate the factors named above, as well as harmonic distortion, frequency, and rise time. While a regular calibration schedule is needed, equipment should additionally be checked any time a problem seems to be present. The daily listening check is a useful way to detect possible problems which indicate the need for more thorough calibration.

STUDY QUESTIONS

1. List the equipment needed for valid administration of the basic battery. What is the purpose of each unit?
2. Refer to Table 2.3 for values to complete the following questions. Remember that dB sound pressure level (SPL) means dB re: 20 μPa, dB hearing level (HL) means dB re: audiometer zero, and dB sensation level (SL) means dB re: an individual's threshold.
   (a) Re: the ASA norms, 0 dB HL at 2000 Hz = ______ dB SPL.
   (b) Re: the ANSI norms, 0 dB HL at 2000 Hz = ______ dB SPL.
   (c) Re: the ANSI norms, 40 dB HL at 2000 Hz = ______ dB SPL.
   (d) Re: the ISO norms, 40 dB HL at 2000 Hz = ______ dB SPL.
   (e) 21.5 dB SPL = ______ dB HL re: the ANSI norms for a 500 Hz tone.
   (f) 1.5 dB SPL = ______ dB HL re: the ANSI norms for a 500 Hz tone.
   (g) If a person has a 30 dB hearing loss for a 4000 Hz tone (re: the ANSI norms), the threshold is ______ dB SPL.
   (h) If a person has a threshold of 40 dB for a 4000 Hz tone (re: the ANSI norms), the threshold is ______ dB SPL.
   (i) At which frequency is there the greatest difference between the ANSI and ASA norms?
   (j) At which frequency is there the least difference between the ANSI and ASA norms?
   (k) If a person has a threshold of 30 dB for a 1000 Hz tone re: the ANSI norms, his threshold for 1000 Hz re: the ASA norms will be ______ dB HL.
   (l) Is the SPL output at audiometric zero less for ANSI or ASA norms?
   (m) At which frequency (re: ANSI norms) does 20 dB HL = 35.5 dB SPL?
   (n) At which frequency (re: ISO norms) does 30 dB HL = 39.5 dB SPL?
   (o) If a person has a 30 dB hearing loss, 20 dB SL = ______ dB HL.
   (p) If a person has a 40 dB hearing loss for an 8000 Hz tone (re: the ISO norms), 20 dB SL = ______ dB HL = ______ dB SPL.
   (q) If a person has a 40 dB hearing loss for a 500 Hz tone (re: the ANSI norms), 30 dB SL = ______ dB HL = ______ dB SPL.
   (r) For a 250 Hz tone, is 25 dB SPL greater or less than audiometric zero according to
      (1) ASA norms ______
      (2) ISO norms ______
      (3) ANSI norms ______
   (s) If a person's threshold for a 250 Hz tone is 10 dB HL (re: the ANSI norms, 20 dB SL = ______ dB SPL.
   (t) The SPL output at audiometric zero for a 6000 Hz tone (re: ISO norms) is equal to the SPL output at 0 dB HL for ______ Hz re: ______ norms.
3. What are the different types of calibration? What equipment is needed for each type?
4. How are an "artificial ear" and an "artificial mastoid" (a) alike? (b) different?

CHAPTER 3 Pure Tone Audiometry

PURPOSE

The purpose of pure tone audiometry is measurement of hearing sensitivity as a function of frequency. People with good hearing sensitivity require relatively less energy for a sound wave to be audible. Those with poor sensitivity require more. Some people use the terms "sensitivity" and "acuity" interchangeably. Ward (1964) pointed out the incongruity of this practice. In vision, sensitivity refers to the ability to detect a single signal, while acuity refers to how well a person can differentiate stimuli. Therefore, while acuity will probably not become a generally used term for the ability to differentiate sounds, it makes sense at least to keep usage of sensitivity parallel for both visual and auditory modalities.

Hearing can be measured as a function of frequency because each pure tone is intended to have energy present at only one frequency. Measurement of sensitivity at different frequencies may reveal that a person can hear some sounds well but has a hearing loss for others. For example, a person may have a high frequency loss of sensitivity with normal low frequency hearing. There are important differences between the problems caused by a uniform loss of sensitivity for all frequencies and a loss for only some frequencies. For this reason it is necessary to obtain a detailed measure of the ear's performance as a function of frequency and intensity. Measurement with a broad band signal, such as speech, gives only an overall indication of sensitivity.

The pure tone audiogram indicates the faintest sounds an individual can hear. These levels are referred to as thresholds of detectibility. Thresholds appear to change by very small amounts from moment to moment for a number of reasons. Therefore, threshold is often defined as the faintest signal which a person can detect half of the time during a given number of presentations. Clinical use of the threshold concept is usually just a little different, as is discussed shortly.

Pure tone thresholds may be obtained with either air conducted or bone conducted signals. To obtain air conduction thresholds, tones are delivered via an earphone mounted over the test ear. For bone conduction thresholds, signals are sent to the inner ear by means of a vibrator placed against the skull. Air and bone conducted signals of several different frequencies constitute the basic test of hearing sensitivity, the pure tone audiogram.

THE AUDIOGRAM

The audiogram is the graph on which pure tone thresholds are recorded. It usually has provision for recording thresholds at octave and some half-octave intervals from 125 through 8000 Hz. Sometimes thresholds are recorded in tabular form, as shown in Figure 3.1. Audiometric records of this sort are common in industry, where results of serial hearing tests must be stored for long periods.

More commonly, test results are recorded on an audiogram similar to that shown in Figure 3.2. A complete Audiologic Record usually includes the pure tone audiogram form and space for the results of speech and impedance tests and other auditory tests not routinely included in the basic battery.

The ASHA (1978a) recommended a pure tone audiogram form with the following characteristics. Frequencies in Hz should appear along the abscissa on a logarithmic scale, and hearing levels in dB should appear along the ordinate on a linear scale. The dimensions of the audiogram form should be such that the distance between octaves on the frequency scale is equal to the distance of 20 dB on the hearing level scale.

From the pure tone audiogram, the audiologist can generalize about the probable effect of the hearing loss on the patient's auditory behavior. The audiologist can predict listening conditions where difficulty is to be expected and the probable magnitude of difficulty. Of course, such variables as intelligence, age at onset of the loss, cause of the loss, and patient motivation influence the effect of a given hearing loss. Two people with the same audiogram will not, in all respects, function the same way. Therefore, some people have advocated "ignoring the audiogram and concentrating on the patient." To do so is to fail to understand the purpose of the audiogram. No single test can tell everything about a person's behavior. The audiogram precisely describes hearing sensitivity as a function of frequency and, in conjunction with other information, permits a general prediction of handicap and rehabilitative needs.

To obtain valid audiograms the student must be thoroughly familiar with audiometric equipment and procedures. Once the equipment and procedures have been mastered, all the clinician's attention can be centered on the patient. Astute observation of patient behavior is called

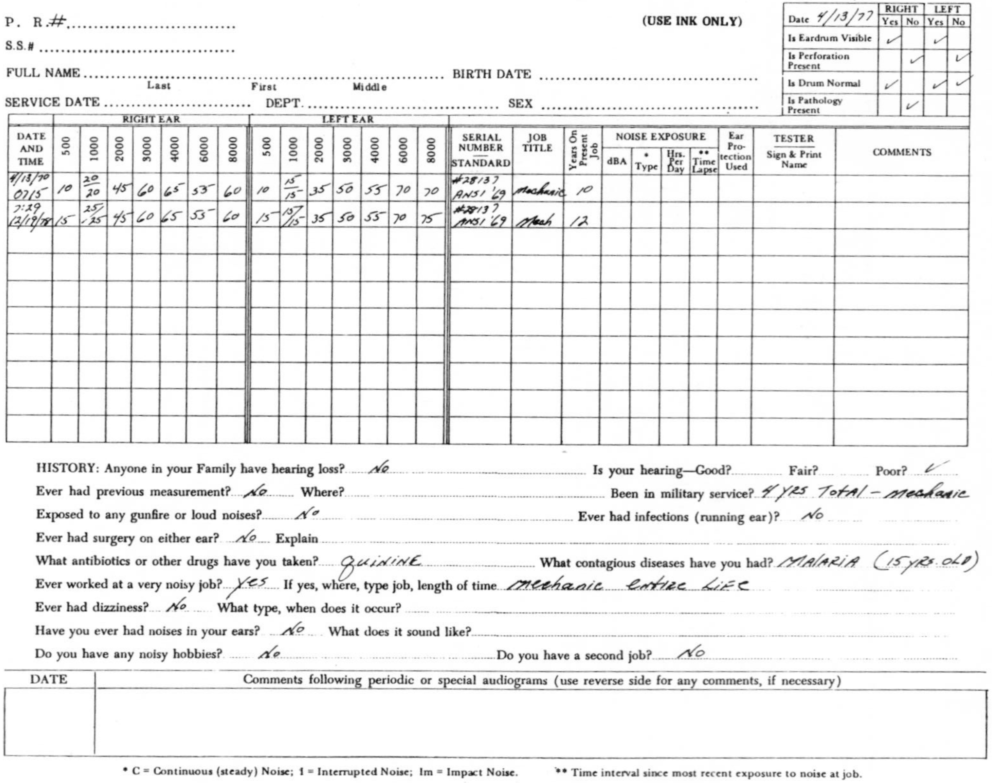

P. R.# ....

S.S.# ....

FULL NAME (Last, First, Middle) .... BIRTH DATE ....

SERVICE DATE .... DEPT. .... SEX ....

(USE INK ONLY)

Date 4/13/77	RIGHT Yes	RIGHT No	LEFT Yes	LEFT No
Is Eardrum Visible	✓		✓	
Is Perforation Present		✓		✓
Is Drum Normal	✓		✓	
Is Pathology Present		✓		

DATE AND TIME	RIGHT EAR 500	1000	2000	3000	4000	6000	8000	LEFT EAR 500	1000	2000	3000	4000	6000	8000	SERIAL NUMBER / STANDARD	JOB TITLE	Years On Present Job	NOISE EXPOSURE dBA	* Type	Hrs. Per Day	** Time Lapse	Ear Protection Used	TESTER Sign & Print Name	COMMENTS
4/13/70 0715	10	20/20	45	60	65	55	60	10	15/15	35	50	55	70	70	#28137 ANSI '69	Mechanic	10							
7:29 12/19/78	15	25/25	45	60	65	55	60	15	15/15	35	50	55	70	75	#28137 ANSI '69	Mech	12							

HISTORY: Anyone in your Family have hearing loss? No Is your hearing—Good? Fair? Poor? ✓

Ever had previous measurement? No Where? Been in military service? 4 YRS Total – mechanic

Exposed to any gunfire or loud noises? No Ever had infections (running ear)? No

Ever had surgery on either ear? No Explain

What antibiotics or other drugs have you taken? Quinine What contagious diseases have you had? Malaria (15 yrs. old)

Ever worked at a very noisy job? Yes If yes, where, type job, length of time mechanic entire life

Ever had dizziness? No What type, when does it occur?

Have you ever had noises in your ears? No What does it sound like?

Do you have any noisy hobbies? No Do you have a second job? No

DATE	Comments following periodic or special audiograms (use reverse side for any comments, if necessary)

* C = Continuous (steady) Noise; I = Interrupted Noise; Im = Impact Noise. ** Time interval since most recent exposure to noise at job.

Fig. 3.1. Form for recording pure tone air conduction thresholds in tabular fashion.

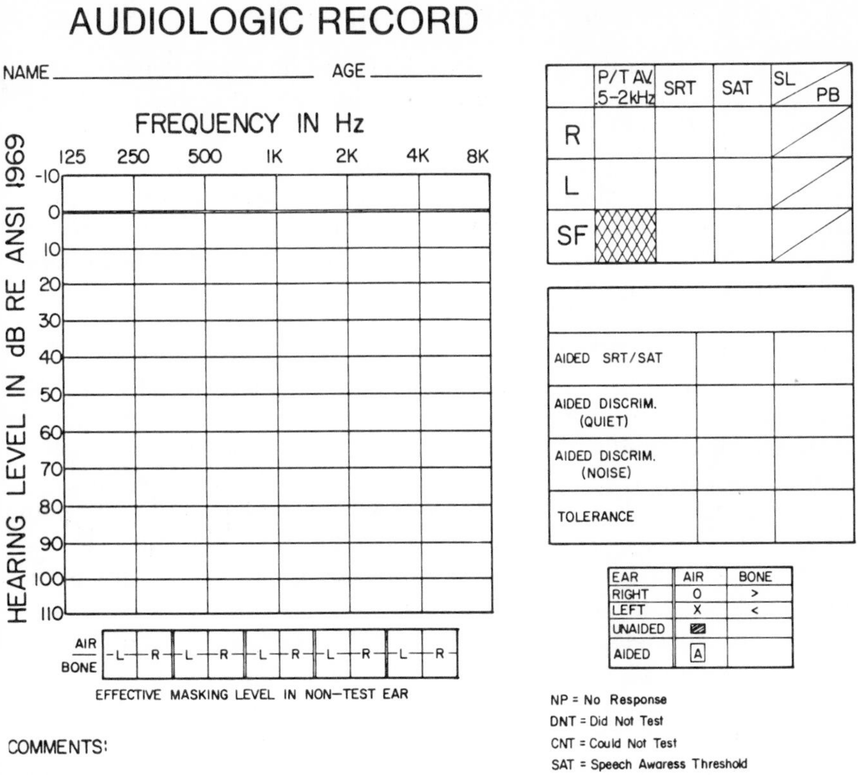

Fig. 3.2. Audiologic Record. In addition to the pure tone audiogram, there is space for identifying information, speech test results, and evaluator comments. Although not seen here, Audiologic Records often include provision for recording impedance measures and site-of-lesion test results.

for, as is the knowledge of how behavior can affect test results. It is necessary to be aware of the interaction between evaluator, patient, and audiometer.

The difficulty of consistently obtaining valid pure tone audiograms is not generally understood. Price (1978) explains:

> Pure tone tests ... for hearing sensitivity are usually thought of as "routine audiometry" and practically everyone, professional and nonprofessional alike, feels competent ... to administer them. As a result there are many inaccurate audiograms floating around. The administration of valid pure tone hearing tests requires (a) a basic knowledge of the anatomy and physiology of the auditory system, (b) some fundamental concepts about how sounds are generated, transmitted, and controlled, and (c) an understanding of the influence of certain procedural variables and pathologic conditions upon the results of the tests.

PREPARATION FOR TESTING

The pure tone audiometer is described in Chapter 2. Before reading further, you should review that description. The listening check, also described in Chapter 2, is a prerequisite to testing. This check provides final assurance that, just prior to starting the test, the equipment is working properly. Always perform a listening check prior to an audiometric session. Of course, equipment can malfunction during the test, and you should be alert to this possibility whenever patient behavior or test results are unusual.

Observing the Patient's Behavior

There will be great variability in the patients you will test. They will differ widely in age, intelligence, language level, education, magnitude of hearing loss, motivation, and willingness to cooperate. Most will be able to respond readily to spoken directions. However, gesture and demonstration will be necessary in some cases because of age, intelligence, or language level. Some adults with normal intelligence and language capability will require written instructions because of the magnitude of hearing loss.

Patients will demonstrate a wide range of knowledge and attitudes regarding hearing testing. Some will understand the purpose of the test. Others will be unaware of the service the audiologist provides. Some will be friendly and cooperative. Others will be questioning and doubtful. A few will be hostile. Some will work hard to follow instructions and will give accurate responses. Others will not. A few will work to convince you that their hearing is different from their actual thresholds.

Astute ongoing observation of the patient is essential for accurate testing. You must quickly assess the effect a patient's behavior may have on the test. Doing so permits you to direct your behavior, the patient's behavior, and the test procedures toward the goal of complete and accurate test results.

You must learn to estimate the patient's overall hearing sensitivity during the pretest observation. You can then select an appropriate means of instructing the patient. An idea of the patient's hearing sensitivity will also permit you to begin testing at an appropriate presentation level. Most important, it will provide a basic reference for assessing the validity of your test results. The patient who responds accurately to faint conversational speech but who shows bilateral flat 80 dB thresholds right across the audiogram is obviously suspect.

Considerable skill and experience are required to estimate magnitude of loss when observing a patient. There are these confounding factors: visual clues, familiarity of the topic under discussion, unilateral loss, configuration, and etiology of the loss. Visual clues may permit a person with large loss to respond well. Be sure you are not providing these clues when estimating sensitivity. As a rule, you should not hold your hand over your mouth when talking with a hearing impaired person. However, violate this rule when communicating to estimate sensitivity. You should also realize that the familiarity and predictability of the topic of conversation will affect how easily the patient understands. For example, after a request for the patient's address, asking for the telephone number is a fairly predictable question. On the other hand, asking next if the room is too warm may be an unexpected question which will permit a more accurate estimate of hearing function.

A person with normal hearing in one ear will manifest no communication difficulty under good listening conditions, nor will someone with a bilateral high frequency loss and normal sensitivity through a part of the speech range. A person with hearing loss caused by outer or middle ear deficit will ordinarily perform better than someone with an inner ear disorder of the same magnitude. In the former case, the normal sensory mechanism can take better advantage of low level clues. Finally, remember that hearing impaired people usually become adept at guessing what others say. Inappropriate responses to questions may alert you to this practice.

Establishing Rapport

Rapport is defined as a harmonious working relationship. An effective working association is needed to obtain maximum cooperation from the patient during testing and for the patient to accept and follow recommendations after testing. The test situation is more pleasant for both evaluator and patient if a climate of amicability is established.

Because of the time consuming nature of the audiologic evaluation and the work load of most clinics, rapport must be established quickly. The most effective type of relationship will certainly vary from patient to patient, as will the time and effort needed for its establishment. Most patients are ready for a pleasant and directed relationship, and the desirable climate is readily established. For some, barriers of ignorance or negative attitude must be removed.

Those attributes of the clinician which promote rapport are difficult to isolate. One may be genuine interest in the well-being of the patient with a desire to help. Such an interest implies an emotional relationship which must be channelled and controlled. Clinician concern is certainly no substitute for training and ability. The audiologist must take care that concern about the patient does not destroy objectivity. In spite of this potential danger, I believe that concern for the patient's well-being can be used in a positive way which will be discernible by most patients and will advance the desirable working relationship.

A uniform approach is not appropriate for all patients. Some react best to a structured and formal setting. Others prefer a casual, less structured situation. Some patients may even enjoy a little humor. Flexibility is important. The audiologist should utilize the clues given by the patient and conduct the evaluation accordingly, within the bounds permitted by good audiologic procedure. Regardless of the desirability for ease and informality, the audiologist must at all times control the test procedure. If the control can be reminiscent of the iron fist in the velvet glove, so much the better.

Finally, the degree of rapport and the best methods for its establishment depend not only on the particular patient involved but also on the individual audiologist and the setting where the testing is done. Audiologists, too, are individuals. It is not practical for each of us to try to fit a universal mold. Regardless of the method employed, the essential purpose of establishing rapport is to reduce apprehension and to establish a working atmosphere which will elicit cooperation and induce the patient to accept and follow recommendations. You should remember that the establishment of rapport is an ongoing process which begins when you meet the patient and continues throughout your association.

Pretest Interview

In addition to observation of patient behavior and establishment of rapport, a pretest interview should serve other purposes. You should learn exactly why the patient has come to you and to whom the results of the evaluation should be sent. You should get information about the patient's history, as described below, which may be helpful in testing, assessing validity of results, and explaining results to the patient.

In many clinical situations, a Preliminary Information or Case History form is filled out by the patient before the interview to facilitate taking of information. From clinic to clinic the length and detail of these forms vary. Generally, after reading patient responses on the Preliminary Information form, you will need to talk further with the patient about questions (1) left blank, (2) answered unclearly, or (3) answered in a way that suggests the need for more information. For example, Northern and Downs (1978) suggest that answers which have been erased and rewritten several times should be given additional consideration. Do not converse aimlessly: have a purpose for all questions. At the conclusion always ask, "Is there anything else I should know?" Usually the Case History form is divided into these sections:

Identifying Information. This section deals with personal information such as the patient's name, address, age, and occupation. The latter may suggest possible job related hearing problems and indicate if the patient needs help paying for the evaluation or for a hearing aid should one be needed. The name and address of the referring source is also included in the identifying information. Be sure you know, from the answers given on the form or from additional questioning, exactly what the patient and the referring source want to learn from the evaluation.

Hearing History. In this section the patient is asked to recall the onset and progression of the problem. From the written answers or those you solicit during the interview, you should learn about possible family history of hearing loss. This information is sometimes difficult to bring out. It is not inappropriate to ask more than once, using different terminology, if a patient indicates that no relatives have hearing problems. You should learn from the patient which ear is involved and to what extent. Knowing which is the better ear will be useful when testing starts. Solicit the patient's concept of the cause of the loss. In addition to the probability of getting factual information, misconceptions may be revealed which will require correction in order for the patient to understand the problem and what can be done about it. The more you know about the hearing history, the better you can predict the type and configuration of the loss and the better you can assess the validity of your test results.

Amplification History. A history of the kind and duration of hearing aid use is helpful. In this section the patient is asked about satisfaction with hearing aid use. This information provides insight into the person's reaction to amplification. Misconceptions and unrealistic attitudes toward hearing aid use may become evident.

Health History. This section relates to medical problems associated with the hearing loss. You may learn of past examinations and diagnoses which lend insight into the problem or, if the diagnoses are incorrect which may reveal misconceptions held by the patient. There may be information about medication the patient has taken or is taking that is either hazardous to hearing or could affect the way the patient responds to the upcoming test. The patient may associate the hearing problem with an accident. In accident associated losses, when claims for compensation are pending, the possibility of functional (nonorganic or feigned) hearing loss should come to mind. Of course, in this instance, as is the case with all hypotheses you form prior to testing, you must keep an open mind as you compare your test results with the impressions gained during the initial observation and interview.

Previous Evaluations and Training. Particularly when there is the possibility of progressive loss, or questions about the hearing level prior to an accident or illness, it is necessary to have access to results of earlier evaluations. It is also important, for the sake of continuity, to learn about previous training. The patient may be able to give these details, but it is more likely that reports should be requested from centers where the evaluation or training was done. A Release of Information form, signed by the patient, should accompany your request.

The Case History form for children is ordinarily filled out by the parents. In addition to the sections described above, the Case History form for children usually contains the following:

Educational History. It is important to learn of the school-age child's progress. Information about special educational needs and provisions is required. In cases of small hearing loss, the child's performance in school may be the determining factor in recommending amplification.

Developmental History. Language and speech development, in addition to being important considerations in their own right, are useful because they correlate with magnitude of hearing loss. Slow language and speech development in hearing impaired children may be the symptoms which first cause parents to seek hearing evaluation. Conversely, normal language and speech in a child found to have significant hearing impairment alerts us to the possibility that the loss may be of recent origin and possibly progressive.

In summary, preparation for testing involves observing the patient, establishing rapport, and soliciting information. These preparations should give an estimate of hearing sensitivity and establish a good working relationship. Remember, however, that rapport is an ongoing process that should continue throughout the evaluation. The information you solicit should help plan and control the evaluation and give data against which to check the validity of test results. No Case History form, regardless of length and detail, can give you all the information that is important in a particular case. Therefore, be alert for other information or for clues that suggest additional questions you should ask. Above all, be receptive to information offered by patients or parents. If accurate, it will help you in testing. If inaccurate it will indicate areas of misconception where counseling is needed.

Because of the usual press for time, the pretest preparation must be accomplished quickly. In other than exceptional cases, the activity should take little more than 10 min. Obviously, skill, experience, and a tightly planned procedure are necessary to meet this criterion.

Seating the Patient

The patient should be seated comfortably, preferably in an armchair. Some audiologists prefer to have the patient facing completely away from them, to prevent the patient from receiving visual clues. It is important that these clues be prevented, because perception of even minimal eye, hand, or body movements made by the audiologist may result in conscious or unconscious alteration of the patient's response. I prefer to see the patient's face during testing to assess attention and attitude and to help score speech tests. The ideal arrangement permits the audiologist to see the patient in profile. Even in this arrangement, patients accustomed to looking at those with whom they are communicating may turn to look at the audiologist. When this happens, the audiologist should simply request, "Don't watch me, please." In addition to not being able to see actions of the audiologist, the patient must not be afforded, either directly or by reflection, a view of the face of the audiometer.

Otoscopic Observation

There are a number of reasons for observing the ear canals prior to testing. Wax occluding the canal will affect the pure tone test results and tympanometric measures. You must observe the size of the canal opening in order to select a tip for tympanometry, as explained in Chapter 7. Additionally, for our immediate purposes, you must decide if there is danger of the ear canals collapsing under the pressure of the earphones. Such collapse will introduce an artifact, a "false conductive component," which will make your patient's hearing appear poorer than it really is. This artifact occurs because the test tone must be increased to overcome the sound-blocking effect of the collapsed external canal. Audiometric results of a collapsing ear canal are shown in Figure 3.3. Ways to detect and prevent the problem will be discussed shortly.

Of a number of possible methods for observing the ear canal, the most convenient for our purpose is the use of an illuminated otoscope. This instrument incorporates a flashlight and a head with a tip which is inserted into the canal. Usually some magnification is afforded to facilitate viewing details in the canal. Use of the otoscope is shown in Figure 3.4.

Select the largest tip which seems to fit comfortably into the canal, and place it on the otoscope head. Turn on the light. As you bring the otoscope close to the patient's head, keep a couple of fingers free to extend against the patient's head. This precaution will help steady the otoscope, facilitate comfortable insertion into the canal, and, should the patient's head suddenly move, prevent injury by the tip of the otoscope. During the observation make all movement slowly and carefully and be alert for signs of discomfort from the patient.

Begin the otoscopic observation by determining the probability that pressure of the earphones might collapse the canals and cause the kind of artifact described above. Hold the otoscope with its tip just at the external opening of the canal. Observe the configuration of the opening. In its natural state, the opening is oval in shape, and fairly narrow. In some individuals the opening is quite narrow, almost a slit, and the course of the canal is very crooked. These are the patients with whom you must be most alert to the possibility of collapsing canals. While viewing the canal opening, use your free hand to push the pinna against the head, as the earphone cushion will do when the headset is in place.

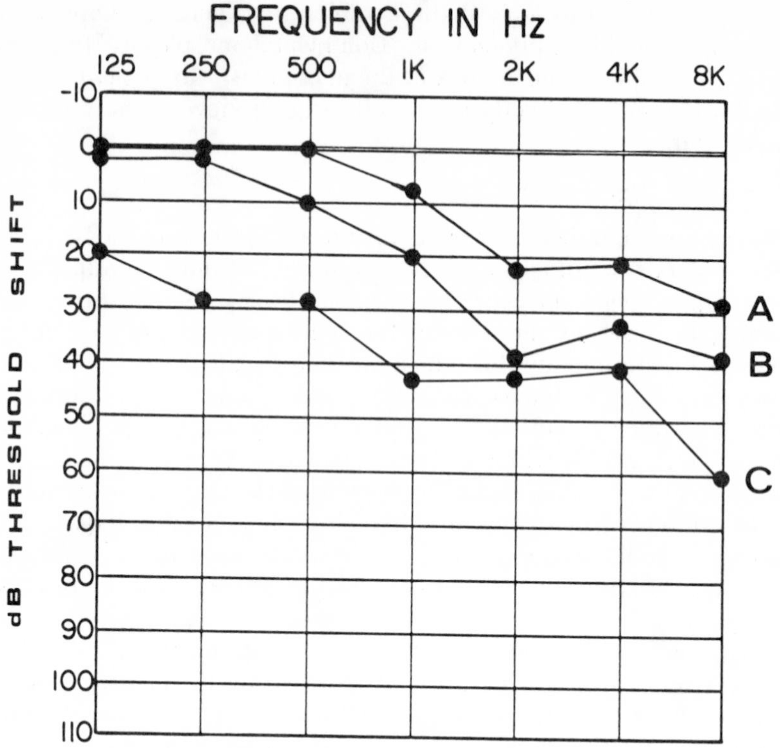

Fig. 3.3. Mean effects on pure tone air conduction thresholds in four normal ears of occluding the external ear canal. *A*, 91.6% occlusion; *B*, 98.3% occlusion; *C*, 100% occlusion. (Data from Chandler, 1964.)

In all patients this action will cause observable narrowing of the canal opening. However, in those most prone to collapsing canals, you can see the canal walls meet. No residual opening will be observable. Canal walls usually collapse bilaterally. However, on occasion you will see only unilateral collapse.

If collapsing canals are suspected, several procedures may be used for confirmation and to obtain valid results. The simplest is to reduce cushion pressure by holding the earphone slightly away from the pinna while retesting. If canals are in fact collapsing, you will see threshold improvement. The resulting threshold probably will not be exactly accurate, since the standard coupling arrangement is disrupted by pulling the earphone-cushion combination away from the head.

Another procedure is to place an insert, or hollow tube, into the external opening of the canal to hold it open during testing. A problem here is that the earphone pressure may tilt the insert so that its opening is against the wall of the canal, resulting in an even more substantial blockage. The insert least likely to create this problem is a standard hearing aid earmold, the kind that snaps onto the external receiver of a body-worn hearing aid. Stock earmolds of various sizes are available in most hearing clinics.

Having checked for the probability of collapsing canals, our primary purpose for looking into the ear canal is to ascertain the amount of wax in the canal. Because this condition is of utmost importance in tympanometry, discussion of otoscopic observation for this purpose is deferred to Chapter 7.

Instructing the Patient

Instructions should be simple and brief. Giving the patient too much detail regarding the test procedure may cause confusion and will use valuable time. Instructions will depend on the response preferred by the audiologist. There are several satisfactory easy-to-make and to-observe responses. The important thing is for the patient to understand that the task is to respond immediately, the same way each time, and even when the test signal is barely audible. Instructions for some common response systems are described below.

Raising a Finger. Instruct the patient as follows: "Place your arm upright with your elbow on the arm of the chair. Make a fist. Each time

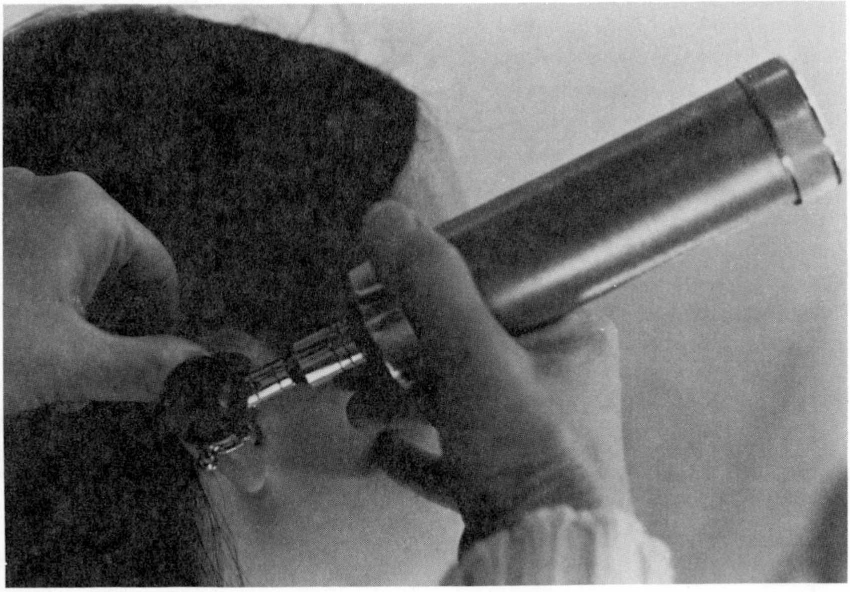

Fig. 3.4. Use of the otoscope.

you hear a tone raise your finger immediately. Put your finger down at once when the tone goes away. I want to find the faintest sound you can hear, so always raise your finger, even when you can just barely hear the tone." During the test, some patients will automatically raise a finger on the left hand when they hear the signal in the left ear and on the right hand when the right ear is being tested. Some audiologists request patients to do this, feeling it gives additional information about the ear in which the test signal is being heard. Reassurance is gained that the earphones are on correctly, that the output controls are in the right position, and most importantly, that the tone is not crossing the head and being heard by the nontest ear. You will learn much more about this last problem in the next chapter. Unfortunately, some patients are quite unreliable in reporting the ear in which the tone is heard. Moreover, accurate lateralization of the test tone grows more difficult as it approaches threshold (Tonndorf, 1972). Therefore, never take the unsupported word of the patient to indicate the ear in which the signal is heard. Always check the placement of the earphones and the position of the output control to be sure you are testing the appropriate ear. Techniques for determination and prevention of crossover hearing are discussed in Chapter 4.

Responding with "Yes." An alternative response is to tell the patient to say "yes" when the tone is heard: "Listen carefully and you will hear a series of tones. Each time you hear a tone, please say 'yes' out loud right away. I want to find the faintest sound you can hear, so always say 'yes' even when you can just barely hear the tone." The advantage of this response is that, since it is audible, you need not watch the patient at all times. Since you may need to look at the audiometer each time the hearing loss dial is changed between signal presentations, audible responses can save you a lot of head movement and, if the patient can see you at all, can save you from giving some visual clues causing anticipatory responses. In theory, you lose the definitiveness of the "on and off" response afforded by the patient raising the finger when the tone comes on and lowering it when the tone goes off. Actually, it is difficult, especially near threshold, to be specific about the onset and offset of the tone. If you use this response system and are relieved of the need to look at the patient's responses, you are still obligated to observe carefully for signs of boredom, fatigue, or discomfort. Personally, I prefer the verbal response for most patients. Of course, it necessitates, with a two room setup, a talk-back system. Actually, this circuitry, along with a talk-forward provision, is necessary anyway to answer the patient's questions, for reinstruction if there is confusion, and to deliver reinforcement.

Pushing a Signal Button. Some audiometers are equipped with a button which, when pushed, activates a light on the face of the audiometer. The patient can be instructed as before, only told to push the button when the tone is heard. I see no advantage to this procedure and feel that it puts an unnecessary piece of instrumentation between audiologist and patient. Manipulation of the button may be difficult for children, the elderly, or those with motor problems.

Play Audiometry. This procedure involves the patient in some motor responses, such as dropping a block in a can when the tone is heard. Other commonly used responses are putting rings on a peg or pegs into a pegboard. Commonly associated with testing of very young children, play audiometry may be useful for older inattentive children, retarded individuals, or others who are difficult to test. The response of play audiometry may be a more concrete and interesting task than raising a finger or saying "yes." Instructions may be given verbally or by gesture and pantomime, showing the child what is expected. Correct responses are reinforced verbally and sometimes with tangible (edible) reinforcement. For a more thorough discussion of play audiometry, refer to Hodgson (1978).

Positioning the Earphones

First, remove obstacles. Eyeglasses should come off since the pressure of the earphones may cause discomfort, or the glasses may prevent adequate seating of the earphone cushions. Earrings should be removed if they will cause discomfort or improper earphone placement. Some hair styles or wigs may cause problems and must be manipulated for a snug fit of the phones directly over the ears.

I prefer to stand in front of the patient when placing the headset. This position permits better observation of the ears and the patient's face, in case something in the process causes discomfort. Standing thus, the right earphone is held in the audiologist's left hand. Earphones are usually color coded: red for the right ear, blue for the left. Hold the phones firmly so they do not slip loose while being placed and strike the patient's head. Enlarge the headband by slipping the phones until it will fit over the head. Push hair aside and place the phones, one at a time, directly over the ears. With your thumbs, tighten the headband by slipping the phones until the phones are snug. Pull each phone lightly away from the ear to observe that there is no hair or other obstruction, that the pinna is not folded over by pressure of the cushion, and that the earphone diaphragm is directly over the ear canal. Make any necessary corrections. Finally, ask the patient if the headset is comfortable. This precaution is important. If you do not ask this question, you may waste time getting invalid results while the patient experiences discomfort from improperly placed earphones.

As a last step before starting the test, visually confirm that the earphones are placed on the ears correctly (red phone on the right, blue phone on left). Repeat this double check each time the earphones are removed and replaced.

OBTAINING AIR CONDUCTION THRESHOLDS

Pure tone audiometry requires integration of the knowledge acquired in earlier courses. As you begin your clinical practice remember that the good clinician must combine knowledge, skill, and experience. Store in your mind, for future use, what you learn about audiometric procedure, patient behavior, and the meaning of test results. Remember what you learn in each evaluation, to help you do the next one better. Benefit from errors; remember not to commit *that* one again! Remember the procedures that worked well and use them again when similar conditions recur.

Three methods of obtaining pure tone thresholds have been suggested: first, an *ascending* method, in which thresholds are determined by gradually increasing the intensity of the test tones, moving from an inaudible to an audible signal; second, a *descending* procedure, wherein intensity is reduced until the patient can no longer hear the signal and threshold is taken to be the last audible level; third, an *ascending-descending*, or bracketing, procedure in which both ascending and descending threshold search is employed, and threshold is taken as the average of the minimum response levels.

Carhart and Jerger (1959) described an ascending procedure which has been accepted as standard by ANSI (1978). Carhart and Jerger found the procedure accurate and quick. They discussed two auditory phenomena which should be considered when evaluating a procedure for obtaining threshold. The first is the on-effect, which they defined as the initial most vigorous response of the auditory system. The on-effect is elicited by a signal which has a brief rise time. Such a signal is produced by depressing the tone interruptor of today's audiometers. The second phenomenon is auditory adaptation. After the on-effect there is adaptation, reduction in responsiveness of the auditory system even though the stimulus is too weak to produce auditory fatigue. If there is pathology of the auditory nerve, the adaptation resulting from continuous stimulation, even near threshold, may be severe and may result in large change in threshold. However, even in ears with extreme adaptation, the auditory system recovers its responsiveness after the briefest rest (Hallpike and Hood, 1951). A threshold finding procedure which considers these factors will encourage response at the minimal level of which the patient is capable and will minimize variability of response.

To investigate feasibility of the ascending procedure, Carhart and Jerger obtained thresholds of 36 normal hearing adults using the ascending, the descending, and the ascending-descending procedure. Mean differences between methods were always less than 2 dB. Furthermore, variability among subjects was about the same from one method to another. Threshold audiometry ordinarily uses changes in intensity of 5 dB. Carhart and Jerger concluded that, because of this relatively large intensity increment in standard clinical use, the differences they found in thresholds determined by the three methods were not clinically meaningful. In other words, thresholds obtained by the three methods were indistinguishable, from a practical point of view. They recommended the ascending method because it was quick and simple and had the advantage of long time clinical use.

There are several points to keep in mind when using the Carhart-Jerger procedure. First, tone presentations are always 1–2 sec in duration. An interstimulus interval of 3 sec, during which no signal is presented to the patient, was recommended by Carhart and Jerger. However, the more recent ANSI (1978) standard specifies a minimum interstimulus time no shorter than the test tone (1–2 sec). These conditions promote elicitation of the on-effect, minimize auditory adaptation, and permit recovery from the adaptation which may occur.

Second, the search for threshold always involves an ascending procedure: a series of increasing intensity steps. The intensity decreases mentioned below occur only for the purpose of getting below the patient's threshold to start the threshold search.

Third, intensity changes *while seeking threshold* are always made in 5 dB steps. These 5 dB changes are always in the direction of greater intensity. A 5 dB reduction in intensity is never employed in the Carhart-Jerger procedure. The only exceptions occur when the patient responds to a tone at 0 or 5 dB HL, and a 10 dB decrement is not possible. Otherwise, intensity decrements are always 10 dB in magnitude, making the next presentation 10 dB below that at which the patient last responded. Reducing intensity 10 dB below the level of the last response ensures that you are below threshold and ready for another ascending series.

Fourth, threshold is defined as the minimal level at which response occurs in 50% or more of the ascents. The operational criterion for threshold is the first level at which three responses are obtained. These three responses need not be consecutive, but often they are. You will often find one level at which the patient never responds, while at a level 5 dB higher, a response always occurs.

After the patient is instructed and earphones are in place, there are three basic steps in the ascending procedure. The first step is to present an easily discernible tone of no more than comfortable loudness. This tone alerts the patient and permits the audiologist to see if instructions are understood and appropriate responses are forthcoming. You must estimate the patient's hearing sensitivity and present an appropriate tone. If the patient does not respond, present a higher level tone, ascending in 10 or 15 dB steps. Carhart and Jerger recommend that the first tone presentation be at 30–40 dB HL if the patient appears to have normal hearing and at 70 dB HL if a moderate loss appears to be present. Patients with sensory loss and loudness recruitment may be startled by a tone appreciably above their threshold. The closer the initial presentation is to threshold, providing that the tone is adequate to alert and prepare the patient, the sooner you can get below threshold. Testing will proceed quickly if you learn to present the first tone at about 10 dB above threshold.

The second step, after obtaining an initial response, is to decrease intensity until the tone is no longer audible. Descend in 10 or 15 dB steps, presenting a 1–2 sec tone at each level, until the patient no longer responds. The purpose of this step is to reach an inaudible level so the threshold search can begin. For efficient testing, the ideal is to get just below threshold. Therefore, let the size of the decrements you select be determined by how far you think your initial alerting presentation was above threshold. You want to get just below threshold utilizing as few presentations as possible.

The third step is to start the ascending search for threshold. This search consists of a series of ascending presentations, with a 1–2 sec tone presented at each level. Beginning the threshold search, you must strictly follow this procedure: each increment in intensity must be 5 dB and when the patient responds, you must decrease intensity 10 dB.

Visualize this sequence: when the patient fails to respond as you reduce intensity and present a signal, turn your hearing loss dial up 5 dB and present another tone. Continue to ascend in 5 dB steps until the patient responds. Then descend 10 dB. This 10 dB descent will put you back below the patient's threshold and permit you to begin another ascending series of signals. Continue this "up 5, down 10" process until you accumulate three responses at a given presentation level. That level is the patient's threshold. Perhaps you can visualize the process better by working your way through the example shown in Table 3.1.

To summarize, the ascending procedure consists of the following steps, which occur after the patient has been seated and instructed and the earphones have been properly positioned.

1. Present a comfortably loud tone of 1–2 sec duration.
2. Descend in 10 dB or larger steps, presenting a signal at each level until the patient fails to respond.
3. Start the threshold search. Ascend in *5 dB* steps, presenting a signal at each level, until the patient responds.

Table 3.1
Determining Auditory Threshold With an Ascending Procedure

Presentation Level in dB	Response	Cumulative Response
50	yes	
40	yes	
30	no	
35[a]	yes	1 response at 35 dB
25	no	
30	no	
35	no	
40	yes	1 response at 35 dB 1 response at 40 dB
30	no	
35	yes	2 responses at 35 dB 1 response at 40 dB
25	no	
30	no	
35	no	
40	yes	2 responses at 35 dB 2 responses at 40 dB
30	no	
35	yes	3 responses at 35 dB threshold is 35 dB

[a] Threshold search starts.

4. When the patient responds, descend *10 dB* and repeat step 3.
5. Threshold is the first level at which three responses are obtained.

When testing, you should vary the intervals between signals. Avoid a regular rhythm. Otherwise, through anticipation of an upcoming signal the patient may make a false response. Actually, the Carhart-Jerger procedure is not very susceptible to this problem, since many of the tone presentations are below the patient's threshold, and do not contribute to the establishement of an audible rhythmic pattern. Be particularly alert for this problem, though, if you ever use a descending procedure for threshold determination.

It is customary to begin air conduction testing with evaluation of the better ear. Having tested the better ear, you can estimate the possibility of crossover hearing when testing the poorer ear. This problem is discussed in the next chapter. Ascertain the better ear by asking the patient before testing. Most people can identify their better ear if there is a difference in sensitivity of perhaps 10 dB or more. Even so, if you begin to test the reportedly better ear and find you are obtaining thresholds which seem poorer than the patient's observed ability to respond, switch your signal to the other ear and ascertain if the patient is perhaps confused about the better ear. If not, you should look for other problems which are giving you incongruous and perhaps invalid results. If the patient cannot report a better ear it is customary to begin with the right ear.

Conventionally, 1000 Hz is the first frequency to be tested. Carhart and Hayes (1949) reported better reliability for 1000 Hz thresholds than for other frequencies. The 1000 Hz signal may have better alerting features than very high or low frequency tones. However, it may be advisable to start at 500 Hz if you suspect a profound hearing loss. The usual configuration of most hearing losses is such that, with profound losses, 500 Hz is more likely to be audible than 1000 Hz.

After establishing threshold at 1000 Hz, it is conventional to proceed to 2000 Hz, 4000 Hz, 8000 Hz, a retest of 1000 Hz, 500 Hz, and 250 Hz. The 1000 Hz retest provides an important measure of reliability of response, although it is sometimes omitted if all results are highly reliable. Some audiologists record on the audiogram both test and retest 1000 Hz thresholds, labeling them "1" and "2" to provide a record of response reliability. The frequency of 125 Hz is not ordinarily tested. Half-octave tones (750 Hz, 1500 Hz, 3000 Hz, 6000 Hz) should be tested if there is a difference in sensitivity between adjacent octave points of 20 dB or more. This practice gives additional information, in cases where there is a large change in sensitivity, about where the change begins. The information can be useful in estimating handicap, particulary when the drop occurs in the range critical for speech intelligibility: between 1000 and 2000 Hz, for example. When obtaining audiograms associated with industrial hearing conservation, or when there is the possibility of claim for compensation because of hearing damage, you should always test 3000 Hz and 6000 Hz regardless of sensitivity at adjacent frequencies. In such instances these frequencies may be used for baseline establishment or for estimation of hearing impairment.

When testing patients with substantial losses you may reach the maximum output limits of the audiometer without eliciting a response. In such cases, some audiologists record the usual threshold symbol on the audiogram at the level of the audiometer's maximum output, then draw an arrow from the symbol pointing downward to indicate there was no response at the maximum available output. Others prefer to enter nothing on the audiogram and write below the audiogram those frequencies at which a response could not be elicited. Whichever procedure is used, be sure you have a method to differentiate between those frequencies at which you could not get a response and those frequencies which were not tested, for whatever reason. It is usual practice to enter DNT (did not test) or CNT (could not test) over the frequencies which were not tested. The particular practices you follow should be those of the clinic where you work. *Be sure that your method of recording is consistent with the key on the audiogram which explains the symbol system and that your results are entered clearly in a way that leaves no room for misinterpretation.*

Be alert to the fact that the maximum audiometer output varies across frequencies. Most audiometers have a maximum air conduction output of 110 dB HL in the range from 500 through 6000 Hz. The usual air conduction maximum output is 70 dB HL at 125 Hz and 90 dB HL at 250 and 8000 Hz. Maximum output limits are ordinarily noted on the audiometer's frequency selector. Be sure you do not exceed these limits. When testing 8000 Hz, for example, if the maximum output is 90 dB HL, never turn the hearing loss dial to 95 or 100. To do so will not result in a tone of 95 or 100 dB HL, since the audiometer is incapable of producing a hearing level above 90 dB at 8000 Hz. Instead, record that there was no response at the maximum output of 90 dB HL, and continue with the test.

Having finished the evaluation of the better ear and recorded the results, turn your attention to the other ear. No additional instruction of the patient is necessary. Testing of the poorer ear usually proceeds in the same fashion as for the ear just completed. A difference which may arise, however, relates to the need for masking noise to prevent participation of the better ear. Without masking, the test tone may be heard in the nontest ear if difference in sensitivity between ears is sufficiently large to overcome interaural attenuation. Interaural attenuation is defined as the reduction in the level of a signal as it crosses the head from one ear to the other. The reduction for an air conducted tone is expected to be about 50 dB, although there is considerable variation from person to person. Therefore, if the difference between ears approaches or exceeds 50 dB, introduction of masking noise to the nontest ear is needed. The masking procedure is discussed in the next chapter.

MAINTAINING A CONTINUOUS ASSESSMENT OF VALIDITY

Errors which are not detected may produce results which appear quite plausible when the audiogram is reviewed. These mistakes, in addition to causing erroneous results, may form the basis for additional mistakes. In audiometry, there are three levels of competency: the audiologist who does not make mistakes, the audiologist who recognizes and corrects mistakes, and the audiologist who does not recognize mistakes. While we should try to operate in the first category as much as possible, it is critical that we stay out of the third category if we are to deliver acceptable clinical services.

You must continuously assess the validity of your results. Errors accumulate into these groups: malfunctioning equipment, improper audiometric procedure, and invalid responses from the patient. Therefore, you must repeatedly ask these questions: Is the equipment working correctly? Am I working correctly? Is the patient working correctly? Some common errors and techniques for correction are discussed below.

Equipment Problems

Most problems of this sort will be avoided with a good maintenance program, a thorough listening check prior to testing, and the immediate correction of any shortcomings detected in the listening check. Exceptions have to do with equipment malfunctions which occur during the test and with intermittent problems not detected during the listening check. Equipment problems of this sort will usually result in illogical patient behavior, which should alert you to check your equipment. For example, if a patient shows a unilateral loss which was not mentioned in the pretest interview, you should, by listening, recheck the output of the test earphone, even though it seemed all right during the listening check. Another procedure is to reverse the earphones on the patient's head and double check your results with the other earphone.

To illustrate an equipment problem which may escape detection in the listening check, you may someday have a patient who responds reliably when one ear is being tested but whose responses become variable when the signal is switched to the other earphone. Through wear it is possible for the wiring of the earphone cord to break without visually observable damage to the covering insulation. When this happens, the result is likely to be an intermittent signal. The signal will be on from time to time when the broken ends of the wires come into contact but will be erratically off, depending on movements of the patient's head. Thus, the observed reliability will deteriorate, simply because the signal either is not always on when you think it is on or else does not meet the temporal requirements necessary for obtaining valid thresholds.

Procedural Problems

Correct placement of the earphones is important for valid audiometry and will help to avoid potential problems. First, always double check to be sure that the earphones are placed on the correct ears—red phone on the right, blue phone on the left. Recheck this placement each time you remove and replace the phones. Second, be sure the phones are comfortably and correctly centered over the ear. There is some unavoidable variability associated with earphone placement. Shaw (1966) reported test-retest variability, with earphones removed after the first test and carefully replaced, of less than 1 dB at 1000 Hz. Substantial variability occurred above 3000 Hz, with almost 10 dB at 8000 Hz. Green

(1978) estimated that poor earphone placement can cause threshold variability of 15 dB or more.

At the start of each day's testing be sure all controls are set properly. During testing, quickly check before you record each threshold to see that the most commonly used controls are set as you wish them to be. Be certain input and output controls are set properly. Be sure the frequency selector is at the desired frequency. Finally, look again at the hearing loss dial to verify the level of the threshold just obtained. A check of these four control settings—input, output, frequency selector, and hearing loss dial—will help you to record consistently correct thresholds.

Be alert to the possibility of error when testing 8000 Hz. At this frequency, standing waves may reduce effective signal intensity. If you obtain a large difference in sensitivity between 4000 and 8000 Hz, ask the patient to "readjust the test earphone to make it more comfortable." Then reobtain the 8000 Hz threshold. If the first threshold was invalid, the standing wave may be broken up when the patient moves the earphone, and a large improvement in 8000 Hz threshold may result.

Patient Problems

Consciously or unconsciously, the patient may fail to follow your directions, and, unless correction is undertaken, invalid results may occur. The patient may simply fail to hear or understand your instructions. If this appears to be the case, reinstruct the patient, taking pains to correct the problem which prevented the original instructions from being effective.

False responses made by the patient are a serious threat to audiogram validity. A committee of the American Speech and Hearing Association (1978) defined two types of false responses. A *false positive* response is one which occurs when the tone is not present or not audible. A *false negative* response is a failure to respond when the tone is present and audible. Most patients make a few false responses. Some make so many that valid testing becomes a problem.

False positive responses presumably occur when the patient's imagination works overtime. The patient is told to listen carefully, that some tones will occur, and to respond to those tones even if they are very faint. The patient may very well imagine that a nonexistent signal has occurred and respond. The problem is compounded if a signal, though inaudible, is presented at about the time the patient makes the false positive response. Suppose the clinician accepts the false response (remember it is at a level already below the patient's threshold) and attenuates the signal 10 dB before the next tone presentation. Now with signal intensity ascending in 5 dB steps, considerable time would pass before an audible tone occurs. Long periods of silence may increase false positive responses, as the patient's anticipation builds while waiting for a signal. If another false positive response occurs and is accepted, the signal will be attenuated still further. The result could be a cycle which will cause the signal to be reduced far below the patient's threshold. The uncritical clinician may record a threshold much better than the patient's true hearing, perhaps along with a comment that test reliability was poor.

False positive responses can be differentiated from valid responses only by careful observation of the temporal relationship between stimulus and response. You must observe this relationship initially as the individual patient responds to suprathreshold tones. Some patients respond quickly when the tone is presented, others slowly. Once you have established the response pattern in a patient, do not accept any response that violates the pattern. The only qualification to this rule is that there is in general a slight increase in response latency as stimulus intensity approaches threshold.

When a false positive response occurs, ignore it. Continue with your pattern of tone presentation just as if it had not happened. If you are not sure whether it was a false response or not, present one or two additional tones at the same level. See if responses to those tones occur. If you are not sure whether a less than 100% pattern of responses at a given level represents false positive responses or the approximately 50% behavior indicating threshold, increase the intensity of the signal 5 dB and present a few tones. If the responses you are observing are real, consistency should now go to 100%, for you will have reached a suprathreshold level. On the other hand, if you are observing false positive responses, the timing between stimulus and response will remain poor and the response pattern will still be less than 100%.

There are a number of ways to reduce false positive responses if the frequency of their occurrence becomes a problem. One way is to reinstruct the patient. Indicate that the patient is trying a little too hard, or guessing too much, and should be a bit more certain that the signal is actually there before responding. However, these instructions may not solve the problem, or may even create new problems. Surprisingly, some patients go right on making false responses, even after being cautioned not to do so. On the other hand, instructions may inhibit responses unduly, particularly in children, and in effect create the problem of false negative responses.

It is better to prevent large numbers of false responses than to try to reduce their prevalence after they have already started. False positive responses tend to be increased by presenting stimuli too quickly or too slowly for a given patient. If the stimuli are presented too rapidly for the patient to handle adequately, a state of overpreparedness to respond can occur. The patient's set can be placed on a "hair-trigger," and increased anticipation can lead to false responses. On the other hand, long periods of silence between signals can also lead to anticipatory false response. For each patient there is a rate of presentation that is just right, not too fast and not too slow. It behooves the clinician to observe the patient's behavior and to establish this rate to prevent the development of numerous false responses.

False positive responses may be associated with the presence of pure tone type tinnitus. A reliable patient may become erratic when the test tone approximates the pitch of the tinnitus. This problem is demonstrated in the Bekesy-type tracing shown in Figure 3.5. To generate this audiogram, the patient listened to a tone of continuously changing frequency while operating a handswitch to control intensity and to trace his own threshold. The threshold trace was reliable until the frequency approached 4000 Hz, approximating the pitch of the patient's tinnitus, and then reliability deteriorated. As the tone moved above the pitch of the tinnitus, reliable tracing resumed.

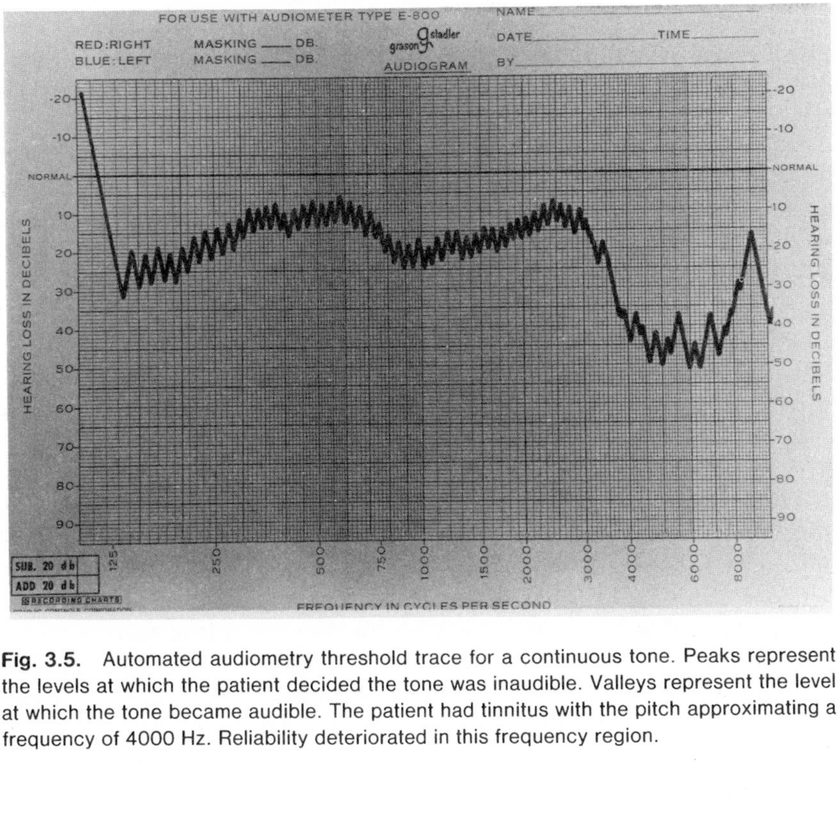

Fig. 3.5. Automated audiometry threshold trace for a continuous tone. Peaks represent the levels at which the patient decided the tone was inaudible. Valleys represent the level at which the tone became audible. The patient had tinnitus with the pitch approximating a frequency of 4000 Hz. Reliability deteriorated in this frequency region.

In your conventional audiometry, if tinnitus associated variability is suspected, it may help to change the test signal from continuous to an interrupted tone, or to a warble tone. Many audiometers provide these signals. An interrupted (pulsed) tone is usually on for 200 or 500 msec and off for the same amount of time. A warble tone is a frequency modulated signal, with small, rapid changes in the frequency of the carrier signal. The patient may find either the pulsed or warble tone easier to differentiate from tinnitus, and reliability may improve. There is evidence that thresholds obtained with interrupted and warble tones are not, because of the nature of the stimulus, different from those obtained with conventional pure tone signals (Staab and Rintelmann, 1972). However, Barry and Resnick (1978) reported slight improvement of warble tone thresholds over those for pure tones as the frequency deviation from the center of the warble tone frequency increased. They concluded that possible differences between warble tone and pure tone thresholds could be minimized by limiting frequency deviations to no more than ± 10% of the carrier frequency and using a modulation rate of no less than 20 times/sec.

Conductive hearing loss may also affect reliability of the pure tone threshold. The clinician expects individuals with conductive loss to have "spongy" or slightly variable thresholds. The line between inaudibility and audibility seems not as sharply drawn as in patients with sensory loss. At a level approaching threshold patients with conductive loss may express doubt about the audibility of the signal.

Patients with sensory loss seldom show doubt about the audibility of a signal. More often than not they will never respond at one level but will respond consistently and with confidence when the next 5 dB increment is provided. This sharp demarkation between inaudibility and audibility is consistent with disorders of cochlear origin.

Patients with retrocochlear (VIIIth nerve) disorders may exhibit marked threshold adaptation in response to a continuous tone. They may respond variably if the test procedure taps their tendency to threshold adaptation. However, use of the ascending procedure, moving from inaudibility to audibility and using tones of short duration, should avoid this problem.

You will probably encounter an occasional apprehensive individual for whom reinstruction or careful timing does not reduce the high incidence of false responses. In a few cases, use of a descending method when obtaining threshold may reduce false positive responses. The reduction probably occurs because, with the descending procedure, the patient does not have to wait in silence as long as when the ascending procedure is used. Audible signals occur more often.

The threshold search in the descending procedure is made as follows. First, present an audible tone and observe that the response is satisfactory. Then, descend in 5 dB steps, presenting a signal at each level, until the patient does not respond. Now, increase intensity 10 dB, and repeat the descending procedure. Continue until you have obtained the same minimum response level three times. This level is threshold.

False negative responses, characterized by a failure to respond to signals exceeding organic thresholds, are less common than false positive responses. False negative responses may be associated with functional hearing loss—the patient who is feigning a hearing loss or who has a psychogenic disorder. A second reason may be simply lack of attention or just a tendency to be absolutely certain that the signal is present before responding. Offenders often reveal themselves by unreliable responses. Fortunately, false responses are probably most common in those who do not pay careful attention. Their problem can often be remedied by maintaining a set to respond. Alert the patient to the upcoming signal. Say, "Ready?" and "Listen, now." Then present the signal. Vary the time between your alerting cue and the signal presentation to prevent development of false positive responses. When the inattentive patient responds, deliver positive verbal reinforcement such as, "Fine," or, "You're doing a good job."

The descending procedure for obtaining threshold, described above to reduce false positive responses, may also reduce false negative responses in the inattentive patient. When the descending procedure is used, the interval between audible tones is reduced, possibly making it easier to maintain the patient's attention.

If you suspect that false negative responses are occurring because of malingering (feigned hearing loss), do not stay with the ascending procedure. The patient may know or learn the steps of this procedure and make reliable responses by counting the supposedly inaudible signals leading up to the level of admitted threshold. If other clues are not available, malingerers must use perceived loudness as a yardstick for the level they will admit hearing. For most, judgment of loudness is not precise enough to permit reliable response. Therefore, lack of reliability may provide a clue that the admitted thresholds are not valid.

A bracketing or ascending-descending procedure may be useful for exploring reliability in suspected functional loss. Thresholds obtained on an ascending run should not vary more than 5 dB from those of a descending run. Greater variability suggests invalid responses. The same generalization applies to the retest of a frequency, such as 1000 Hz after the intervening test of a number of other frequencies. Thresholds should be repeatable within ± 5 dB.

RECORDING RESULTS

If, in spite of all your efforts, you cannot obtain reliable indications of thresholds and good intertest agreement, do not record test results uncritically. If you do, those who look at those test results thereafter will have no indication that the patient's responses were unreliable and that you question the validity of your test results. Indicate the confidence you place in the results and the limitations which reduce your confidence.

Results must be recorded completely, accurately, and clearly. Once your memory of the testing has faded, only the results you have recorded will exist as a record of the test. The way you have recorded the results will determine the usefulness and the accuracy of what you have learned.

Identifying Information

Record accurate and complete identifying information. Those who examine the record later need clear and complete information about who was tested, by whom, on what date, and with which test equipment. The identity of the referring source and those to whom reports of test results were sent should be included. You should enter clearly and completely all information for which space is provided on the Audiologic Record. Avoid the following pitfalls: (1) spaces left blank, (2) information entered illegibly, (3) incorrect information, or (4) incomplete information. Avoid using initials instead of the evaluator's name. Especially in large clinics after some time has passed, the use of initials makes identification of the evaluator difficult. Always include the year of the test as well as the day and month. Otherwise, comparison of serial audiograms and estimation of progression of loss will not be possible.

Thresholds

There is no universal or completely standard method of recording thresholds. The conventional red circle and blue X for right and left air conduction thresholds are probably in universal use. Beyond that, variations abound. Therefore, it is important that the Audiologic Record contain a *key* explaining the symbols and abbreviations used and that you follow this key in recording your test results. Only through careful adherence to this practice can you be sure you have done everything possible to communicate effectively and prevent misinterpretations.

The ASHA (1974) and the ANSI (1978) recommend audiometric symbols for standard use. These symbols are shown in Figure 3.6. The recommended system has separate symbols for the right and left ear and for air and bone conduction thresholds. There are also separate symbols to indicate thresholds obtained with and without the use of masking. There are symbols for less commonly used procedures and for the indication of "no response" when the patient does not respond at the maximum output of the audiometer.

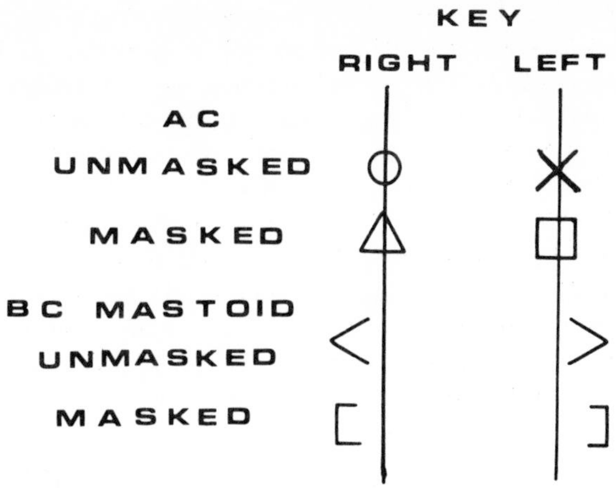

Fig. 3.6. Threshold symbols recommended by the ASHA (1974).

Table 3.2
Symbols Used by 50 Hearing Clinics to Record Auditory Thresholds

	n	*n* Who Record Amount of Effective Masking Used
Use all ASHA recommended symbols	31	23/31
Use ASHA recommended AC but not BC symbols	10	6/10
Use same symbols for masked and unmasked thresholds	9	9/9

A survey asking 50 clinics about the symbols used for threshold resulted in the information shown in Table 3.2. Separate symbols for masked and unmasked thresholds make audiometric interpretation more complex and may confuse referring sources. It may also discourage recording of the *amount* of effective masking used. As indicated by the survey, various bone conduction threshold symbols remain in use.

Regardless of the symbol system used, the important thing is that a key to interpretation be provided on the audiogram and that the key be followed in recording the test results. In addition to an explanation of symbols, the key should explain abbreviations in common use at a given clinic. Examples are "NR" for "no response," "DNT" for "did not test," and "CNT" for "could not test."

Comments

The Audiologic Record usually provides space for evaluator comments. Depending on the philosophy of the individual clinic, this space may be intended to contain the entire audiologic report which interprets the test results and makes recommendations or for the more limited purposes discussed below. Report writing is discussed in Chapter 8.

The "comments" section should include a statement about the confidence the evaluator had in the test results. Inconsistencies between results and observed behavior should be noted as well as special procedures or retesting necessary to obtain complete and valid results. The patient behavior which necessitated this additional testing should be recorded. Other tests not routinely administered, for which there is no space on the form, should be recorded here. In this section, and throughout, the content and form of what you record should be guided by this rule: the person who next looks at the audiogram should be able to get all the valid information about the patient which you obtained during testing.

BONE CONDUCTION AUDIOMETRY

Bone conduction thresholds are sometimes described as "direct" measures of the sensitivity of the inner ear. There are important qualifications to this description, as you will learn later in this chapter.

To obtain bone conduction thresholds, a pure tone oscillator, or vibrator, is placed against the skull and the signal vibrates the skull. Thus, the sound does not take the normal air conduction route through the external ear canal, the middle ear, and into the cochlea. Rather, the intent is to stimulate the cochlea directly, by bone conduction, bypassing the conductive mechanisms of the outer and middle ear. Bone conduction testing is intended to measure cochlear functioning independent of any defect in the outer or middle ear. If the sensorineural system is normal, normal bone conduction thresholds should be obtained. I used "sensorineural system" in the sentence above rather than "inner ear" because bone conduction measures assess auditory nerve as well as cochlear sensitivity. Bone conduction thresholds are not always entirely normal when the sensorineural system is normal because, unfortunately, the status of the outer and middle ear does contribute to bone conduction results under certain circumstances. These problems are discussed later in this chapter.

Purpose

Bone conduction tests are not tests of functional hearing sensitivity. Although a sensitivity measure, the tests are not designed, as are air conduction tests, to determine how intense an everyday sound must be for audibility. Rather the purpose of bone conduction testing is diagnostic. The *type* of hearing loss can be determined through air-bone comparison. To explain, air conduction tests are sensitive to deficits in all three of the ear's parts: outer, middle, and inner. Bone conduction tests, bypassing the outer and middle ear, are sensitive to deficits only in the sensorineural system. Therefore, the difference between air and bone conduction thresholds in a given ear represents the amount of conductive hearing loss: the amount of loss caused by disorder of the outer or middle ear. Stated differently, the magnitude of conductive loss is equal to the magnitude of the air-bone gap, or the air conduction threshold minus the bone conduction threshold.

Audiograms showing normal bone conduction with reduced air conduction thresholds indicate *conductive* hearing loss. Audiograms showing equally reduced air and bone conduction thresholds indicate *sensorineural* hearing loss. Audiograms showing bone conduction thresholds reduced, but with a greater reduction of air conduction thresholds, represent an ear in which there is both a conductive and a sensorineural component: a *mixed* hearing loss. In both sensorineural and mixed losses the reduction in bone conduction sensitivity represents the amount of sensorineural hearing loss. Figure 3.7 shows examples of the three types of hearing loss: conductive, sensorineural, and mixed.

Mechanisms of Bone Conduction

To help you understand some of the clinical procedures associated with bone conduction testing, a brief discussion of the mechanisms of bone conduction is necessary. Many investigators have studied the process of bone conduction and have proposed various mechanisms which contribute to bone conduction sensitivity. Conclusions have not always been harmonious. However, it is clear that inertial and compressional bone conduction are two major factors (Kirikae, 1959; Bekesy, 1960). A third factor is associated with energy radiating from the walls of the external ear canals.

Inertial bone conduction is so named because it arises from the inertia of structures not rigidly attached to the skull. The ossicular chain is the most important of these structures. When the skull vibrates as a unit, the inertia of the ossicular chain causes it to lag behind. The result is relative movement between the footplate of the stapes and the oval window. Thus, energy is sent into the cochlea just as it is in air conducted hearing.

Compressional bone conduction results when forces are transferred from the skull into the cochlear fluid. The result is movement of the membranes of the oval and round windows. Movement of the cochlear fluid also causes deformation of the basilar membrane, and stimulation occurs. Because of the fashion in which the skull vibrates, inertial bone conduction is more important for low frequencies, and compressional bone conduction makes a greater contribution to transmission of high frequency signals.

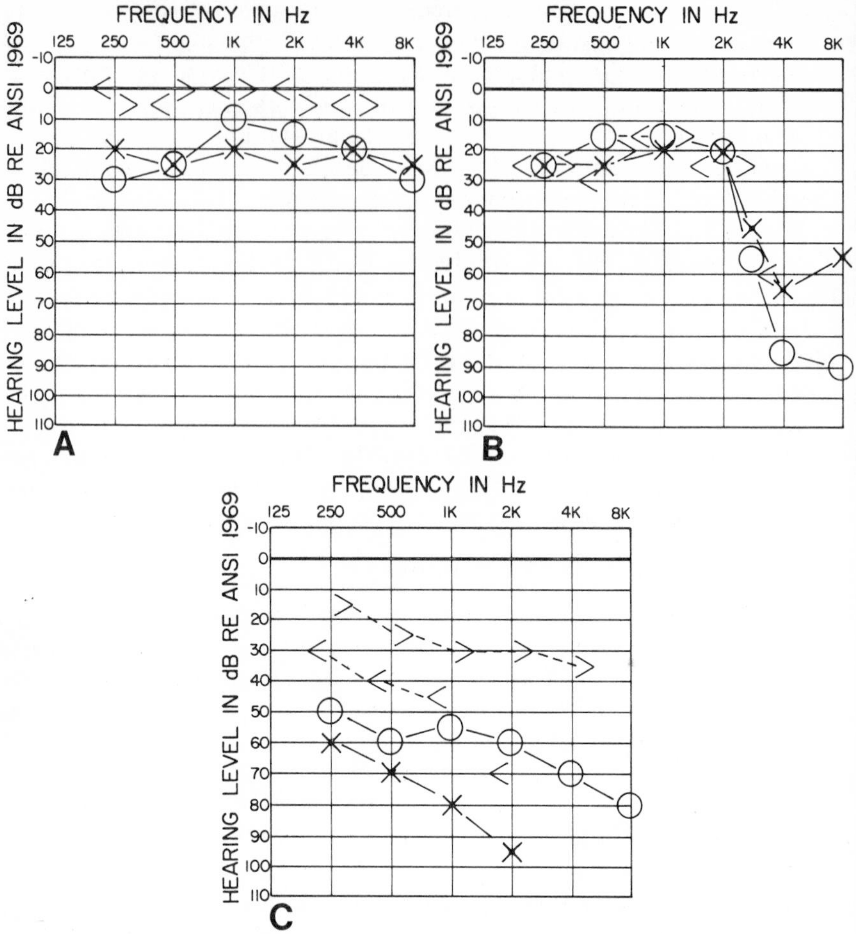

Fig. 3.7. Audiograms illustrating three types of hearing loss. *A*, conductive loss. Audiometric indicators of a pure conductive disorder are normal bone conduction thresholds and reduced air conduction sensitivity. The size of the resulting air-bone gap represents the magnitude of the conductive blockage. *B*, sensorineural loss without a conductive component is represented audiometrically by equally reduced air and bone conduction thresholds. Such results indicate that the deficit is in the sensorineural mechanism. There is no bone conduction response on the right ear at 4000 Hz because the sensorineural level at that frequency exceeds the maximum bone conduction output of 70 dB HL. *C*, mixed loss. When there is both a conductive and a sensorineural component in the same ear, bone conduction thresholds will be reduced and air conduction thresholds will be reduced even more. The reduction of bone conduction thresholds reflects the sensorineural loss and the air-bone gap indicates the conductive component. Thresholds on the left ear at 4000 Hz and 8000 Hz (AC) and 4000 Hz (BC) exceed maximum output limits.

A third mechanism of bone conduction which has important clinical implications is discussed by Tonndorf (1966, 1972). Vibrations of the skull radiate energy from the walls of the external ear canals. This energy may create sound waves which travel to the inner ear via the regular air conduction route: external canal, eardrum, and ossicular chain. Therefore, as you would expect, the effect of this mechanism is *increased* if the external ear canal is covered, directing the energy inward. The effect is *decreased* if there is a conductive deficit which reduces the efficiency of the air conduction system. This mechanism is associated with the occlusion effect, which is discussed below.

In summary, three mechanisms have been discussed which are important to bone conducted hearing. First, the inertial response of the ossicular chain transmits energy into the cochlea. Second, compressional stimulation occurs when distortion of the skull transmits energy into the cochlear fluid. Third, varying amounts of energy may reach the inner ear by radiation from the walls of the external canals, depending on the state of occlusion of the canals and the status of the conductive mechanism.

The maximum conductive loss, that is, the maximum air conduction loss in the presence of normal bone conduction, is 60–70 dB re: 1969 ANSI norms (Goetzinger, 1978). Vibration of the skull afforded by contact with a TDH 39-MX 41/AR earphone-cushion combination which is producing a signal of 60–70 dB HL is sufficient for audibility if the cochlear is normal, even in the absence of an air conduction mechanism. Thus, purely conductive losses should not exceed 70 dB and, in practice, should rarely reach that magnitude.

Principles of Bone Conduction Which Affect Audiometry

Here are some points which may help you to obtain and interpret bone conduction thresholds. If you understand these points clearly, it will probably make your reading of the rest of this chapter easier.

People with normal air conduction thresholds have normal bone conduction thresholds. The inner ear and auditory nerve are part of the system measured when determining thresholds by air conduction. Therefore, any deficit in these structures will be reflected in air conduction thresholds, as well as in bone conduction thresholds. Bone conduction thresholds are ordinarily not tested if air conduction thresholds are found to be entirely normal (0 dB HL).

You cannot have significantly poorer bone conduction thresholds than air conduction thresholds. Since the system measured by bone conduction is also part of the system contributing to air conduction sensitivity, it follows that bone conduction thresholds cannot validly be poorer than air conduction thresholds. Bone conduction thresholds 10 dB "poorer" than air conduction thresholds may be seen because of allowable variability. Greater differences suggest invalid air or bone conduction thresholds, or both. Retesting, with careful attention to transducer placement and test procedure, may resolve this problem.

Interaural attenuation for a bone conducted tone is essentially 0 dB. Earlier you learned that "interaural attenuation" means the amount by which the intensity of the tone is reduced as it travels across the head from the test to the nontest ear. Remember that the interaural attenuation of a tone introduced to the test ear by air conduction is expected to be about 50 dB. No such attenuation is expected for a signal which is impressed directly on the skull. Regardless of the point of contact of the vibrator on the skull, the signal may stimulate each cochlea with approximately the same energy. Some interaural attenuation of bone conducted signals may occur, especially for higher frequencies. However, because its occurrence is not dependable, the clinician must always assume that the interaural attenuation of a bone conducted tone is essentially zero. Valid bone conduction audiometry can be assured only by introducing masking noise to the nontest ear in all instances of bone conduction testing when there is any possibility that the nontest ear can contribute importantly to test results. The procedure for masking during bone conduction testing is explained in the next chapter.

People with unilateral sensorineural loss lateralize bone conducted sound to the better ear while those with unilateral conductive loss lateralize bone conducted sound to the involved ear. With unilateral sensorineural loss, there is a normal cochlea only on one side. It follows that such an individual would have the sense of hearing a bone conducted tone via the ear with the normal cochlea. This phenomenon involves the Stenger effect, which dictates that, when tones identical in all ways except loudness are introduced simultaneously to a person's two ears, the person will have the sense of hearing the tone only in the ear where the loudness is greater. In unilateral conductive loss, both cochleas are normal. The sense of lateralization to the impaired ear may relate to a phase lead introduced by the conductive disorder (Allen and Fernandez, 1960; Tyszka and Goldstein, 1975) or to interaural intensity differences resulting in relatively greater stimulation of the cochlea associated with the conductive impairment (Naunton and Elpern, 1964). These lateralization phenomena are the basis for the Weber test, discussed in the next section.

Tuning Fork Tests

The Weber is a classic tuning fork test which can also be performed with the audiometer bone vibrator. The test gives supportive information to differentiate conductive and sensorineural loss. To perform the audiometric Weber, the bone vibrator is placed on the forehead and held in place by the regular headband. Ask the patient to tell you in which ear the sound is heard. Testing is usually done at 250, 500, and 1000 Hz. An efficient procedure is to pulse the bone conducted tone and, beginning at 0 dB HL, increase the level until the patient responds. Then, test at the next frequency. Finally, go back and retest each frequency as a reliability check. It is convenient to record results in the space above each audiometric frequency by indicating "left" or "right," according to the patient's response. In unilateral loss, the Weber is expected to lateralize to the involved ear if the loss is conductive and to the normal ear if the loss is sensorineural. In bilateral loss, the Weber is expected to lateralize to the ear with the greater conductive component. The Weber test has a poor clinical reputation for reliability and should be used only as a preliminary indicator of type of hearing loss or to gain corroborative information in a battery of tests. More is said about interpretation and recording of Weber test results in Chapter 8.

Other tuning fork tests, usually performed by physicians, include the Schwabach test, during which a tuning fork is held against the mastoid process and the length of time the patient can hear it is compared to normal. The patient with conductive loss should hear the tone for a normal period of time. The duration of audibility is reduced in sensorineural loss.

In the Rinne test, determination is made of comparative ability to hear the tuning fork by air conduction (fork near the ear canal) and by bone conduction (fork on the mastoid process). With normal hearing or sensorineural loss, the tone should be heard better by air conduction or equally well by air and bone conduction (positive Rinne). Patients with conductive loss should hear the tone better by bone conduction (negative Rinne).

To perform the Bing test, the examiner holds a low frequency tuning fork against the mastoid process while alternately covering and uncovering the test ear canal with a finger. Patients with normal hearing or sensorineural loss should hear a louder tone when the ear is occluded. For patients with conductive loss there should be no change in loudness.

The Bone Conduction Vibrator

It is difficult to generalize from research about factors that affect bone conduction testing. Vibrators of different styles have been used in various experiments, and the findings derived with one type of vibrator may not generalize to others. Early bone vibrators were of the "grenade" type, large hand held units with a small vibrating surface. "Hearing aid type" vibrators are in current audiometric use. They are attached to the head, usually by a springy metal clip. Such a bone vibrator and its head

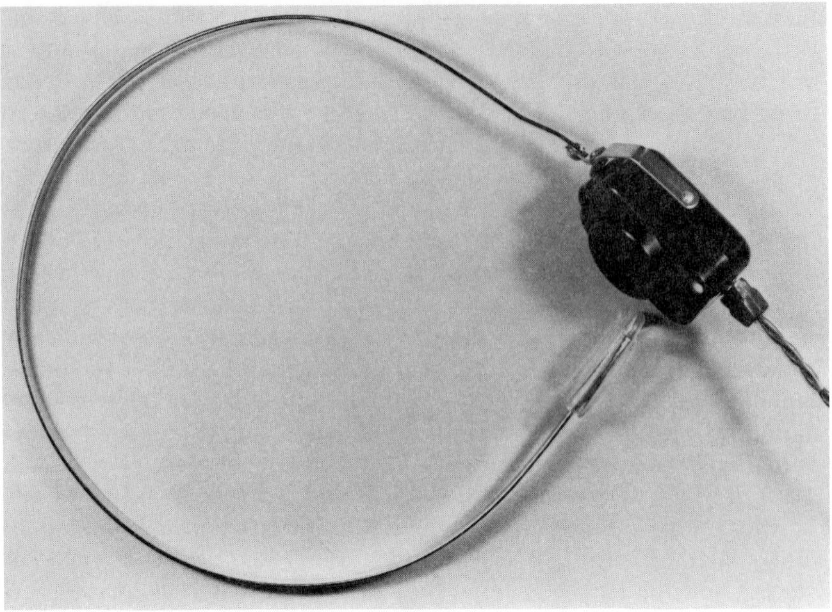

Fig. 3.8. Bone conduction vibrator and headband.

band are shown in Figure 3.8. Vibrators used clinically include the Sonotone B-9, the Radioear B70A, and the Radioear B71 and B72. The latter two meet the configuration recommended in a standardization move by the IEC (1971) and the ANSI (1972). These specifications stipulate a circular contact tip with a surface area of 1.75 cm^2.

Placement of the Vibrator

Traditionally the bone vibrator has been placed against the mastoid process on the side of the ear under test. There is some evidence that forehead placement is more satisfactory. Mastoid placement may give clinicians a false sense of security, it is said, since it may appear that the ear being tested is the one closest to the vibrator. Actually, since the interaural attenuation for a bone conducted tone is expected to be zero, the unmasked bone conduction threshold is likely to represent sensitivity of the better cochlea, regardless of vibrator placement. Therefore, forehead placement, with appropriate masking to prevent participation of the nontest ear, will prevent the false sense of security. As it turns out, forehead placement may offer other advantages as well. Experimenters have found that placement of the vibrator on the forehead is less critical than on the mastoid. That is, changes in placement result in smaller changes in threshold when the vibrator is on the forehead than on the mastoid. Another possible advantage of forehead placement is increased test-retest reliability. A third reported advantage is a decrease of the contribution of the middle ear to bone conduction thresholds when the vibrator is on the forehead rather than on the mastoid. Dirks (1964) did, in fact, find less variability and better test-retest reliability with forehead rather than mastoid placement but concluded that differences were small when a hearing aid type vibrator was used. Dirks and Malmquist (1969) and Goodhill, Dirks, and Malmquist (1970) reported that forehead placement resulted in bone conduction thresholds more representative of cochlear function in certain middle ear lesions. They felt that mastoid placement added an artifact of middle ear origin whose magnitude at some frequencies was as large as 20 dB. They recommended that forehead placement be considered in difficult cases with mixed hearing loss, where accurate determination of cochlear levels is critical.

In addition to finding only small improvement in reliability of forehead over mastoid placement, Dirks (1964) pointed out a disadvantage of forehead placement. More intensity is required to reach threshold with forehead placement than with mastoid placement. Dirks reported that the difference was about 5 dB at 4000 Hz, ranging to 15 dB at 250 and 500 Hz. This reduction in the practical range of bone conduction testing can be a real problem, particularly at 250 Hz, where output in dB HL is more limited than at the higher frequencies.

Research has suggested advantages of forehead placement of the bone vibrator. However, the advantages are small and most clinical procedures still involve testing of bone conduction with the vibrator on the mastoid. The data which have revealed the variability of responses with the vibrator in that position dictate that you place the vibrator carefully and be alert for any slippage resulting in deterioration of placement during testing. If you obtain results which appear incongruent, reposition the vibrator and retest the suspect frequency.

Figure 3.9 shows a bone vibrator in place on the mastoid. To position the vibrator, move aside hair and place the test surface of the vibrator against the mastoid prominence. Because the B70A vibrator is attached to the headband with a swivel arrangement, it is possible to put this vibrator on backwards, with the casing rather than the slightly concave test surface against the mastoid. The casing also vibrates. Of course, it is not calibrated for accurate output, so if you make this erroneous placement and do not correct it, inaccurate results will occur. Since the casing does vibrate, it is preferable that it not touch the back of the pinna. If it does, additional clues may be given to the patient.

Position the headband so that the vibrator exerts an even force across its entire surface. If most of the force is concentrated on one side of the vibrator, invalid results may occur. Hair oil or perspiration may create a slippery mastoid surface, causing the vibrator to slip. If you have

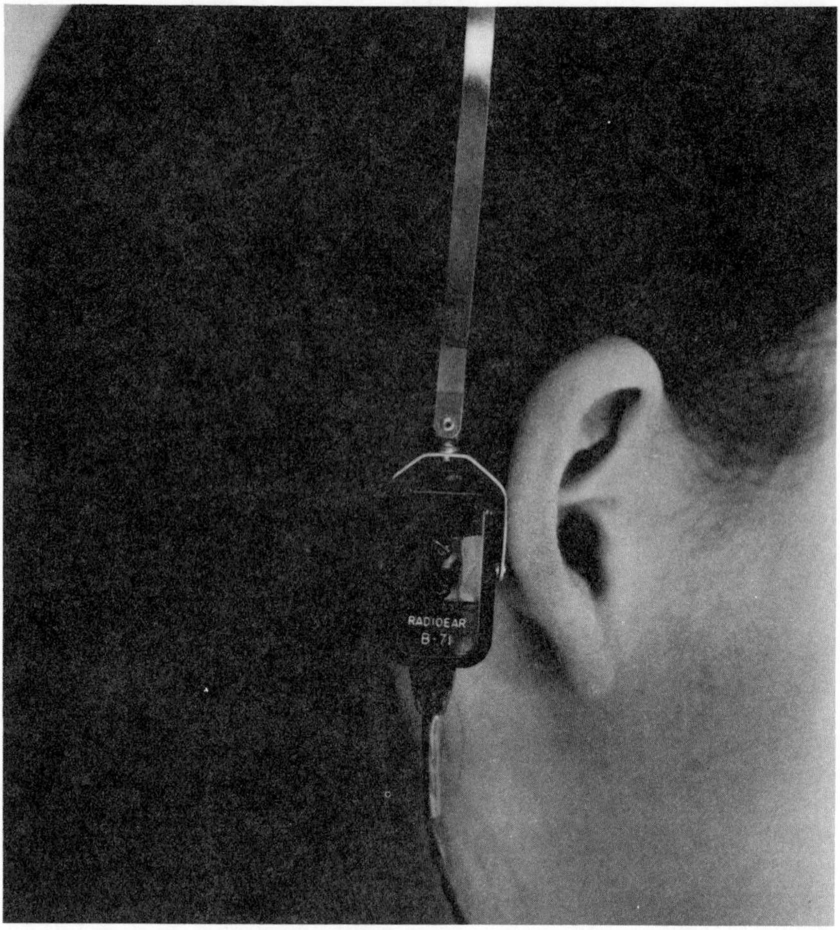

Fig. 3.9. Mastoid placement of the bone vibrator.

reason for concern, ask the patient to inform you if the vibrator moves during testing.

Placement is a greater problem with some patients because of variations in mastoid anatomy. Persons who have undergone mastoid surgery with resultant deformation of mastoid area, may present a particular problem. Finally, removal of wigs or hair decorations may be necessary to secure adequate placement. If the patient is wearing a hairnet you should request its removal, since the headband may otherwise become entangled and tear the net.

Force of the Vibrator

The force which the vibrator exerts against the skull is a source of variability in bone conduction testing. In general, the greater the force, the less the energy required to reach threshold. However, this generalization is affected by the amount of force, the test frequency, and the type of vibrator involved. Konig (1957) reported substantial improvement in threshold for some vibrators until a force of 1250 g was reached. However, he recommended that a force of 1000 g was adequate for clinical evaluation. Actually, this amount of force is uncomfortable, and it is unlikely that clinical patients will tolerate it for any prolonged period. Other investigators have not demonstrated the need for as much force to obtain clinically acceptable results. Harris and associates (1953) recommended a force of 200–400 g. Goodhill and Holcomb (1955), working with animals, reported good reliability between 300 and 600 g. Investigators agree that, for the frequencies used in clinical bone conduction, variability in force will cause the greatest change in threshold for the lower frequencies. The IEC (1971) and the ANSI (1972) recommend for a vibrator with a contact surface area of 1.75 cm^2 a force against the skull equal to 550 g (5.4 Newtons). Dirks (1964) determined no significant differences between test-retest thresholds when force was or was not replicated. In his experiment, force was always over 400 g, whether replicated or not. Studebaker (1962) reported that the tension of the standard steel bone conduction headband exerted a mean force of 322 g against the mastoid of adult subjects, with a range of 142 g. Dirks (1964) concluded that good reliability can be obtained without meticulous replication of vibrator force as long as at least 400 g of force is maintained and reasonable care is observed in placing the vibrator.

The force is an important variable and the clinician should be alert whenever small heads or loose headbands are involved. It is helpful to have a smaller than standard headband available for bone conduction testing of young children. If, at any time, incongruous bone conduction results are obtained, adjust the force of the vibrator against the head and retest.

Instructions to the Patient

Bone conduction testing is ordinarily done after pure tone air conduction testing is completed. Therefore, little additional instruction is needed. You may tell the patient that the tone will be delivered via the vibrator placed behind the ear and that testing will otherwise be unchanged. It may be helpful to tell the patient to respond even if the signal seems to be in the nontest ear. To do so may prevent confusion on the part of the patient who may be unsure whether to respond or not if the tone seems to be heard in the nontest ear. Masking of the nontest ear will be used much more commonly in bone than in air conduction testing, and brief instructions regarding the masking noise are necessary. These instructions will be covered in the next chapter.

Procedures

The Carhart-Jerger ascending procedure for the determination of threshold lends itself equally well to bone conduction or air conduction audiometry. There are, however, some differences to keep in mind.

It is expeditious to rest the better ear first in air conduction audiometry. Doing so provides information about the validity of test results in light of the patient's observed auditory behavior and gives some information about the probable need for masking when testing of the poorer ear is started. However, it may be more efficient to begin bone conduction testing with the ear which has the poorer air conduction thresholds. As explained in the next chapter, masking is necessary much more often in bone conduction than in air conduction audiometry. If the poorer ear is tested first, masking may establish that the bone conduction thresholds are sufficiently reduced so that they could not contribute to response while the better ear bone conduction is being tested. In this case, masking need not be used when testing the better ear. This concept is discussed more fully in the next chapter.

The initial tone in the Carhart-Jerger procedure should be delivered at a comfortably loud, easy-to-hear level. Within these confines, the closer the first presentation is to threshold the faster the test will proceed. In bone conduction testing, look at the better ear to estimate this starting level. If testing is started without the presence of masking, a level 10–15 dB above the thresholds of the better ear will, because of the absence of interaural attenuation, most likely satisfy these criteria.

Maximum output restrictions are more stringent in bone than in air conduction audiometry. You should observe the limits stated on each audiometer. In general, the limits are likely to be 40 dB HL at 250 Hz and 70 dB HL at 500, 750, 1000, 1500, 2000, 3000, and 4000 Hz. Few audiometers are capable of accurate bone conduction testing below 250 or above 4000 Hz. It may not be necessary to test the interoctave frequencies in bone conduction testing, even though their air conduction counterparts were obtained. Bone conduction testing is a diagnostic measure, not a test of functional sensitivity. A midoctave air conduction threshold may give important information about auditory function. Since the function of bone conduction testing is to search for an air-bone gap, information at midoctave intervals may not be as important.

Finally, one obvious procedural difference will be mentioned. Today's audiometers have two air conduction earphones and the change from testing one ear to the other involves only a change of the output selector. There is only one bone conduction vibrator, so changing from one ear to the other requires moving the vibrator to the other mastoid.

The Occlusion Effect

As mentioned earlier, when the external ear is covered, or occluded, there is an increase of energy directed toward the inner ear by the bone conduction vibrator. In persons with normal hearing or sensorineural loss this increase results in an enhancement of bone conduction measures known as the occlusion effect. However, the occlusion effect is ordinarily not seen in patients with conductive loss, and they present the same bone conduction thresholds regardless of whether the ear is occluded or unoccluded.

The occlusion effect is important clinically because of the changes it dictates regarding the need for masking and the amount of masking needed to prevent participation of the nontest ear during bone conduction testing. When the nontest ear is covered by the usual earphone-cushion combination during bone conduction testing, the occlusion effect is introduced to that ear, providing it has no conductive pathology. The resulting enhancement increases the probability that the test tone will be heard via the nontest ear. Masking must be introduced to prevent this occurrence. Of course, the problem could be solved by leaving the earphone off the nontest ear, except it is necessary for that phone to be in place to deliver masking when there is a real superiority in the bone conduction threshold of the nontest ear. In this case more masking than would otherwise be necessary must be delivered to the nontest ear because of the enhancement afforded by the occlusion effect. The masking procedure is covered in the next chapter. Some details regarding the occlusion effect, discussed below, will be helpful in determining the need for masking and the amount of masking noise which must be used.

The size of the occlusion effect is determined by subtracting the value of the occluded threshold from that of the unoccluded threshold. Figure 3.10 shows that the effect is greater for low frequencies. The magnitude of the effect varies from more than 20 dB at 250 Hz to 0 at 2000 Hz (Hodgson and Tillman, 1966).

The volume of air trapped under the occluding object influences the size of the occlusion effect. As this volume increases, the size of the occlusion effect decreases. Compare the results in Figure 3.10, obtained with the standard TDH 49-MX 41/AR earphone-cushion combination and with a Sharpe HA-10 earphone-cushion combination. The latter, which incorporates a larger volume of air under the earphone, resulted in a smaller occlusion effect. "Pederson enclosures," devices designed

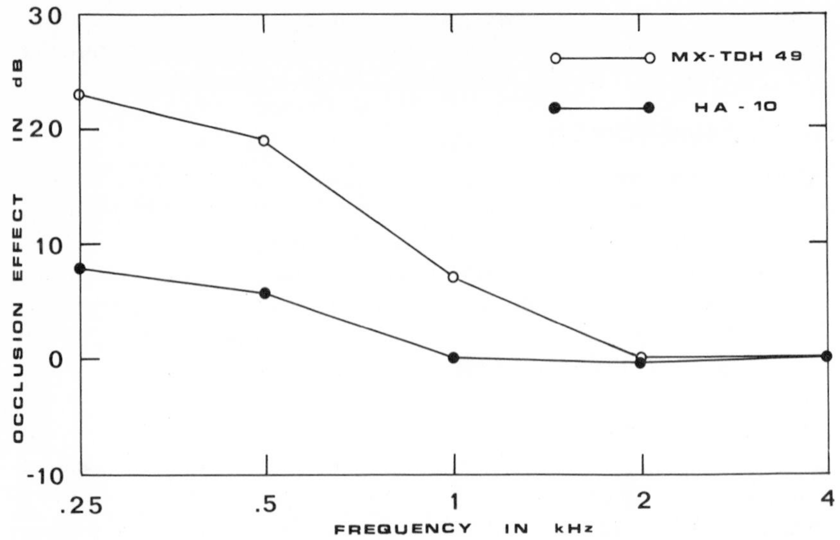

Fig. 3.10. Mean occlusion effects for 16 normal hearing subjects. (Reprinted by permission from: Hodgson, W., and Tillman, T.: *J. Auditory Res. 6:* 141–151, 1966.) Ears were occluded with a TDH 49-MX 41/AR earphone-cushion combination or a Sharpe HA-10 earphone with a circumaural cushion.

to obviate the occlusion effect entirely, consist of 7-inch globes in which loudspeakers are mounted. The generalization that the occlusion effect increases as volume decreases has this exception: If the occluding object is inserted into the ear canal as far as the bony part of the canal, the occlusion effect is greatly diminished (Allen and Fernandez, 1960).

Finally, it should be noted that the occlusion effect shows a good deal of variability. Table 3.3 shows standard deviations of occlusion effects in normals. Hodgson and Tillman (1966) concluded that one source of this variability was the force exerted against the ear by the occluding earphone-cushion combination. Presumably, as this force varies the enclosed volume of air also varies, resulting in changes in the occlusion effect. The clinical implication of the occlusion effect and its role in masking are discussed in the next chapter.

Participation of the Conductive Mechanism

Other conductive phenomena, in addition to the occlusion effect just described, may influence bone conduction thresholds. Experimenters working with animals and humans have shown many effects of surgically or mechanically changing the conductive system. We will concentrate here on clinical observations in which pathological conditions of the conductive system affect bone conduction responses. Obviously, this is an important consideration, since bone conduction testing is

Table 3.3
Standard Deviations of Occlusion Effects Created by Two Earphone-Cushion Combinations in a Group of 16 Normals[a]

Occluding Device	Frequency in Hz				
	250	500	1000	2000	4000
TDH 49-MX 41/AR	7.7	5.5	4.6	3.0	4.0
Sharpe HA-10	8.5	9.5	4.9	3.9	4.0

[a] Hodgson and Tillman (1966).

designed to measure sensorineural function. Error is introduced when the conductive system contributes to bone conduction responses.

Carhart (1950) demonstrated that patients with otosclerosis and stapes fixation may show a reduction in bone conduction thresholds which disappears after successful surgery. He attributed this reduction of the preoperative bone conduction thresholds to the effects of stapes fixation causing a reduction in the mobility of cochlear fluid. The reduction, or "Carhart Notch," introduces an artifact in bone conduction thresholds of approximately the following magnitudes: 5 dB at 500 Hz, 10 dB at 1000 Hz, 15 dB at 2000 Hz, and 5 dB at 4000 Hz. The size of the notch is variable, and may be considerably larger than the figures just given. The magnitude of the Carhart Notch is important since it disappears after successful surgery. The true sensorineural level of an individual, and therefore his candidacy for surgery may be difficult to determine.

Dirks and Malmquist (1969) commented on the effect of the middle ear on bone conduction measurements. Comparing results obtained from frontal bone and mastoid placement of the vibrator, they concluded that stapes fixation resulted in quite similar thresholds between the two placements. However, other middle ear disorders (malleus fixation and ossicular discontinuity) were associated with considerably better bone conduction thresholds via frontal than mastoid placement, when appropriate threshold norms are used for either measurement. Furthermore, the improvement in air conduction thresholds resulting from surgery showed that the forehead measures were the more indicative of true sensorineural function. As mentioned earlier, Dirks and Malmquist recommended that forehead placement of the bone conduction vibrator be considered in cases of mixed loss to specify the sensorineural level as accurately as possible.

Investigators have reported that middle ear fluid, such as that found in serous otitis media, results in characteristic deformation of bone conduction thresholds. Dirks gave the example shown in Figure 3.11. The initial audiogram obtained showed depression of both air and bone conduction thresholds. After treatment of the serous otitis, both air and bone conduction thresholds returned to normal.

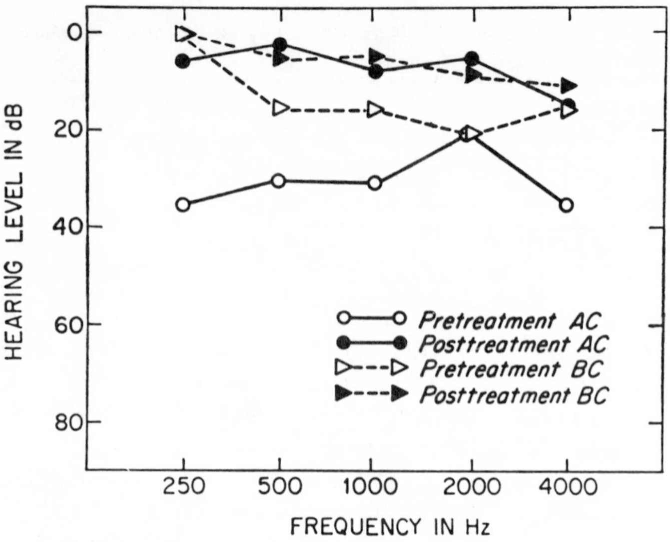

Fig. 3.11. Pre and postoperative thresholds of a patient with serous otitis media (Reprinted by permission from: Dirks, D.: *Handbook of Clinical Audiology*, Ch. 10, Baltimore: Williams & Wilkins, 1978.)

From the foregoing discussion it becomes obvious that there is some error in the assumption that bone conduction thresholds at all times accurately reveal the level of sensorineural function. This error does not obviate bone conduction testing. Rather it necessitates alertness to the possibility of error, caution in the interpretation of bone conduction results, and additional testing in critical cases. These cases are likely to be (1) those with mixed loss for which it is important to determine candidacy for surgery and (2) those with small loss for which the presence of a small air-bone gap suggests the possibility of a conductive component.

Reliability and Validity

The factors discussed above contribute to potential variability of bone conduction measures. Nevertheless, investigators have demonstrated acceptable reliability in carefully controlled bone conduction testing. Carhart and Hayes (1949) demonstrated that the reliability of bone conduction testing was as good as that of air conduction audiometry when appropriate precautions were taken in testing. Dirks and Swindeman (1967) reported that the test-retest reliability of bone conduction thresholds was similar to air conduction with a few exceptions.

Studies assessing bone conduction thresholds have commonly used normal hearing subjects, necessitating presentation of only low level signals. At higher output levels, harmonic distortion produced by the bone vibrator may be a problem. It is not unusual for the second harmonic (500 Hz) of the 250 Hz signal to approach the intensity of the fundamental. In such cases, if the patient's hearing sensitivity is materially better at 500 Hz than at 250 Hz, the patient may respond to the harmonic rather than the fundamental signal. Thus, the actual sensitivity at 250 Hz may not be measured, and some spurious level may be recorded.

Distortion may also arise in bone conduction testing from a source other than the vibrator. Arlinger and associates (1978), using a system with low inherent harmonic distortion, showed distortion apparently associated with nonlinear mechanical properties of the skull. The effect was greatest for high amplitude, low frequency signals, particularly 500 Hz. For example, in one instance, harmonic distortion measured via an artificial mastoid showed the second harmonic to be 35 dB less than the fundamental for a 500 Hz signal of 65 dB HL. However, on the skull, the second harmonic was 5 dB stronger than the fundamental. Based on the use of an audiometer meeting the International Electrotechnical Commission (1971) requirement that each harmonic be at least − 30 dB, the authors recommended these maximum outputs above which skull distortion may cause measurement error: 50 dB HL at 250 Hz, 25 dB HL at 500 Hz, 50 dB HL at 750 Hz, and 65 dB HL at 1000 and 1500 Hz.

Air-bone agreement is an important consideration. Pure tone audiometry is ordinarily conducted using 5 dB intensity steps. It is axiomatic that carefully conducted test-retest procedures (either air or bone conduction) will result in ± 5 dB of variability. Thus, since two tests, each with 5 dB variability, are involved in air-bone comparison, it follows that clinical significance should not be attributed to air-bone differences of 10 dB or less. Bone conduction thresholds 10 dB poorer than air can occur without suspicion of invalidating influences, and a bone conduction threshold 10 dB better than air does not necessarily indicate a conductive component. Two cautions: First, small air-bone gaps across all or much of the audiogram should arouse suspicion of a conductive component, even if the magnitude is no more than 10 dB. Impedance audiometry, discussed in Chapter 7, is valuable in corroborating the significance of small air-bone gaps. Second, if air-bone disagreement (in either direction) consistently occurs at a given frequency in patients who otherwise appear to have purely sensorineural losses, the calibration of the audiometer should be checked; either the air or the bone conduction outputs may be faulty.

To summarize this section, bone conduction testing is an important diagnostic measure. The factors discussed above may influence reliability. Therefore, careful attention to the following is necessary for valid bone conduction audiometry:

1. Correct placement on the mastoid process. Hair should be brushed away from under the vibrator. Wigs, barettes, or other decorations should not be permitted to interfere with the vibrator or its headband. Care should be taken that the headband is positioned to distribute force equally and so that the vibrator will not slip. The casing of the vibrator should not touch the pinna. Be alert for incongruous results which may be associated with vibrator placement. Remember that the force of the vibrator against the skull is a source of variability. Beware of headbands which have lost their spring. It is a good idea to have a smaller headband available for small heads.
2. Remember to observe audiometer output limits, which are considerably restricted relative to air conduction testing. Frequency and intensity limits which usually apply are: 250 Hz, 40 dB HL; 500 Hz–4000 Hz, 70 dB HL.
3. Since the interaural attenuation of a bone conducted tone is essentially zero, it is likely that the patient will hear the unmasked bone conduction signal via the better cochlea. In all instances where that probability can materially affect test results, masking of the nontest ear is indicated. The masking procedure is discussed in the next chapter. Remember that the variable presence of the occlusion effect when the nontest ear is covered by the masking phone must be taken into account.

SUMMARY

The pure tone air conduction audiogram provides a measure of hearing sensitivity as a function of frequency. It establishes magnitude of hearing loss and permits generalization about expected handicap. It is the only auditory test which establishes the configuration of hearing loss, indicating which frequencies the patient can hear well, poorly, or not at all.

Pretest observation of the patient and elicitation of a case history provide information to facilitate testing and assist you in understanding and helping the patient. This is the time, also, to begin the process of rapport, an effective working relationship important not only for testing but to ensure that the patient accepts and follows recommendations.

The Carhart-Jerger ascending procedure is an efficient method for obtaining thresholds. Careful assessment of reliability and validity is necessary. This assessment includes attention to correct audiometric settings, valid procedure, and careful observation of patient behavior. It is important that false positive and false negative responses be identified and that their occurrence not prevent valid audiometry. Test results must be recorded fully, accurately, and clearly.

Pure tone bone conduction audiometry helps to determine the type of hearing loss and is of diagnostic usefulness. An air-bone gap indicates a conductive component, while equal air and bone conduction thresholds indicate a sensorineural loss. Through comparison of air and bone conduction thresholds, three types of hearing loss can be differentiated: conductive, sensorineural, or mixed. Several variables are potentially dangerous to bone conduction validity. These include placement of the vibrator, the force which is exerted against the skull, performance characteristics of the vibrator, and the danger of participation of the nontest ear. Careful attention to these factors is necessary for valid bone conduction audiometry.

Pure tone air and bone conduction threshold audiometry are important parts of the basic audiologic evaluation. Other basic components are speech threshold audiometry, speech discrimination testing, and impedance audiometry. These aspects are discussed in subsequent chapters.

STUDY QUESTIONS

1. Review the following characteristics of the pure tone audiogram form: What are the units and the range of units (a) on the ordinate? (b) on the abscissa? What are the threshold symbols for (a) right ear and (b) left ear (1) air conduction and (2) bone conduction?
2. How can you gain some clues to the patient's probable hearing sensitivity before starting the test? What are some factors which may confound your estimate of the magnitude of loss?
3. Why is it important to establish rapport? How is it done?
4. What should you learn from the case history form? Which of the patient's answers should you talk further about?
5. When doing otoscopic observation, what clues should alert you to possible collapse of ear canals under pressure of the earphones? What can you do to confirm the presence of collapsing canals and to obtain valid air conduction thresholds?
6. Review the steps of the ascending and descending procedures for obtaining threshold. What is the criterion for threshold in each method?
7. How can you identify (a) false positive responses? (b) false negative responses? How can you prevent false responses from invalidating test results?
8. What are three *mechanisms* of bone conduction discussed in this chapter?
9. How can the following factors affect bone conduction thresholds: (a) placement of the vibrator? (b) force of the vibrator against the head? (c) the occlusion effect? (d) participation of the conductive mechanism? How can adverse effects be minimized?

CHAPTER 4 Masking

In air conduction testing, the need for masking arises when there is a large difference in sensitivity between ears. Without masking, if the difference between ears is large enough, the test tone may cross over and stimulate the more sensitive nontest ear. The patient may respond, and an erroneous threshold be recorded. Introduction of masking noise into the nontest ear can determine whether or not a threshold obtained in quiet is a crossover response. The noise causes a temporary shift of threshold in the nontest ear. The test ear threshold is then re-established in the presence of the masking noise. If threshold remains the same, we conclude it was the test ear which was responding all along, since shifting the threshold of the nontest ear with masking noise did not change the threshold of the test ear. On the other hand, if the threshold on the test ear changes by an amount similar to the threshold change caused in the nontest ear by the masking noise, there is strong evidence of crossover response.

An understanding of masking is necessary to evaluate hearing and to interpret audiograms. Your grasp of the process may depend on how well you understand concepts relating to air and bone conduction hearing and to factors which determine conductive and sensorineural loss. Perhaps you should at this time review, at least in your mind, the route which signals follow for air and bone conduction hearing. Think about the effect of conductive and sensorineural loss on air and bone conduction thresholds. Specifically, a conductive loss makes air conduction thresholds poorer but leaves bone conduction thresholds essentially unchanged. A sensorineural loss reduces air and bone conduction thresholds equally. These considerations affect (1) the conditions under which crossover of the test tone to the nontest ear occurs and (2) the amount of masking necessary to prevent participation of the nontest ear.

PURPOSE

The purpose of clinical masking is to prevent the participation of the nontest ear in the hearing evaluation. Audibility of the test signal in the nontest ear is called "crossover hearing." The audiometric correlate of crossover hearing is the shadow curve shown in Figure 4.1. The shadow curve is prevented by introducing a masking noise to the nontest ear during the hearing test when there is a possibility that the nontest ear could participate. The effect of the masking noise is to give the nontest ear a temporary threshold shift.

RULES GOVERNING CLINICAL MASKING

The factors which determine if the test tone will be heard in the nontest ear are (1) the intensity of the test signal, (2) the sensitivity of the nontest ear, and (3) the reduction of the signal as it travels across the head. As you learn about masking, it will help to keep in mind the following generalizations.

The crossover route ordinarily is by bone conduction. Zwislocki (1953) established that, even for a signal which originates from an earphone, the crossover route to the nontest ear is by bone conduction. That is, vibration of the earphone-cushion combination impressed against the

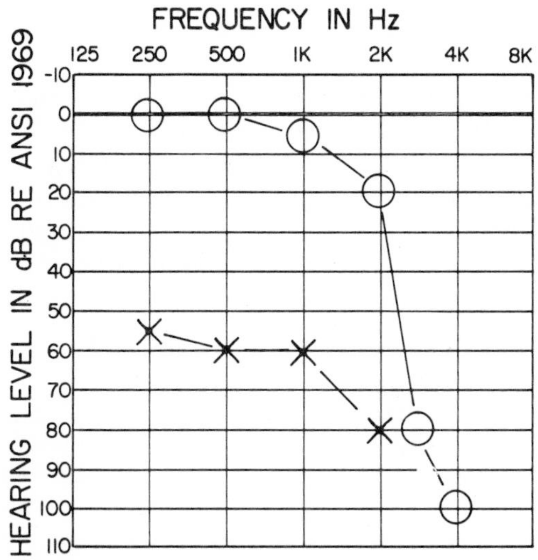

Fig. 4.1. Air conduction shadow curve for a patient with a dead left ear. Note that the crossover thresholds are 50–60 dB poorer than the thresholds of the better ear and that the configuration of the shadow curve approximates that of the better ear. In effect, this patient's right ear has been tested twice, once with the head in the way.

skull stimulates the cochlea of the nontest ear by bone conduction. Therefore, even when we try to stimulate the test ear by air conduction, crossover, if it happens, is by bone conduction. Thus, the *bone conduction threshold* of the nontest ear is the critical value contributing to whether or not crossover hearing will occur.

The interaural attenuation of an air conducted tone may range from 40 to 80 db. The difference between the effective intensity of the signal emanating from the earphone and the signal at the nontest cochlea may be anywhere from 40 to 80 dB, depending on interaural attenuation characteristics. Table 4.1 shows means and ranges of interaural attenuation. There is a good deal of variability. Therefore, while you would expect interaural attenuation to be about 50–60 dB, occasionally it may be as little as 40 dB, or as much as 80 dB. As a result, crossover hearing is most likely when the test signal is 50–60 dB above the bone conduction threshold of the nontest ear. However, crossover hearing may happen when the test signal is no more than 40 dB above the bone conduction threshold of the nontest ear. In other instances, crossover may not occur until the test signal is as much as 80 dB above the bone conduction threshold of the nontest ear. The data of Zwislocki (1953) suggest that there is some frequency effect on interaural attenuation, with less attenuation for low frequency tones. However, because the effect is small, and attenuation so variable, it is probably just as well to ignore the frequency effect and conservatively generalize that the expected interaural attenuation for any air conducted tone is about 50–60 dB, ranging from 40 to 80 dB.

The interaural attenuation of a bone conducted tone is essentially 0 dB. The bone oscillator, vibrating against the skull, is likely to stimulate the better cochlea regardless of the mastoid on which the vibrator is placed. There may be a small amount of interaural attenuation, particularly for higher frequencies. However, the attenuation is quite variable and for clinical purposes 0 dB attenuation should be expected. Indeed, if the nontest ear is covered by an earphone, the occlusion effect may

Table 4.1
Interaural Attenuation in dB for an Air Conducted Tone

Frequency in Hz	Investigator	
	Zwislocki (1953) Mean	Liden *et al.* (1959) Range
250	45	40–75
500	50	45–75
1000	55	50–70
2000	60	45–70
4000	65	45–75
8000		45–80

be induced, as described in the previous chapter. In this case, the bone conduction response of the nontest ear will be enhanced and the result may be an apparently negative attenuation value.

The crucial values which determine the need for masking are (1) the bone conduction threshold of the nontest ear and (2) the presentation level to the test ear at which threshold is obtained without masking. The bone conduction rather than air conduction threshold of the nontest ear is the important value, since it is by the bone conduction route that crossover occurs. The presentation level required for threshold response is the other important value. If the difference between the two (presentation level minus bone conduction threshold) is larger than the expected interaural attenuation, crossover hearing is a possibility. Masking should be used to prevent possible participation of the nontest ear. Through masking, we can learn whether the threshold obtained in quiet is a valid measure of the test ear or a crossover response.

Keeping in mind the rules discussed above which determine the need for masking, you should have no difficulty understanding the examples in Figures 4.2 and 4.3, which show how crossover hearing occurs in patients with different HLs. Figure 4.2 illustrates crossover in air conduction testing and Figure 4.3 shows crossover in bone conduction testing. In each instance the stimulus delivered to the test ear is the

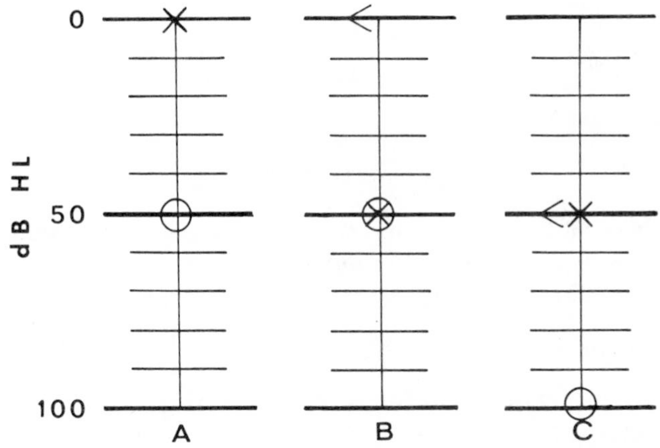

Fig. 4.2. Examples of crossover hearing during air conduction testing. In each case the right test ear has no hearing. *A*, the left nontest ear is normal and crossover hearing occurs when the stimulus reaches 50 dB HL; *B*, the left nontest ear has a 50 dB conductive loss. Crossover hearing still occurs when the test signal reaches 50 dB HL, since the bone conduction threshold of the nontest ear is normal and audibility occurs as soon as the test signal exceeds the interaural attenuation. *C*, the left nontest ear has a 50 dB sensorineural loss. Now crossover does not occur until the test signal reaches 100 dB HL. Assuming 50 dB of interaural attenuation, at 100 dB HL the signal reaches the nontest ear at an effective level of 50 dB: the bone conduction threshold of the nontest ear.

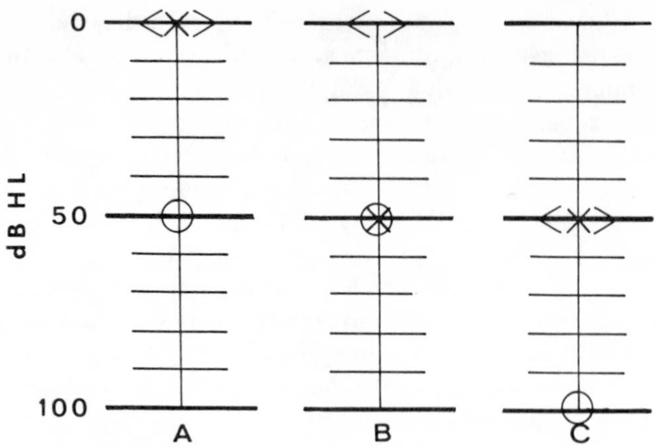

Fig. 4.3. Examples of crossover hearing during bone conduction testing. In each case the right test ear has no hearing and air conduction crossover occurs when the test signal is 50 dB above the nontest ear bone conduction thresholds. *A*, the left nontest ear is normal. Since no interaural attenuation is expected, crossover hearing occurs when the test signal is at 0 dB HL. *B*, the patient has a 50-dB conductive loss. Crossover hearing still occurs at 0 dB HL, since that is the bone conduction threshold of the nontest ear. *C*, there is a 50-dB sensorineural loss in the left nontest ear. Now crossover hearing occurs when the test signal reaches a level of 50 dB HL.

expected level to elicit the crossover response. Notice that the bone conduction threshold of the nontest ear always determines the level necessary for crossover.

MASKING PROBLEMS

Among the problems associated with masking are the possible occurrence of *overmasking* and *central masking*. Each shifts the threshold of the test ear when masking is introduced to the nontest ear.

Overmasking

Overmasking occurs when the level of masking noise introduced to the nontest ear is high enough for the noise to cross over and shift the threshold of the *test* ear as well as that of the nontest ear. The interaural attenuation for masking noise can be expected to approximate that of pure tones, about 50–60 dB, although it may be a little less or a little more. Thus, when the masking noise is about 50–60 dB above the bone conduction threshold of the test ear, the danger of overmasking is present. The result of overmasking, of course, is to make the threshold of the test ear look poorer than it really is. Some methods to detect or prevent overmasking are considered in the section on masking procedure.

Central Masking

Central masking is blamed when a shift in the threshold of the test ear occurs, relative to its threshold in quiet, and the level of the masking noise is insufficient for physical crossover (overmasking) to occur. Thus, a threshold shift observed when the level of the masking noise is less than the magnitude of interaural attenuation is attributable to central masking. Presumably the origin of central masking is in the higher pathways of the central auditory nervous system where the neural interaction "between the ears" causes a threshold shift of the test ear because of the noise introduced to the nontest ear. The amount of central masking increases as the masking level increases. The clinical effect of central masking is often negligible but may change threshold by 5–15 dB. Zwislocki (1953) estimated the maximum threshold shift from central masking at 5 dB. However, Dirks and Malmquist (1969) reported central masking of 10–12 dB and Liden *et al.* (1959) found as much as 15 dB of central masking. Some few individuals seem so confused by the addition of masking that reliability deteriorates. The possibility of central masking dictates that no more masking than necessary be used. Determination of the minimum effective masking level is discussed in the section on masking procedures. When there is a difference between unmasked and masked thresholds it probably makes sense to record the masked threshold even though central masking is suspected. Presumably the masking would not have been introduced unless crossover hearing was possible, and it seems preferable to record a test ear threshold made a few decibels poorer by central masking than to risk recording a nontest ear crossover response.

TYPES OF MASKING NOISE

Audibility of a signal is best prevented by the presentation of another signal of the same frequency. When a pure tone is masked by broad band noise, only the energy of frequencies adjacent to the tone supplies masking. Fletcher (1940) explained this phenomenon in terms of the *critical band* concept. There is a critical band of noise for a tone of any frequency which supplies maximum masking with minimum intensity. If the bandwidth of the masking noise is narrower than the critical band, greater intensity will be required for masking. Energy above or below the critical band does not contribute to masking of the test tone, although this energy does contribute to perceived loudness. The critical band concept is important in assessing the value of the masking noises described below.

Complex Noise

Complex noise was available on many early pure tone audiometers. The various types of complex noise consist of a low fundamental frequency and amplified harmonics. A type called sawtooth noise is most common. Complex noise has a buzzing, low pitch quality. The typical complex noise concentrates energy in the low frequencies and is a good masker of low frequency tones but a poor masker of high frequency tones. In the presence of a high intensity complex noise generating great loudness, crossover hearing can still occur for high frequency tones. Dependence on complex noise, because of this shortcoming, may result in invalid audiograms.

A nonlinear masking function is another problem with complex noise. The masking sources described below will, once a minimum level is reached, supply an equal increase in masking for each like increase in masking noise level. Such is not the case with complex noise, and this fact may create problems, as discussed below under the heading of effective masking.

Complex noise is no longer commonly supplied as the sole masking source on an audiometer. The typical complex noise must be used with caution, and one must assume it is not likely to be an adequate masking source for pure tones above 1000 Hz.

White noise

White noise is so called because its distribution of energy is random, analogous to the distribution of light waves which produce white light. In theory white noise has equal energy per cycle; that is, an equal distribution of energy across its bandwidth. In clinical use, the spectrum is shaped by the earphone. Because of its broad and nearly flat spectrum, white noise is an efficient masker of all the pure tones used in clinical audiometry. However, there are two problems with white noise as a masking source.

Remember that only the energy in frequencies immediately surrounding the test tone are useful in masking that tone. There is a great deal of unused energy in white noise below and above the critical band for a given test tone. This unused energy contributes to perceived loudness. On occasion, patients will object to the loudness of white noise at an intensity level necessary to prevent crossover hearing.

Another problem with the clinical use of white noise is related to the differential sensitivity of the ear across frequency. As you know, a different SPL is required in normal ears for audibility of each test tone. White noise has equal energy at each test frequency, and its masking ability differs for each of the audiometric test tones. Therefore, a given level of white noise will produce different amounts of masking for each test frequency and will be least effective for low frequency signals, where sensitivity in normals is poorest. It is very helpful to have the masking control dial of the audiometer calibrated in decibels of effective masking. Effective masking means the level to which an ear's threshold will be shifted by a given amount of masking noise. Since the effectiveness of white noise varies for each audiometric frequency, the dial controlling the intensity of the noise is not calibrated in decibels of effective masking. The implications of this problem, and the solution, are discussed further in the section on effective masking.

Narrow Band Noise

Narrow bands of noise can be obtained by filtering white noise. These bands, centered around each audiometric test frequency, contain energy that masks efficiently. The result is extensive threshold shift without objectionable loudness. To demonstrate, Figure 4.4 shows how the three

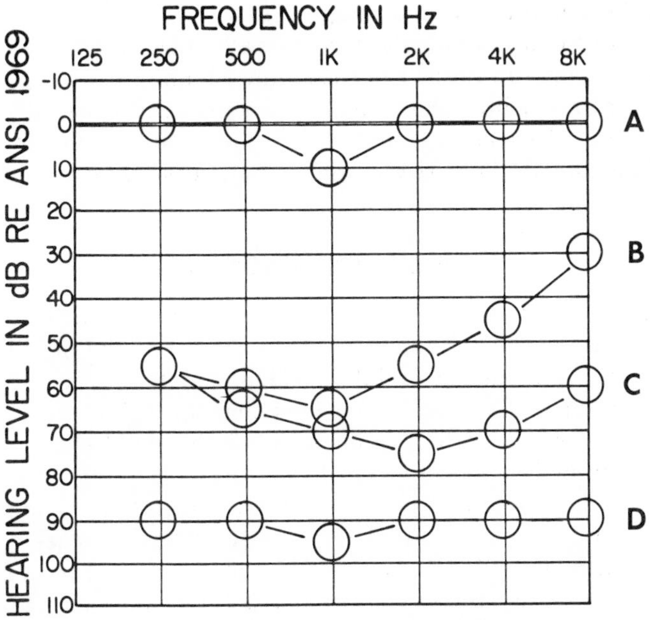

Fig. 4.4. Threshold shift achieved in a normal ear by the complex, white, and narrow band masking sources of one audiometer. All masked thresholds were obtained with the tone and the noise directed to the same ear. For all masked thresholds, the hearing loss dial on the noise channel was set at 90 dB, the maximum output setting for noise on this particular audiometer. *A*, unmasked thresholds; *B*, thresholds shifted by complex noise reveal inefficiency for masking high frequency tones; *C*, greater threshold shifts result from white noise masking, but masked thresholds are not uniform, with less shift for low and high frequency tones; *D*, essentially uniform shift results from use of narrow band noise calibrated to equal effective masking levels. The white and narrow band noise sources, at maximum output, are more than adequate to prevent crossover hearing in this example. However, it is quite possible that crossover could occur in the presence of complex noise when testing frequencies above 1000 Hz.

masking sources we have discussed shifted thresholds for a normal ear. Note that the complex noise was quite inefficient in shifting high frequency thresholds. The white noise was more efficient throughout but shifted mid frequencies more than high and low frequencies. The narrow bands, calibrated to uniform effective masking, were essentially equivalent in masking effectiveness.

There is another advantage of narrow band noise. The band used to mask each pure tone is an individual noise source. Therefore, the masking level control can be calibrated in decibels of effective masking. That is, output can be regulated to compensate for difference in sensitivity across the audiometric frequencies. The result is a masking control dial which, at any given setting, shifts threshold for all frequencies to the same level. The convenience of such a control is explained further in the section on effective masking.

White and narrow band noise have this advantage relative to complex noise: for clinical purposes their masking function can be considered linear. Therefore, within the limits of test variability, each 5 dB increase in the level of the masking noise will result in a 5 dB threshold shift. Our reliance on the linearity of this function is important in clinical masking.

EFFECTIVE MASKING

Informed use of masking in audiometry requires that the clinician know the HL to which the nontest ear is shifted by the masking noise. Coupled with knowledge of interaural attenuation, this information permits assurance that crossover is not occurring. Clinically, masking is described in terms of effective masking, or threshold shift. "Z" is the common symbol for "effective masking." Decibels of effective masking describe the HL to which the air conduction threshold is shifted by a given amount of noise. Stated differently, effective masking equals threshold shift re: 0 dB HL. Notice that the effective masking concept does not necessarily relate to *how much* threshold shift occurs as a result of the introduction of a given amount of masking noise; rather it indicates the *level to which* the masked ear is shifted. Thus, "50 dB effective masking" will shift an ear's air conduction threshold for a given tone to 50 dB.

Effect on Normal Versus Impaired Ears

A given amount of effective masking will shift the air conduction threshold of anyone to essentially the same level, regardless of the unmasked threshold. The preceding generalization excepts, of course, those individuals whose unmasked hearing thresholds are poorer than the level of effective masking in question. With this exception you can expect all ears to be shifted to approximately the same HL by a given amount of effective masking. Examples are shown in Figure 4.5. Notice that the air conduction thresholds of all three ears are shifted to the same effective level by the same amount of masking noise. The masking noise cannot, however, change the relationship between air and bone conduction thresholds. If an air-bone gap exists in the unmasked condition, it will persist in the masked condition. Therefore, the masking only shifts the bone conduction threshold in example *C* to 20 dB, and the 40 dB air-bone gap is retained. It is important to remember that the effectiveness of masking to shift the bone conduction threshold of the nontest ear is affected by a conductive component in that ear. The effectiveness of the masking to shift the bone conduction threshold will be reduced by the size of the conductive component. That amount of masking is dissipated by the conductive component and does not reach the inner ear. As a result, ears with conductive components may be troublesome cases for masking. Two problems may arise: (1) because of the masking dissipated by the conductive component there may not be enough masking available at the maximum audiometer output to assure that crossover is not occurring; (2) the increased masking necessitated by the conductive component in the nontest ear increases the probability of overmasking: crossover of the masking noise to shift the threshold of the test ear. In cases of bilateral hearing loss, probability of the latter

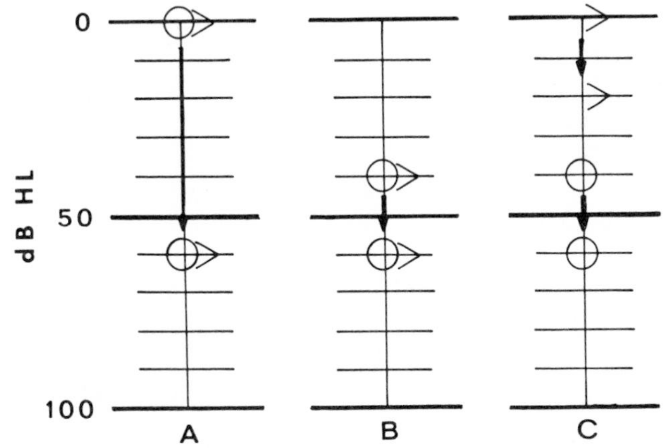

Fig. 4.5. Threshold shift resulting from 60 dB of effective masking applied to a normal ear (*A*), an ear with 40 dB sensorineural loss (*B*), and an ear with 40 dB conductive loss (*C*). Since the masking is an air-conducted signal, the air conduction thresholds of all three ears are shifted to the same level. However, since 40 dB of the masking are dissipated by the conductive blockage in example *C*, the bone conduction threshold is shifted to only 20 dB. The effective air-bone gap present in the unmasked condition is retained in the masked condition.

problem is increased if there is also a conductive component in the test ear. The crossover route, you remember, is by bone conduction, and the better the bone conduction threshold of the test ear, the lower the level at which crossover can be expected.

Determining the Amount of Effective Masking

The relationship between masking dial setting and amount of effective masking must be determined for each audiometer. This determination must be made before the audiometer is placed in use and periodically thereafter. Two methods are available.

For white noise, effective masking can be determined by computation if these values are known: (1) the bandwidth of the noise and (2) the overall sound pressure level. For clinical purposes a method which involves the use of real ears is satisfactory, and it is discussed below. If you are interested in more information about the computation procedure, Sanders (1978) gives a clear description.

A second method to determine the effectiveness of a masking noise requires directing the noise and test tone into the same earphone and finding the thresholds of a number of subjects in the presence of the noise. By establishing the level to which threshold is shifted by the noise, the relationship between masker dial setting and masking effectiveness can be determined.

For most two channel audiometers, you need only turn the output selector to the appropriate setting to deliver both signals to the same earphone. However, most portable audiometers do not include this setting on their output selectors. If your audiometer does not provide for this output, the same effect can be achieved with a "Y" patch cord which delivers both pure tone and noise to a single earphone. This arrangement is shown in Figure 4.6. It is necessary to follow the details shown in the circuit to avoid changing the normal relationship between tone and noise signals. This arrangement will cause a small reduction in the output of both signals, but since the reduction is equal for each signal, effective masking results will be unchanged.

Narrow band masking generators are generally, though not always, calibrated in decibels effective masking. That is, if the narrow band generator's attenuator dial is set to 60 dB, the output will cause a threshold shift to 60 dB for the frequency at which the generator is set. Therefore, your use of the calibration procedure will be limited to making sure that the Z levels indicated by the dial are accurate.

The attenuator of a broad band masking source does not read directly in Z, since a different noise level is required for a given Z at each pure tone audiometric frequency. Therefore, to use broad band noise, either an effective masking table or a correction chart must be made up as follows. First, determine that the attenuator itself is linear. The proce-

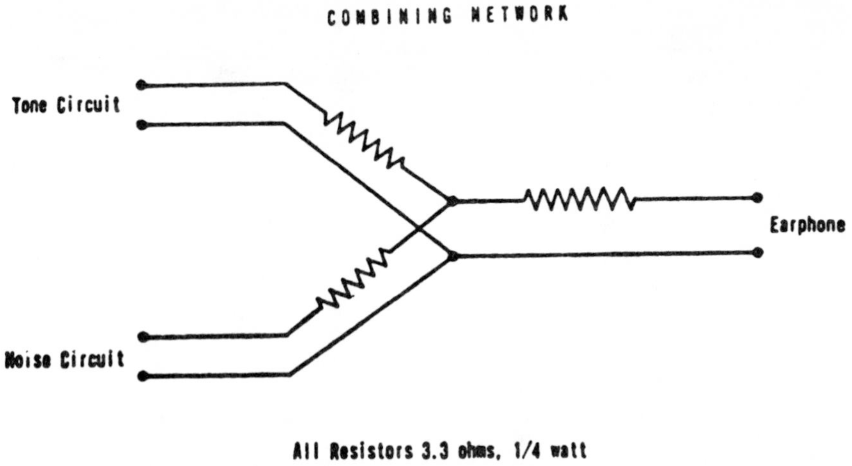

Fig. 4.6. "Y" arrangement to direct noise and tone into a single earphone (Reprinted by permission from: Studebaker, G.: *J. Speech Hearing Dis.* 32:360–371, 1967).

dure for measuring attenuator linearity is described in Chapter 2. Next, determine masking effectiveness.

1. Turn the output selector so that both tone and noise are delivered to the same earphone.
2. Set the noise attenuator to a reasonably high level, such as 60 dB.
3. Obtain, at each audiometric frequency, the thresholds in noise for 5–10 reliable normal hearing subjects.
4. Compute the mean masked thresholds of those subjects.
5. Prepare a masking table based on these threshold shifts.

If white or narrow band noise is the masking source, it is necessary to obtain masked thresholds at one level only. The other Z figures in the masking tables are projections justified by the essentially linear masking function. An example of a masking table is shown in Table 4.2. After a masking table has been prepared for a given audiometer it is used as follows:

1. Select the Z desired (for example, 30 dB).
2. Find that number in the column under the frequency being tested (for example, 1000 Hz).
3. Follow the row in which the number (30) is located over to the number in the "masking control dial setting" column (in this example, "50").
4. In the current example, setting the masking control at 50 will result in 30 dB of effective masking for a 1000 Hz tone.

As an alternative to a complete masking table, a masking correction chart can serve the same purpose. K (correction) factors are shown in

Table 4.2
Effective Masking Table

Masking Control Dial Setting	Z (Threshold Shift Re: 0 dB HL)						
	125	250	500	1000	2000	4000	8000
				Hz			
0							
10							
20				0	0		
30		0	5	10	10	5	0
40	5	10	15	20	20	15	10
50	15	20	25	30	30	25	20
60[a]	25	30	35	40	40	35	30
70	35	40	45	50	50	45	40
80	45	50	55	60	60	55	50
90	55	60	65	70	70	65	60
100	65	70	75	80	80	75	70
110	75	80	85	90	90	85	80

[a] 60 dB is the only level at which Z was actually determined.

Table 4.3
Masking Correction Chart

K Factor (Noise Control Dial Setting Required for 0 dB HL Effective Masking)						
125	250	500	1000	2000	4000	8000
			Hz			
35	30	25	20	20	25	30

Table 4.3. If a masking correction chart is used, observe the following procedure.

1. Select the Z desired (for example, 30 dB).
2. From the correction chart, determine the K factor for the frequency being tested (for example, 1000 Hz K factor = 20 dB).
3. Add the K factor and the desired Z (20 + 30 = 50).
4. In the current example, setting the masking control at 50 will result in 30 dB of effective masking for a 1000 Hz tone.

In summary, Z can be determined by:

1. the dial setting of the NB generator calibrated in dB of effective masking;
2. a masking table that has been prepared for the broad band noise generator; and
3. a correction chart that has been prepared for the broad band noise generator.

WHEN TO MASK

The following rules for masking are based on evidence that the minimum expected interaural attenuation for an air conducted tone is

40 dB (Zwislocki, 1953). Remember that the interaural attenuation will usually be larger: 50–60 dB or even more. The conservative minimum is used in the belief that it is better to mask many times when not necessary than to fail to mask once when necessary. For bone conduction testing, the interaural attenuation is assumed to be essentially zero.

Air Conduction Testing

Masking is indicated during air conduction testing of the poorer ear when the better ear is normal or sensorineural and there is a difference of 40 dB or more between the air conduction thresholds. Masking is also indicated during air conduction testing of the poorer ear when the better ear has a conductive loss and there is a difference of 40 dB or more between the bone conduction thresholds of the better ear and the air conduction thresholds of the poorer ear. These situations are illustrated in Figure 4.7. In each case, when the illustrated relationship between better ear thresholds and poorer ear responses is obtained, masking is indicated to validate the response. Of course, you can see from studying Figure 4.7 that a simpler way of saying when masking is needed in air conduction testing is this: regardless of the status of the nontest ear, masking is indicated in air conduction testing when there is a difference of 40 dB or more between the bone conduction thresholds of the nontest ear and the responses obtained in quiet from the test ear.

Bone Conduction Testing

In the usual clinical situation utilizing mastoid placement of the bone vibrator, masking is ordinarily supplied by one of the air conduction

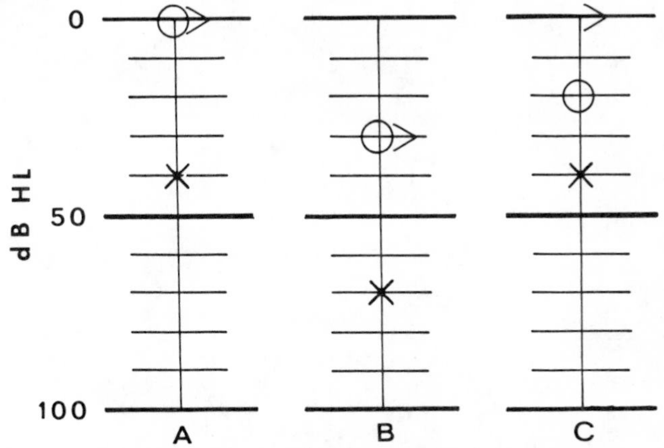

Fig. 4.7. During air conduction testing, masking is indicated in each of the above cases when there is a difference of 40 dB or more between the response in the left test ear and (*A* and *B*) the air conduction thresholds of the right nontest ear or (*C*) the bone conduction thresholds of the right nontest ear.

earphones. Of course, this necessitates placing the headset and the bone vibrator on the head. The nontest ear must be covered to receive the masking noise but the test ear must be uncovered to prevent a possible occlusion effect. The occlusion effect on the nontest ear can be handled through proper masking procedures, as explained below. The result is the rather awkward arrangement shown in Figure 4.8. Observe the following precautions:

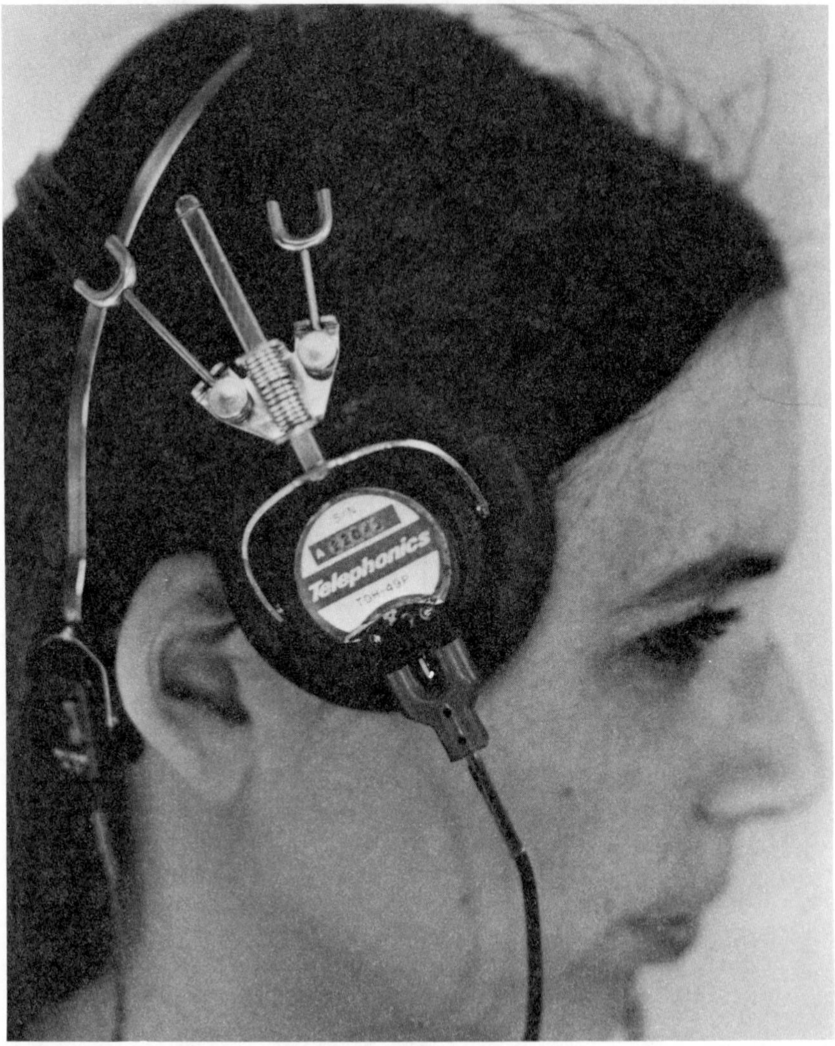

Fig. 4.8. Placement of the headset for masking during bone conduction testing. The masking phone covers the nontest ear.

Be sure that the correct earphone is placed on the nontest ear. Audiometers differ. Some will deliver the noise only to one earphone when the output selector is on bone conduction, so that phone must be used for all masking, regardless of which ear is being tested. Other audiometers permit delivery of the noise to either phone during bone conduction testing and you may select the phone you wish to use.

Be sure that the transducers are placed properly and that putting on the air conduction headset does not displace the bone conduction head band. Position the unused earphone against the side of the head, not over the test ear. Make it as comfortable and secure as possible. The arrangement is awkward, increasing the possibility of patient discomfort. Ask if the apparatus feels all right before you start testing.

Because of the expected absence of interaural attenuation, the feature in air conduction testing which usually prevents crossover, masking is needed in bone conduction testing much more often than in air conduction testing. Some sources recommend masking during all bone conduction testing (Glorig, 1965; Lybarger, 1966; O'Neill and Oyer, 1966; ANSI, 1978). Bone conduction norms are ordinarily generated while testing normals with masking in the nontest ear to prevent binaural response. Therefore, when patients are tested using audiometers calibrated to these norms, use of masking replicates the condition under which the norms were obtained. The effect of central masking is probably the most important variable. Its presence during generation of the norms and its absence in unmasked clinical thresholds may result in bone conduction thresholds better than the patient's actual sensorineural level. However, a low level of masking is used to prevent crossover hearing in normal subjects. Therefore, the expected central masking effect is small. Unmasked bone conduction thresholds will not result in appreciable error because of the central masking variable.

Masking is necessary in bone conduction testing of all unilateral losses. The normal ear must be masked while obtaining bone conduction thresholds on the poorer ear. Bone conduction thresholds are ordinarily not obtained on ears with normal air conduction thresholds. Therefore, the question of masking the poorer ear while testing the better ear does not arise when one ear is normal.

Masking is needed in bone conduction testing of bilateral losses if the air conduction sensitivity of the ears is unequal *or* if a preliminary unmasked bone conduction threshold shows an air-bone gap. Figure 4.9 illustrates these situations. Refer to Figure 4.9 while reading the discussion below.

During bone conduction testing, masking is needed (*A*) in the left ear to prevent its participation while establishing the bone conduction threshold of the right ear, which may be anywhere between 0 and 40

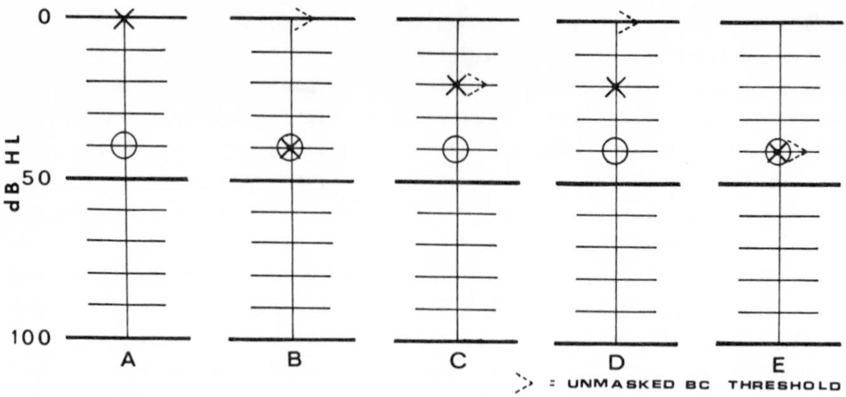

Fig. 4.9. Various conditions which, except for *E*, require masking during bone conduction testing of the right ear. Refer to the text for additional explanation. *A*, in this unilateral loss masking is needed while testing the right ear; *B*, in this bilaterally equal loss in which a preliminary unmasked bone conduction threshold shows an air-bone gap, masking may be necessary while testing both ears, depending on whether or not there is a conductive loss in both ears; *C*, in this bilaterally unequal loss, masking is needed while testing the right ear; *D*, in this bilaterally unequal loss wherein the unmasked bone conduction threshold is potentially attributable to either ear, masking may be necessary during testing of both ears; *E*, in this bilaterally equal loss wherein a preliminary unmasked conduction threshold shows no air-bone gap, masking is not necessary.

dB. *B*, air conduction thresholds are bilaterally equal, but a preliminary unmasked bone conduction threshold establishes an air-bone gap potentially attributable to either ear. Several conditions are possible. Bone conduction sensitivity is normal in at least one ear. It may be the right ear. It may be the left ear. It may be normal in both ears. Masking is needed to differentiate these possibilities. If, with sufficient masking to the left ear, the test ear bone conduction response remains at zero, that ear's bone conduction thresholds are normal (a conductive loss is present). It will then be necessary to mask the right ear while testing the left ear to determine if the left ear's bone conduction thresholds are normal. On the other hand, if masking the left ear shows that the right ear has a sensorineural loss, it will not be necessary to mask the right ear while confirming the normal left ear bone conduction thresholds. *C*, air conduction thresholds are bilaterally unequal. The preliminary unmasked bone conduction threshold establishes a potential air-bone gap only on the right ear. If the left ear bone conduction thresholds were, in fact, better than the air conduction thresholds, the unmasked bone conduction threshold (by crossover hearing) would reflect that fact. Therefore, masking is needed on the left ear while establishing the right ear bone conduction threshold. It will not be necessary to mask the right ear while confirming the left bone conduction threshold. *D*, the preliminary unmasked response is potentially attributable to either ear. Bone conduction sensitivity is normal in at least one ear, possibly both. Masking must be introduced to the left ear while establishing the sensorineural level of the right ear. If the right ear loss is sensorineural, with a 40 dB bone conduction threshold, masking will not be needed when testing bone conduction on the left ear. This is true because the left ear bone threshold must be somewhere between 0 and 20 dB, and the 40 dB right ear cochlear sensitivity cannot participate during the left ear bone conduction testing. However, if the right ear is found to be conductive with bone conduction thresholds at 0 dB, then the right ear must also be masked while establishing the bone conduction thresholds in the left ear. Overmasking is possible.

Because masking is so often needed in bone conduction testing, it may be simpler to remember when masking is *not* needed. Keep this rule in mind: masking is always needed in bone conduction testing unless (1) the air conduction thresholds are bilaterally equal and (2) a preliminary unmasked threshold shows no air-bone gap. Remember that *both* conditions must be present, as shown in Figure 4.9 E, before you can forego masking. The unmasked threshold (E) indicates that neither ear has a conductive component, for such would be reflected by an air-bone gap regardless of which ear contained the conductive component.

In the foregoing rules the need for masking depends on the presence or absence of an air-bone gap. Therefore, it is necessary to define the magnitude of difference between air and bone conduction thresholds sufficient to be considered an air-bone gap. Here is a rule of thumb: since 5 dB of variability is considered allowable in both the air and bone conduction thresholds, do not conclude that a true air-bone difference is present unless the gap exceeds 10 dB. The same reasoning would require air conduction thresholds to be more than 10 dB different for them to be considered bilaterally unequal. As is always the case, this rule should not be applied uncritically, without asking if the particular case may be an exception to the rule. For example, if there is indication of an air-bone gap of 10 dB or so across most of the audiogram, the probability of a real conductive component is increased. In this case masking should be used to determine the ear to which the conductive component can be assigned.

You have no doubt noticed by now that decisions regarding the need for masking are based on sensitivity measures of the test and nontest ears, both by air and bone conduction. For example, a decision about masking the poorer ear when testing air conduction depends on the better ear bone conduction sensitivity. You have probably realized that this decision may ask for information not yet available. That is, if you are testing the poorer ear air conduction thresholds, you probably do not have bone conduction results yet. How then, can you know the better ear bone conduction thresholds? Simply stated, you must guess. Consider this situation, and refer back to Figure 4.9C while reading the discussion below. The better ear air conduction threshold is 20 dB. Unmasked poorer ear air conduction threshold occurs at 40 dB. If the better ear is sensorineural, with bone conduction threshold at 20 dB, there is only a 20 dB difference between the bone conduction threshold of the nontest ear and the air conduction response of the test ear. Crossover is not possible. The threshold is valid, and masking is not necessary. On the other hand, if the better ear is conductive, with 0 dB bone conduction threshold, there is a 40 dB difference between the bone conduction threshold of the nontest ear and the unmasked test ear response. Crossover is a possibility, and masking is necessary. In this situation, you may choose to guess that the better ear is sensorineural and not mask. Or, you may guess that the better ear is conductive and mask. Later, bone conduction testing of the better ear will tell you whether your guess was right or not, regardless of your decision. There are some clues which will help you with your guessing. If the history or audiometric configuration suggest a conductive disorder, mask. If a sensorineural disorder is suggested by the patient's history or the audiometric configuration, do not mask. Be alert to accumulate information which will confirm or invalidate your decision. If you decide not to mask, be ready to repeat the test with masking if the need becomes apparent. When the decision to mask or not seems a toss up, err on the conservative side and try some masking even when it may not be necessary.

To summarize, masking is needed in air conduction testing when there is a difference of 40 dB or more between the unmasked threshold obtained on the test ear and the bone conduction threshold of the nontest ear. In bone conduction testing, masking is needed at all times, unless the air conduction thresholds are bilaterally equal and a preliminary unmasked bone conduction threshold shows there is no air-bone gap.

HOW TO MASK

A knowledge of the effectiveness of the masking noise, as discussed above, is necessary for any informed masking procedure. You must know the level to which the nontest ear will be shifted by any dial setting available on the masking level control. Given this information, two useful procedures are available. Used correctly, either will tell you (1) whether or not sufficient masking was available and used to prevent participation of the nontest ear, or (2) if overmasking is a danger, causing possible threshold shift of the test ear and resulting in an invalid test.

Begin masking as soon as the first unmasked threshold indicates that masking is needed. Do not obtain an entire unmasked audiogram for the poorer ear before masking is used. By establishing masked thresholds as you progress across frequency, you accrue more information to assess the validity of your results and to judge if masking is actually needed.

The Hood Procedure

The Hood procedure has also been called the shadowing or plateau procedure. It was suggested by Hood (1960) for masking in bone conduction testing, but it is equally applicable to air conduction testing. I believe it is the best procedure for difficult masking cases or when obtaining the first threshold on an ear about which you have little information.

Because it is time consuming, the formula procedure discussed below may be preferable to the Hood procedure in the most routine masking cases or after the use of the Hood procedure at one or two frequencies has determined the basic characteristics of the loss.

The Hood procedure may be applied at any time when the need for masking, as discussed in the previous pages, arises. The procedure, as it is used in clinical audiometry, follows:

1. Obtain threshold in quiet.
2. Shift the air conduction threshold of the nontest ear 10 dB. For an ear with a threshold of 0 dB, 10 dB Z will be required to accomplish the 10 dB threshold shift.
3. Re-obtain threshold in the test ear while masking the nontest ear. One of the two eventualities should occur.
   (a) the masked threshold will be the same as the threshold in quiet; or
   (b) there will be a 10 dB shift in the masked threshold.
4. The next step is determined by whether eventuality (a) or (b) above occurs.
   (a) If there was no shift assume that the obtained threshold is probably valid; but to be sure, introduce one additional 10 dB shift to the nontest ear and again establish threshold in the test ear. If that threshold remains the same as the original measure in quiet, accept it as a valid test ear threshold. Stated differently, the threshold of the test ear as initially obtained in quiet has remained unchanged during the time that the threshold of the nontest ear was shifted 20 dB. This procedure eliminates the possibility of a crossover response.
   (b) If introducing the masking noise resulted in a shift of the threshold of the test ear, proceed as follows: shift the nontest ear an additional 10 dB; that is, introduce an additional 10 dB

of masking to the nontest ear. Reestablish threshold. Continue this alternating procedure until

(1) the threshold of the test ear stabilizes, resulting in a plateau wherein there is no shift of the test ear threshold over an increase of 20 dB in effective masking; or

(2) the maximum output of the test tone is reached, and with the addition of 10 dB of noise to the nontest ear, there is no response from the test ear.

In either case, record the result on the audiogram. Record also the amount of effective masking required to obtain the response.

The following is an example of the use of the Hood procedure to establish an air conduction threshold at 1000 Hz in a patient who has a good ear threshold of 0 dB and a poor ear threshold of 70 dB. It may help you to obtain a blank audiogram form and enter the responses indicated below as you read through this example.

1. The good ear is tested first.
2. The 1000 Hz threshold in quiet is established on the poor ear. Assume crossover response occurs at 50 dB.
3. Shift threshold of the good ear to 10 dB.
4. Threshold of the poor ear will shift to 60 dB.
5. Shift threshold of the good ear to 20 dB.
6. Threshold of the poor ear will shift to 70 dB.
7. Shift threshold of the good ear to 30 dB.
8. Threshold of the poor ear will remain unchanged.
9. Shift threshold of the good ear to 40 dB.
10. The threshold of the poor ear will remain unchanged. A 20 dB plateau has been achieved.
11. Record the poor ear threshold and amount of Z used and proceed to the next frequency.

The Hood procedure is equally effective for masking during either air conduction or bone conduction testing. For either test, the procedure is the same. Of course, the rules governing the need for masking are different for air and bone conduction testing. In difficult masking cases, the use of 5 dB, rather than 10 dB, masking increments may be helpful.

Three phenomena sometimes complicate masking: (1) overmasking, (2) central masking, and (3) the occlusion effect.

The effect of *overmasking* is seen in the Hood procedure when a test ear which does, in fact, retain some sensitivity (is not a dead ear) never plateaus during but continues to shift to and beyond audiometer limits. Overmasking becomes a practical problem in large bilateral conductive losses.

Central masking relates to the threshold shift that sometimes occurs in the test ear upon presentation to the nontest ear of a noise level too low to cross over physically. The shift is usually no more than 5 dB but may be as much as 15 dB. The variable response associated with central masking reduces the sensitivity of testing done in the presence of masking noise. As discussed earlier, it is probably best to record the masked threshold even though central masking is suspected.

The *occlusion effect* is the apparent enhancement of bone conduction sensitivity which results in improved bone conduction thresholds when the ear is covered by an earphone or otherwise occluded. The effect may be present when masking is used since of necessity the nontest ear is occluded. According to Tonndorf (1972) the effect results from an increase in transmission of low frequency energy from the occluded ear canal. Because of the effect there is a difference in occluded versus unoccluded bone conduction thresholds of normal ears and those with sensorineural loss but not ears with conductive loss. For audiometric purposes consider the effect of occlusion (when the ear is occluded by an earphone mounted in an MX 41/AR cushion) to operate only at 500 Hz, where its size is about 20 dB, and at 250 Hz, where its size is about 25 dB (Hodgson and Tillman, 1966). The occlusion effect changes the rules for when masking is needed. That is, masking is required *anytime* bone conduction thresholds are obtained from a patient whose nontest ear is either normal or has a sensorineural loss and that ear is covered by an earphone-cushion combination. Under those conditions, at least at 250 and 500 Hz, the occlusion effect can be expected to introduce the appearance of an air-bone gap for unmasked testing. The actual Hood procedure, however, is not changed by the occlusion effect. That is, you should continue to increase masking until a 20-dB plateau is achieved.

The Formula Approach

Formulas have been proposed (1) to determine the need for masking, (2) to compute the amount needed to prevent crossover hearing, and (3) to warn when the danger of overmasking is present. These formulas have logical appeal and are useful to the student in gaining concepts relating to masking. However, as Studebaker (1964) explained, they are not practical as a tool in clinical masking. This is true because some of the information needed to complete the formula at any given time will probably not be available. Also, the time needed for computation can scarcely be afforded in the clinical evaluation. Besides, as pointed out by Price (1978), if the concepts underlying the formula are understood, the actual use of the formula in clinical evaluation is not necessary. Study the formulas below as a means to help you understand the masking process rather than as tools for routine clinical use.

Formulas use the concepts of *minimum masking* and *maximum masking*. Minimum masking is the least amount of masking delivered to the nontest ear which will prevent audibility of the test tone in the nontest ear. Maximum masking is the greatest amount of masking which can be delivered to the nontest ear without shifting the threshold of the test ear. Obviously a masking signal somewhere between these two extremes is needed. You will find in some instances, however, that the value representing maximum masking is smaller than that of minimum masking. In those cases, conventional determination of a valid masked threshold may not be possible. At other times the maximum output of the masking generator may not be as large as the minimum masking value. In these cases you cannot be sure that crossover is not occurring.

Here are the formulas proposed by Liden and associates (1959) for determining minimum and maximum masking. First for air conduction testing:

$$M_{min} = A_t - 40 + (A_m - B_m)$$

where A_t is the actual air conduction threshold of the test ear, A_m is the air conduction threshold of the masked ear, and B_m is the bone conduction threshold of the masked ear. Minimum masking is equal to the actual air conduction threshold of the test ear minus the smallest possible interaural attenuation (40 dB) plus the difference between the air and bone conduction thresholds of the nontest (masked) ear. In this formula the actual air conduction threshold of the test ear is the value which determines the crossover intensity to the nontest ear. From this value may be subtracted the amount by which the tone is attenuated as it goes across the head (at least 40 dB). To the result must be added any masking which is effectively lost by a conductive component in the masked ear. The result is the minimum masking which will prevent audibility of the test tone in the nontest ear. You should then choose a masking level greater than M_{min} but less than M_{max}. Here is the formula to determine maximum masking in air conduction testing:

$$M_{max} = B_t + 40.$$

Maximum masking possible without danger of crossover is equal to the bone conduction threshold of the test ear (B_t) plus the least possible interaural attenuation (40 dB). When masking is introduced to the nontest ear at a level greater than the sum of these values, it may start to shift the threshold of the test ear.

Here is the formula for minimum masking when testing by bone conduction:

$$M_{min} = B_t + (A_m - B_m)$$

The minimum amount of masking to prevent audibility of the test tone in the nontest ear is equal to the actual bone conduction threshold in the test ear (B_t) plus the difference between air and bone conduction thresholds in the masked nontest ear ($A_m - B_m$). Now, with bone conduction testing, the 40 dB minimum interaural attenuation expected in air conduction testing is gone. The amount of masking effectiveness lost by any conductive component in the masked ear must be added to the bone conduction threshold of the test ear to determine the least masking that can be used. You must remember to include the estimated occlusion effect on B_m if the better ear is normal or sensorineural. To do so, mask as if the bone conduction threshold at 500 Hz were better by 20 dB than the unoccluded threshold and that at 250 Hz better by 25 dB. These values approximate the size of the occlusion effect (Hodgson and Tillman, 1966). For confidence in bone conduction results, you should choose a masking level greater than M_{min} but less than M_{max}.

The formula for maximum masking in bone conduction testing is the same as for air conduction:

$$M_{max} = B_t + 40.$$

Maximum masking that can be used without danger of crossover is equal to the actual bone conduction threshold of the test ear plus the minimum 40 dB of interaural attenuation expected to apply to the air conducted masking noise. Once the noise exceeds the sum of these values, the bone conduction threshold of the test ear may be shifted. Figure 4.10 shows usage of these formulas.

The relationship between undermasking, the range of adequate masking, and overmasking is shown in Figure 4.11. The example *A* shows a normal left ear and a 70 dB mixed loss on the right ear, 20 dB of which is sensorineural and 50 dB conductive. Assuming 50 dB interaural attenuation during air conduction testing, the unmasked crossover air conduction response will occur at 50 dB, as indicated in *B*. Minimum masking will be reached with 20 dB Z in the nontest ear. There is then a wide range of adequate masking, between 20 and 70 dB Z. Maximum masking is reached at 70 dB Z. Above that level the expected 50 dB of interaural attenuation afforded by the head will be overcome and the masking will start to shift the test ear threshold. This example portrays an easy masking situation, with a wide range of adequate masking reducing the probability of under- or overmasking.

The example shown in Figure 4.12 is not so easy. The actual audiogram (*A*) reveals a conductive component on each ear, with an additional sensorineural loss on the right. Masking during air conduction testing will be no problem. But the clinician will find there is not enough masking available at maximum audiometer output to verify the bone conduction thresholds of the right ear. The masking function (*B*) is all undermasking. The unmasked right ear bone conduction responses will be at zero, resulting from crossover hearing. Sixty dB Z is needed to

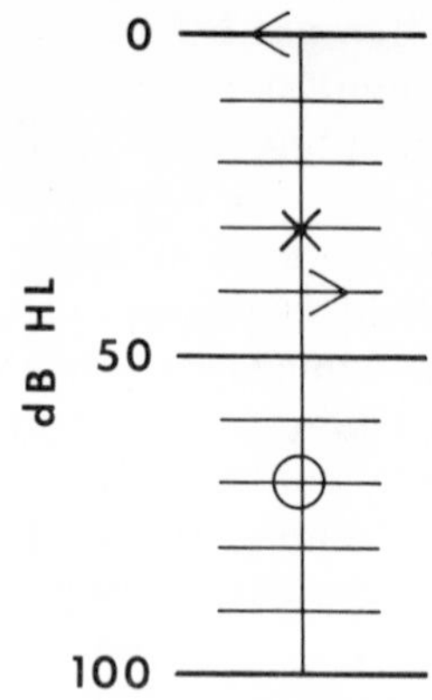

Fig. 4.10. Example of use of formulas to determine minimum and maximum masking. The left is the nontest ear and the right is the test ear. For air conduction,

$$M_{min} = A_t - 40 + (A_m - B_m) = 70 - 40 + (30 - 0) = 60 \text{ dB}.$$

$$M_{max} = B_t + 40 = 40 + 40 = 80 \text{ dB}.$$

For bone conduction,

$$M_{min} = B_t + (A_m - B_m) = 40 + (30 - 0) = 70 \text{ dB}.$$

$$M_{max} = B_t + 40 = 40 + 40 = 80 \text{ dB}.$$

Notice that minimum masking is the amount required to shift the nontest bone conduction threshold to a level where, considering interaural attenuation, it cannot participate in the test. Maximum masking is the greatest amount which can be used, considering interaural attenuation, without shifting the threshold of the test ear. Since the crossover route which results in overmasking is by bone conduction, M_{max} is the same during both air and bone conduction testing.

afford a 10 dB shift in the crossover response. Ninety dB Z, the usual limits of audiometric masking generators, will be reached before adequate masking is available to document the right ear bone conduction thresholds.

A final example (Fig. 4.13) shows a case where overmasking may occur before minimum masking is reached. In this instance there is a large conductive loss on both ears and an additional large sensorineural loss on the right. Sixty dB Z will be needed for the initial 10 dB threshold shift of the left (masked) ear. By the time the masking shifts the left ear 30 dB (80 dB Z), the effective level in the masked ear will be 50 dB above the bone conduction thresholds of the right test ear. At that level, overmasking may start, shifting the bone conduction thresholds and, of course, also the air conduction thresholds of the test ear. The only fortunate thing in this example is that the interaural attenuation of air conducted signals is often larger than 50 dB, and it may be possible through using the Hood procedure to see some evidence of a plateau representing adequate masking.

Clinicians must try to avoid both undermasking and overmasking. We must try to deliver masking to the nontest ear between minimum masking and maximum masking, the range of adequate masking. During undermasking both the tone and the noise are stimulating the nontest ear, creating invalid results. During overmasking both the tone and the

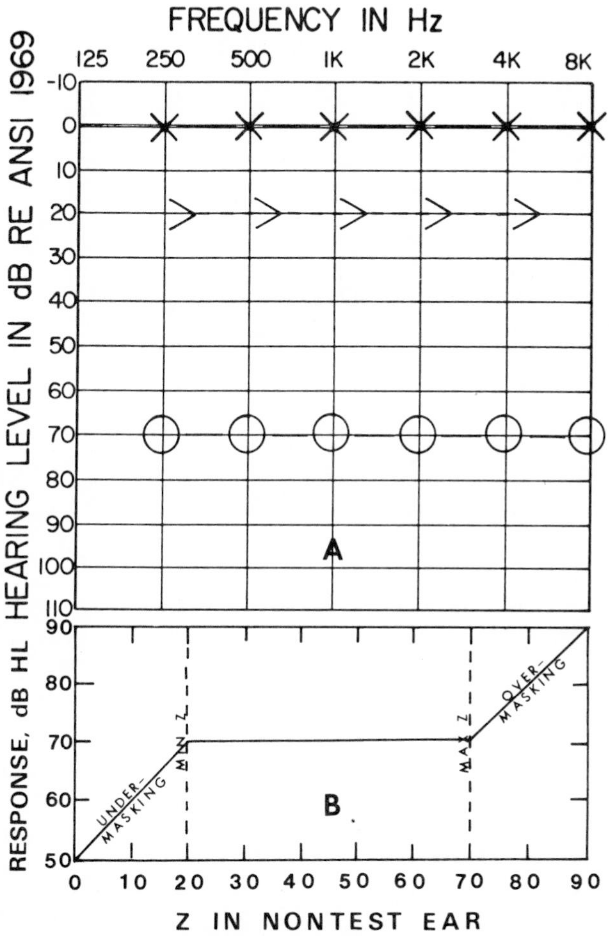

Fig. 4.11. Relationship between undermasking, the range of adequate masking, and overmasking when masking the left ear and testing the right ear with a mixed loss as shown in *A*. Refer to text for explanation of the masking function shown in *B*.

noise are stimulating the test ear, creating invalid results. Only during adequate masking are things as they should be, with the noise stimulating the nontest ear and the tone stimulating the test ear, permitting valid results. In addition to learning how to achieve adequate masking whenever possible, we must learn to recognize the occasional instances when it is not possible, and valid results cannot be assured with conventional audiometry.

In these cases, other procedures may be helpful. For example, in Figure 4.12, where undermasking is a problem, the issue is whether or not there is a conductive component on the right ear. Tympanometry,

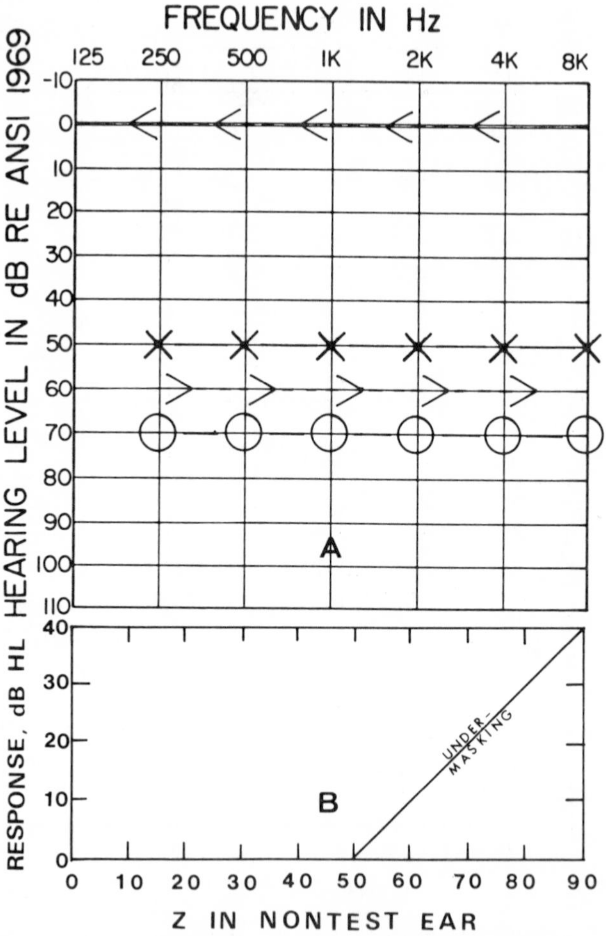

Fig. 4.12. When attempting to establish air conduction thresholds shown in *A*, insufficient masking (undermasking) will result as indicated in *B*, even at maximum audiometer output because of the conductive components.

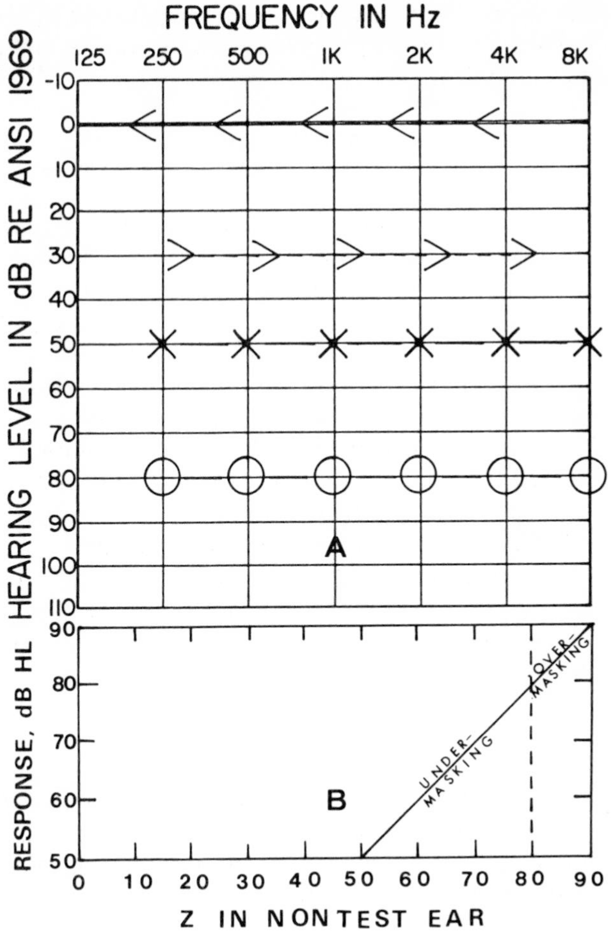

Fig. 4.13. The large conductive components shown in *A* may result in overmasking before adequate masking occurs, as indicated in *B*. Refer to text for explanation.

discussed in Chapter 7, will probably indicate the conductive component. Another procedure, the Sensorineural Acuity Level (SAL) test (Jerger and Tillman, 1960), might be helpful. Problems with the SAL test prevented it from being a universal substitute for bone conduction testing (Tillman, 1963). However, in cases such as that shown in Figure 4.13, the SAL test should give useful qualitative information about the presence of the conductive component.

In Figure 4.13, the problem is with probable overmasking. As stated earlier, adequate masking may be possible in this case unless interaural attenuation is near the low end of the range. Tympanometry should indicate that there is in fact a conductive component in both ears. In this case, too, the SAL test might give qualitative information indicating a conductive component.

SUMMARY

The purpose of clinical masking is to prevent the participation of the nontest ear. If masking is not used when needed, a shadow curve, or crossover hearing, results. Crossover occurs when there are large differences in sensitivity between the two ears. The crossover route is ordinarily by bone conduction. Even when the test signal emanates from an air conduction receiver, vibration of the earphone-cushion combination against the skull may create a bone conducted signal which can stimulate the nontest cochlea. The interaural attenuation of an air conducted tone may range from 40 to 80 dB. The interaural attenuation of a bone conducted tone is essentially zero. It follows that crossover may occur in the absence of masking when the presentation in air conduction testing is 40 dB or more greater than the bone conduction threshold of the nontest ear. In bone conduction testing, crossover may happen when the test tone is at any value above the bone conduction threshold of the nontest ear. The crucial values which govern possible crossover and the need for masking are (1) the bone conduction threshold of the nontest ear, (2) the presentation level to the test ear, and (3) interaural attenuation.

Various types of masking noise have been used—complex noise, white noise, and narrow band noise. Narrow band noise delivers more masking with less loudness and presents fewer calibration problems. For accurate work, the effectiveness of the masking noise must be known, and the masking control dial calibrated in decibels of effective masking.

The Hood masking procedure is often the method of choice. It gives more information than other methods about what is happening as increments of masking are introduced and successive thresholds are established. Obtaining a 20 dB plateau across which increments of masking result in no additional threshold shift assures that adequate masking is being used.

The Hood procedure is time consuming. In simple cases or after one or two frequencies tested with the Hood method have established the basic nature of a case, a single adequate masking level may be used. This method utilizes what we know about crossover to estimate minimum and maximum masking levels for a given test frequency. Between these extremes is a range of adequate masking which permits valid determination of threshold.

For a valid test these conditions must obtain: (1) the difference between the masked bone conduction threshold of the nontest ear and the threshold obtained on the test ear must be less than interaural attenuation (a minimum of 40 dB for an air conducted signal; essentially 0 dB for a bone conducted signal); *and* (2) the effective masking level should not exceed the bone conduction threshold of the test ear plus the interaural attenuation (a minimum of 40 dB). If criterion (1) is not met, undermasking and a shadow curve may result. If criterion (2) is not met, overmasking and a spuriously poor threshold may result.

STUDY QUESTIONS

1. In testing the right ear at 1000 Hz by air conduction, responses are obtained at 60 dB. Assume left ear air and conduction responses are normal. Should masking be used or not? Why?
2. In testing the right ear at 1000 Hz by air conduction, you obtain responses at 55 dB. The left ear, already tested, has an air conduction threshold at 35 dB and a bone conduction threshold at 0 dB at 1000 Hz. Should masking be used or not? Why?
3. In testing the right ear at 1000 Hz by air conduction, you obtain responses at 60 dB. The left ear has air and bone thresholds at 35 dB. Should masking be used or not? Why?
4. You have obtained a bone conduction threshold (vibrator on right mastoid) of 30 dB at 1000 Hz. Right and left ear air conduction thresholds at 1000 Hz are also 30 dB. Is masking necessary or not? Why?
5. Use the following information to fill in the correction factors on the chart:

	Frequency in Hz					
	250	500	1000	2000	4000	8000
Average threshold shift obtained with masking dial at 60	20	30	40	45	45	35
K factors for effective masking	250 ___	500 ___	1000 ___	2000 ___	4000 ___	8000 ___

CHAPTER 5 Speech Threshold Testing

Carhart (1951) defined speech audiometry as a technique wherein standardized samples of language are presented through a calibrated system to measure some aspect of hearing ability. Speech threshold testing is a measure of hearing sensitivity and the results are expressed in dB HL.

PURPOSES

Speech threshold testing provides a *direct* measure of *overall* hearing for speech. Pure tone thresholds are a measure of sensitivity as a function of frequency. Pure tone threshold averages are useful for predicting the level of speech necessary for audibility. However, the speech threshold is a direct measure of how loss of sensitivity affects the audibility of speech.

Speech thresholds serve as a basis for determining the presentation level of other tests. They are commonly used to help select the level at which discrimination tests, discussed in the next chapter, are presented. Aided and unaided sound field speech threshold tests help determine the effectiveness of amplification by indicating the effective gain of a hearing aid.

Most importantly, the speech threshold is a tool for confirming pure tone thresholds or for alerting the audiologist to invalid pure tone results. Hughson and Thompson (1942) reported a stable relationship between speech threshold and the average of pure tone thresholds at 500, 1000, and 2000 Hz. Lack of the expected relationship may suggest functional (nonorganic) disorder or other invalidating patient behavior. Alternately, the problem may be associated with the examiner or equipment error. At any rate, poor pure tone-speech threshold agreement is an important sign that further exploration of thresholds is called for.

SPEECH THRESHOLDS DEFINED

The speech threshold in most common clinical use is the threshold of intelligibility. It is defined as the level at which the listener can identify 50% of a simple speech signal. Remember that the threshold of *intelligibility* is intended to be a sensitivity measure, even though the word, intelligibility, implies a test of discrimination ability. The key word is *threshold*, the level at which speech becomes intelligible. Of course, because intelligibility is the criterion, discrimination ability is involved even though we take steps, described below, to minimize this variable.

On occasion another speech threshold is preferable for clinical use. The threshold of detectibility is the level at which the listener can *detect* the presence of speech 50% of the time. The patient is not expected to identify the speech signal, merely to detect its presence. For various reasons discussed below, the threshold of intelligibility cannot always be obtained. In these instances, the threshold of detectibility for speech provides a stable and useful alternative.

There are various common clinical names for the two thresholds discussed above. The threshold of intelligibility is usually called the "speech reception threshold," and commonly abbreviated SRT. The threshold of intelligibility may also be called "spondee threshold" or "spondaic threshold" (ST) since disyllabic words (spondees) are the usual test material. In clinical use the threshold of detectibility is probably most often called the "speech awareness threshold" (SAT).

SPEECH THRESHOLD TEST MATERIAL

The words used to establish SRT should be easily understandable and equally understandable. High intelligibility is important because the test is intended to be a measure of sensitivity, not of discrimination ability. Therefore, words are needed which minimize the influence of discrimination disorder. As you shall see later, poor auditory discrimination ability does occasionally frustrate efforts to obtain speech thresholds, in spite of efforts to use easily understandable words.

Homogeneity of intelligibility is important for quick, precise determination of threshold. If words used to obtain threshold are equally intelligible, then the patient's response should not vary as a function of the test words but only as a function of the presentation level. Therefore, threshold can be determined quickly with few words.

There are other attributes of good speech threshold test material, in addition to being easily and equally intelligible. Hudgins *et al.* (1947) specified that test words should be dissimilar in phonetic composition and constitute a normal sampling of English speech sounds. Making the test signal more nearly representative of every day speech may increase the practicality of the measure.

Spondee words are the most common speech threshold materials. Spondees are defined as two syllable words spoken with equal stress on each syllable. Actual spondees are not common in English, since we ordinarily stress the first syllable of disyllabic words. However, there are many words which still serve if care is taken to place equal stress on each syllable. "Hotdog," "baseball," and "cowboy" are examples. Figure 5.1 shows the performance-intensity (PI) function for a group of spondee words obtained from a normal hearing listener. The graph indicates the growth of intelligibility (percentage correct) as intensity of the words is increased. PI functions are discussed further in Chapter 6. The function shown in Figure 5.1 indicates that two basic requirements of good speech threshold material are met: the high intelligibility is indicated by the low presentation level at which audibility starts; and homogeneity of intelligibility is indicated by the steepness of the function. Once audibility begins, the words become 100% intelligible with only a small increase in presentation level.

Although not clinically common in routine testing, other speech material in addition to spondees is satisfactory for obtaining speech thresholds. Carhart (1946) compared thresholds obtained with spondees

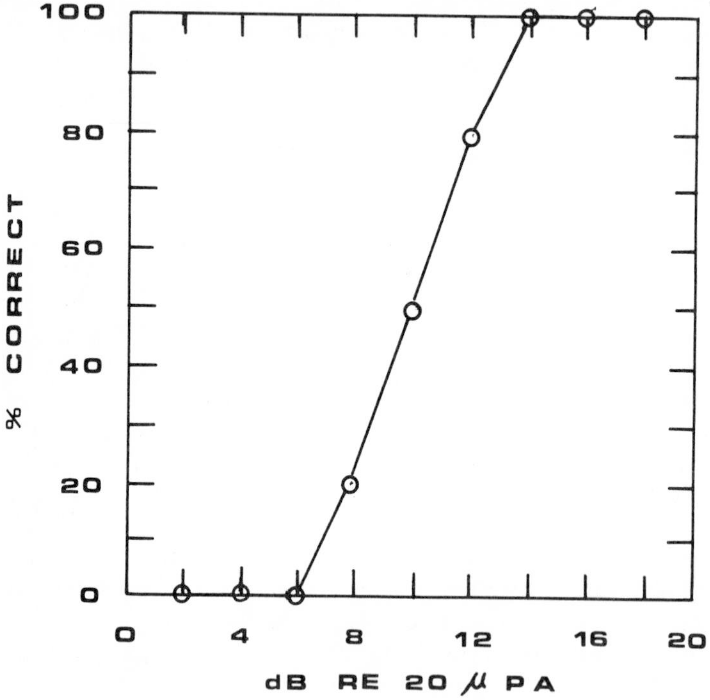

Fig. 5.1. Performance-intensity function for spondees.

and with sentences developed at the Bell Telephone Laboratories. He concluded that the two were essentially equivalent in determining speech thresholds. However, the ease, speed, and reliability of thresholds obtained with spondees make them the almost unanimous choice for routine testing

Keaster's (1947) speech threshold test is composed of sentences containing nouns derived from the first thousand words on the International Kindergarten Word List. The sentences are shown in Appendix A. Since the sentences require no verbal responses you may find them useful for establishing threshold with children who cannot or will not repeat spondees.

INSTRUMENTATION FOR SPEECH AUDIOMETRY

A two-room test environment is preferable for speech audiometry. This arrangement consists of a test room in which the patient is seated with the transducers—earphones, bone vibrator, and loudspeakers—which deliver the signal. The audiometric equipment and the audiologist are located in an adjacent control room. If speech testing must be done in a one-room setup, testing is limited to recorded procedures to assure that the patient does not receive clues except via the audiometer circuit. The audiometer, as well as the test rooms, should meet the requirements described in the standards section of Chapter 2.

Some audiometers combine pure tone and speech circuitry. Others are designed for speech testing only. In either case, the speech portion of the audiometer will contain the elements shown in Figure 5.2. Refer to this figure as you read the sections below.

Inputs

Use of the input selector permits (naturally enough) selection of the input signal of choice. Generally, the available choices will be a microphone for live voice testing and a phonograph and a tape input for recorded testing. Most speech audiometers are two-channel units which permit simultaneous selection of two inputs: recorded speech from one channel and masking noise from the other, for example.

Correct use of the input gain control and VU meter is necessary for accurate testing. A VU meter is shown in Figure 5.3. The VU meter serves two purposes. First, in conjunction with manipulation of the input gain control, the VU meter permits adjusting the input signal to the correct level. Second, in live voice testing the VU meter serves as a visual monitor to assure consistency of the input level—thus, the term, "monitored live voice," to describe the live voice testing in speech audiometry.

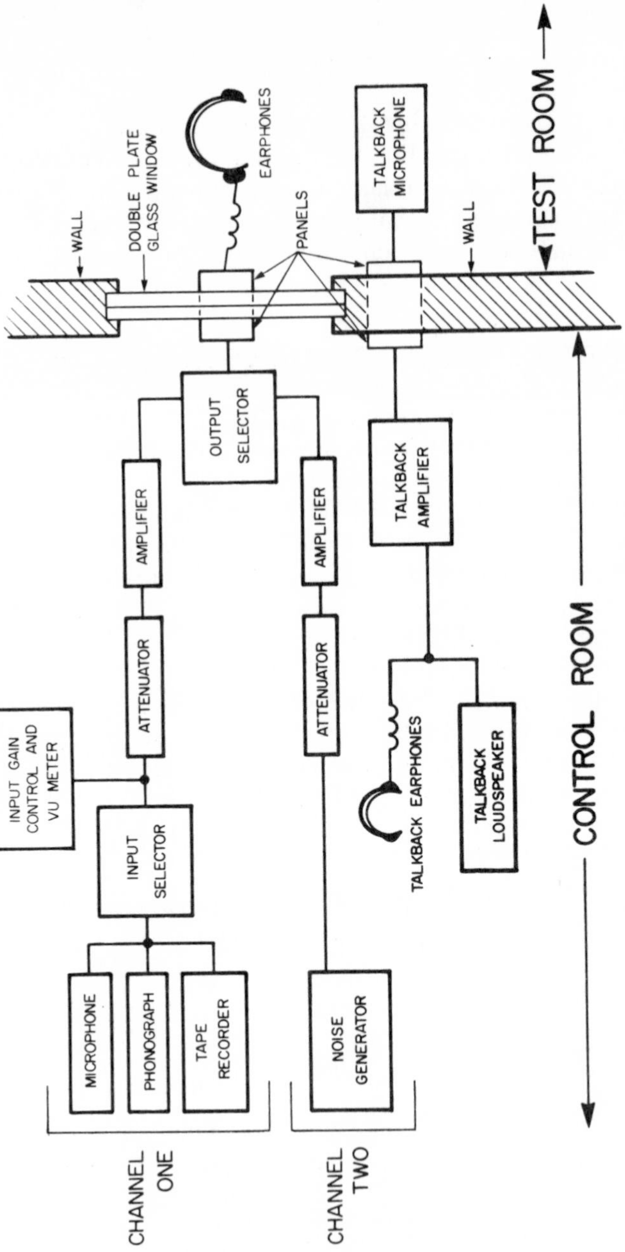

Fig. 5.2. Block diagram of a speech audiometric arrangement.

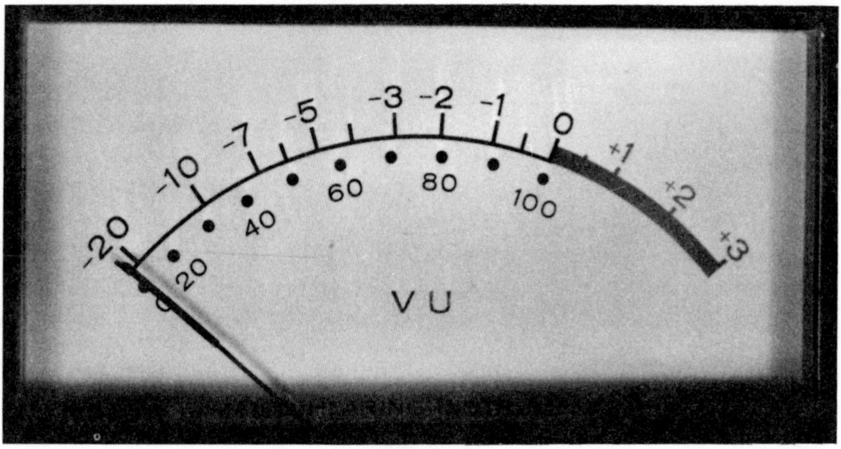

Fig. 5.3. VU meter.

Phonograph discs or audio tapes on which speech tests are recorded ordinarily contain a 1000 Hz calibration tone recorded at a level equivalent to the speech. While presenting this calibration tone to the audiometer circuit, the audiologist should adjust input gain control so that the needle of the VU meter points to zero. This procedure assures an input of correct magnitude. Whether or not the output signal will be correct depends on the calibration of the other audiometric circuitry. Therefore, input calibration is not a substitute for the calibration described in Chapter 2. However, assuming correct output calibration, the signal from the audiometer will be weak or strong by the number of decibels which the needle of the VU meter peaks below or above zero.

For input calibration in live voice threshold testing, the audiologist should peak each syllable of each spondee at zero. To do so requires first of all that each syllable be spoken with equal stress. You will probably have a natural tendency to place more stress on the first syllable. Some practice in consistent presentation is necessary. You may then control the overall strength of the input signal by any combination of these methods: First, the gain control may be rotated while you present spondees until the needle is peaking at zero. Second, you may vary the intensity of your voice until the needle is peaking at zero. Third, you may regulate the distance between your lips and the microphone until the needle is peaking at zero. Certain considerations may influence the procedure you use. During live voice testing into a single wall sound room there is danger that patients with good hearing may hear your voice directly through the wall of the room rather than via the audiometer. Therefore, you must keep your voice at a low level and compensate by using the other two methods to increase input. However, if you hold the microphone extremely close to your lips, distortion may result, especially of unvoiced plosives. A distance of about 6 inches between microphone and lips, with the microphone not quite directly in front of the lips is satisfactory. Finally, if there is some noise in the control room, you can minimize its effect by increasing the level of your voice or holding the microphone closer to your lips, thus permitting you to turn down the input gain control. As you can see, the exact method you use for input calibration during monitored live voice testing must depend on circumstances.

If masking is to be used, the input level of the masking noise, as well as the speech signal, may require calibration. Turn the input gain control of the channel presenting the masking noise until the VU meter peaks at zero.

Outputs

The output selector of a two-channel audiometer can be rather complicated. It ordinarily permits direction of a signal from either channel into any of the audiometer's transducers. Thus, you can simultaneously direct speech to one earphone and masking noise to the other. Two channels with separate attenuators permits independent control of the intensity of each signal. You can also select the desired arrangement to send speech or noise to the loudspeakers if your equipment includes a provision for sound field testing. Obviously it is important that you be familiar with the operation of the output selector and other features of the audiometer for quick and accurate manipulation.

Talkback

In a two-room setup provision must be made to hear the patient's responses. This circuit is also shown in Figure 5.2. It may consist of only a headset for you to wear or may include a loudspeaker so that others in the test room can hear the patient's response. Be alert for feedback. During live voice testing, particularly if the signal is directed to the patient via loudspeaker, a high level of the test signal or talkback gain control may result in uncomfortably loud feedback. Make it a habit to (1) turn hearing level dials down before turning on the test microphone, (2) switch the talkback loudspeaker off and monitor patient responses via earphones when high test levels are necessary, and (3) reduce talkback gain control when you must increase the speech test signal to exceedingly high levels. In addition to talkback, it is quite helpful for an audiometer to have a talk forward circuit so you can communicate with the patient without resetting the test controls each time you wish to speak. This talk forward circuit will also have a gain control and you should remember to set it to an appropriate level, depending on the hearing loss and tolerance requirements of each patient.

MONITORED LIVE VOICE VERSUS RECORDED TESTING

Use of recorded tests for obtaining speech threshold promotes standardization, but they are less flexible and usually take longer to administer than do live voice tests. With cooperative patients either method yields valid thresholds. For the difficult to test—children, elderly persons, and those with language problems—the flexibility of live voice testing is useful. Several studies have supported live voice testing. Siegenthaler and Smith (1961) found no significant differences in speech thresholds obtained with monitored live voice and recorded stimuli. Beattie *et al.* (1977b) found that the reliability of thresholds obtained by monitored live voice was as good as that of thresholds obtained with recorded materials. The studies cited utilized experienced talkers to obtain the live voice thresholds. It is necessary to be competent in test procedure, audiometric manipulation, and vocal presentation to obtain valid live voice thresholds. These competencies require practice.

A survey by Martin and Pennington (1971) found that most audiologists prefer live voice threshold testing. Research evidence and clinical experience justify such usage.

HISTORY

Early equipment, material, and concepts for speech audiometry were developed by Fletcher and his colleagues at the Bell Telephone Labs (Fletcher, 1929 and 1953). The procedures they developed were designed to test telephone systems. Their speech audiometer, the Western Electric 4A, utilized phonographically recorded numbers as material for speech threshold testing. This audiometer was used for group screening of school children.

Hughson and Thompson (1942), using the Bell Telephone sentences, established a clinically feasible method for determining speech threshold. They established the relationship between speech reception threshold and pure tone threshold averages.

During World War II scientists working at the Psychoacoustic Laboratories (PAL) at Harvard University developed additional speech material for testing military communications equipment. They developed recorded tests for obtaining speech threshold (Hudgins *et al.*, 1947). PAL test no. 12 consisted of sentences. PAL test nos. 9 and 14 each contained 42 different spondees. On no. 9, groups of words were recorded at the same level with attenuation of level between groups. Thus, with the attenuation built into the record, speech threshold could be obtained without changing the audiometer's attenuator once the test was started.

No. 14 consisted of all words recorded at the same level so that the audiometrist could obtain threshold by manipulating the audiometer attenuator while the test was under way.

These materials were used in military hospitals where aural rehabilitation centers were established to treat handicapped veterans (Carhart, 1946).

With the aim of eliminating words which were too easy or too difficult, Hirsh *et al.* (1952) selected 36 of the 84 PAL spondees for recording at the Central Institute for the Deaf (CID). Two recordings, W-1 and W-2, were made. Each contains the same words in the same order: 6 scramblings of the 36 spondees. Each spondee is preceded by a carrier phrase, "Say the word." To be sure the patient is alerted for each upcoming test word, the carrier phrase is recorded at the level of the 1000 Hz calibration tone. The test word is recorded 10 dB below that level. While the W-1 words are recorded at a constant level, the spondees on the W-2 are recorded at decreasing levels. The level is reduced by 3 dB after each group of three words. Thus, the last group of spondees is 33 dB below the first group. Because of the attenuation in the record, a speech threshold can be obtained without manipulation of the audiometer attenuator if a level less than 33 dB above the patient's threshold is chosen to start the test. To obtain threshold with the W-2 record, the number of correct responses is subtracted from the starting level and 1.5 dB (½ of the value of the first 3 dB step) is added. The W-1 and W-2 tests are commercially available.[1] The W-1 recording is more common in clinical use, and its administration is discussed in detail in a later section.

Hirsh and his co-workers (1952) were aware of remaining differences in intelligibility of the spondees they chose, even after eliminating the easiest and most difficult items. In fact, they varied the level as they recorded different words to compensate for differences in intelligibility. In live voice testing, this compensation is scarcely feasible. Beattie and associates (1975) reported a 7.9 dB range in the relative intelligibility of the 36 CID spondees. Olsen and Matkin (1979) recommended 15 spondees on the basis of homogeneity as determined in six separate studies. The CID spondees, with those recommended by Olsen and Matkin identified, appear in Appendix B.

There is a tendency for speech threshold to get better as fewer words are used to determine threshold. If only three or four words are used, the speech threshold may be quite close to the threshold of detectibility.

---

[1] *Addresses:* Technisonic Studios, 1201 S. Brentwood Blvd., Richmond Heights, MO 63117 (phonographic disc recordings); Auditec of St. Louis, 330 Selma Ave., St. Louis, MO 63119 (audio tape recording W-1 and W-22).

PROCEDURE

Order of Testing—SRT Versus Pure Tones

It has been traditional to obtain speech thresholds after completion of pure tone testing. Since the basic purpose of speech thresholds is comparison with pure tone thresholds it probably makes sense to get the speech thresholds first. Speech thresholds constitute a quick measure and pure tone air and bone conduction testing requires more time. Speech thresholds, obtained first, are available for comparison as you begin the pure tone audiogram. If, through comparison with speech thresholds, it becomes obvious that the pure tone thresholds are not valid, not much time has been lost. You can quickly begin to look for the problem. On the other hand if the speech thresholds, obtained after air and bone conduction sensitivity has been tested, suggest that the pure tone thresholds are not valid, a great deal of time will have been lost. Therefore, it makes sense, particularly if you have any reason to believe that it may be difficult to elicit valid pure tone thresholds, to obtain the speech thresholds first.

Instructions

Be sure the patient cannot get visual clues by watching you with even peripheral vision. At the same time it will be helpful if you can see the patient's face and, particularly later in discrimination testing, can get visual clues to verify your auditory impression of the patient's response. A good arrangement is to seat the patient so you can see the face in profile, making observation of you difficult. Then, if the patient does turn to look at you, simply say, "Please don't watch me during this test."

Instructions should be brief and simple. Probably you need say no more than, "Please repeat these words." Then, begin the familiarization step described below. After familiarizing the patient with the spondees, it may be helpful, though probably not necessary, to say, "Now I'm going to make the words softer and softer. Please keep saying them as long as you can. Guess if you're not sure."

Special instructions and precautions may be necessary in some cases. You must be sure the patient understands the instructions. If the patient wears a hearing aid, you may want to give instructions before removing the aid. If there is a large loss but the patient does not have an aid, it may be convenient to supply amplification and instructions via the speech audiometer. However, if you do not intend to instruct the patient via the audiometer, do not put the earphones on before giving instructions. To do so would simply reduce the effective level of your voice. It is possible to use written instructions, although it is unlikely that the standard test procedure can be used with a patient whose hearing is so poor that spoken instructions, with appropriate amplification, cannot be understood. With children or individuals with limited language or speech, special instructions and procedures may be necessary. These are discussed in a subsequent section of this chapter.

Familiarization

The patient should be informed of the words which will constitute the test. This familiarization procedure serves two important purposes. First, Tillman and Jerger (1959) established that the threshold will be 4–5 dB better if the individual has prior knowledge of the test vocabulary. The threshold norms reflect this knowledge, so your patient should have it also for valid test results. Additionally, familiarization will stabilize the threshold-finding procedure, since the patient will not need to be learning the vocabulary during the actual test.

A second important function of the familiarization procedure, performed properly, is the elimination of words which the patient cannot identify because of poor discrimination ability. The intent is to measure sensitivity and simple, easy-to-understand words are used. Nevertheless, if the patient's discrimination is really poor, it may become an unwanted influence in the test. To minimize this influence, always read the test words to the patient via the audiometer without visual clues during familiarization. Discard any words which the patient cannot identify at a suprathreshold level. In some cases with very poor discrimination ability, the patient may be able to identify only three or four spondees. If so, indicate on the Audiologic Record the number of selected spondees which were used. The speech threshold so obtained will be closer to the threshold of detectibility than is ordinarily the case. If the patient cannot identify any of the spondees, the threshold of detectibility may be substituted as described in a subsequent section.

Use of a Carrier Phrase

In an early study of speech audiometry, a carrier phrase, "You will write," preceded each test item (Egan, 1948). The carrier phrase has been retained in discrimination testing to alert the patient to the upcoming test item and to assist the audiologist in using the VU meter to monitor the presentation. However, authorities agree that the carrier phrase is not needed in threshold testing (Giolas and Randolph, 1977; Hopkinson, 1978). Since the carrier phrase is time consuming and apparently serves no purpose, its routine use in threshold testing is not indicated.

Size of the Test Increment

The size of the intensity step used in establishing speech threshold will, of course, be influenced by the way the hearing loss dial is calibrated. The pure tone threshold finding procedure has traditionally used 5 dB increments. However, the attenuator of popular speech audiometer in earlier use—the Grason-Stadler 162—was calibrated in 2 dB steps. Later, as combined pure tone and speech audiometers became more popular, use of 5 dB steps consistent with their instrumentation became more common. Chaiklin and Ventry (1964) reported no clinically significant differences in speech thresholds derived through use of 2 or 5 dB steps. Both increments are clinically feasible, and a slightly different procedure is probably justified for use of each. Therefore, two procedures are suggested below, based on 2 dB and 5 dB increments.

Numerous methods for establishing speech thresholds under clinical conditions have been suggested (Chaiklin and Ventry, 1964; Tillman and Olsen, 1973; ASHA, 1977; Hopkinson, 1978). Any of these can be used to obtain valid thresholds with monitored live voice, the W-1 recording, or other spondees recorded at a constant level. The methods given below are suggested for quick and accurate threshold determination.

Monitored Live Voice Procedure Using 2 dB Steps

Instruct the patient and read the list of spondees at a comfortable listening level. Discard any words which are not repeated correctly. During the test do not present words in the same order as when familiarizing the patient. If you must go through the list more than once to establish thresholds rearrange the order of presentation again. It is convenient to have each word typed on a 3 × 5 card. These may be discarded or reshuffled as necessary.

Be sure to set the input gain control and monitor your voice so that the VU meter needle peaks at zero for each syllable of each word. This precaution is critical for accurate thresholds. If the needle peaks 5 dB below zero, the obtained threshold will be 5 dB poorer than the patient's actual sensitivity. If the needle peaks over zero, a better than actual threshold will be obtained.

Plan to get threshold quickly. The process should take less than 1 min. Remember you are finding a threshold, a measure which has some variability, or at least for which we cannot get a single, never changing value. Do not wear yourself and the patient out.

Starting at a level 10 dB below that at which the familiarization was done, descend in 10 dB steps, presenting one word per level, until the patient misses a word (fails to respond or responds incorrectly). Increase the level 8 dB. Now you are 2 dB below the last correct response. Descend in 2 dB steps, presenting one word at each level until the patient misses a word. Because of the steep articulation function of spondees, this level should be ± 2 dB of threshold. Clinically, this rule will not always hold true, but it is useful to remember as a guide.

Present three more spondees at this level. Depending on the response, do one of the following: (1) If the patient repeats two of the four words, take this level as threshold. (2) If three or all four of the words are missed, increase the level 2 dB. (3) If three of the four words are repeated correctly, decrease the level 2 dB. If (2) or (3) is the case, present four more words at the new level. Take threshold as the level at which the patient repeats two of the four words. If it should happen that the patient always repeats less than 50% of the words at one level and always repeats more than 50% at the next highest level, take the latter level as threshold.

Monitored Live Voice Procedure Using 5 dB Steps

Instructions, preliminaries, and precautions are the same as those noted above under discussion of the 2 dB step procedure. Descend in 10 dB steps, giving one word at each level, until the patient misses a word. Give three more words at that level. If the patient gets two of the four words correct, take that level as the speech threshold. If three or all four of the words are missed, increase the level 5 dB. If three of the four words are repeated correctly, decrease the level 5 dB. At the new level, present four more words. Continue until two of the four words are repeated correctly. It is more likely than when using the 2 dB procedure that you will find one level at which less than 50% accuracy will obtain, with 100% accuracy at the next highest level. If so, record threshold as the lowest level at which more than 50% correct response occurs.

Obtaining Threshold with a Recorded Test

Recorded tests will ordinarily incorporate a 1000 Hz calibration tone. Adjust the input gain control until the VU meter needle is deflected to zero. The calibration tone and the carrier phrase on the CID W-1 record are at a level 10 dB greater than the test words. This provision ensures that the patient will hear the carrier phrase even if the test word is near or even slightly below threshold. Because the test words are 10 dB weaker than the calibration tone, and because the input signal is calibrated to that tone, you must make the obtained threshold 10 dB better to compensate for the weakness of the test words. For example, if the hearing loss dial reads 20 dB at the level of 50% response, the patient's threshold is 10 dB, and that is the value you should record. This provision applies only to the W-1 recording. It does not apply to monitored live voice testing or to any recorded test in which the calibration tone and test words are recorded at the same level.

With the exceptions noted above, recorded spondee tests with all words at the same level can be utilized with the same procedure suggested for monitored live voice. Test increments of either 2 dB or 5 dB can be used. The problem of eliminating words which the listener cannot identify is troublesome. You should note those words during the familiarization process and just ignore them when they occur during the test. Actually, while occasions no doubt arise when a recorded threshold test is preferable, it usually makes better sense to use live voice testing with a patient whose discrimination is so poor that all words on the test cannot be identified.

EXPECTED RELATIONSHIP BETWEEN SPEECH THRESHOLD AND PURE TONE AVERAGE

The fundamental purpose of the speech threshold is confirmation of the pure tone audiogram. Therefore, as soon as speech and pure tone thresholds have been obtained you must compare them. Do not wait until the evaluation is completed or until other tests have been done. If speech and pure tone thresholds do not agree, you must re-evaluate your procedure, reinstruct the patient, or do whatever possible to determine what is invalidating test results.

Comparison of speech thresholds with the average of pure tone thresholds of 500, 1000, and 2000 Hz has been the most common procedure. Routinely, the dB value of the speech threshold and this pure tone average should be almost identical. However, as you will see below, there are some qualifications and some exceptions to this rule.

Speech Awareness Threshold

As mentioned earlier, it is not always possible to obtain the commonly used threshold of intelligibility (SRT). If discrimination ability is extremely poor, the patient may not always be able to identify spondees even at suprathreshold levels. In these cases attempts to determine SRT will be invalid. In other instances, reduced language ability or poor speech may prevent establishment of SRT. In these situations, the speech awareness threshold (SAT) may be substituted. SAT is defined as the lowest level at which the patient can detect the presence of speech at least 50% of the time.

The patient is instructed to say "yes" or to raise the hand each time the speech signal is detected. It is conventional to use (bʌ-bʌ-bʌ) as the speech signal in SAT testing. The level is varied in a manner similar to that for obtaining SRT, until the lowest level is found at which the patient can respond at least half of the time.

Expected Relationship between Thresholds of Intelligibility and Detectibility

SRT and SAT represent different criteria: intelligibility versus detectibility. Naturally, for a given individual the threshold values will not be the same. Greater intensity is required for intelligibility than for detectibility. Egan (1948) reported that the difference did not exceed 12 dB. Hirsh *et al.* (1952) found a difference of 10 dB between the two thresholds. Beattie and associates (1978) reported a difference of 8 dB. Frisina (1962), comparing the SAT directly with the pure tone audiogram, found that it agreed closely with the best pure tone threshold across the range, 500–2000 Hz. Thus, when SATs are obtained instead of the more common intelligibility threshold, you should assume for purposes of comparison that the SAT will be about 8 to 10 dB better than the intelligibility threshold should have been, or that the SAT should be about the same as single best pure tone threshold across the range, 500–2000 Hz.

Calibration Norms for Speech and Pure Tone Thresholds

To understand the clinical relationship between speech and pure tone thresholds the standards which specify the SPLs required for thresholds must be studied. These are the levels to which audiometers are calibrated and which represent audiometer zero.

The ANSI (1969) pure tone SPLs (dB re: 20 μ PA) for 0 dB HL are 11.5 dB for 500 Hz, 7 dB for 1000 Hz, and 9 dB for 2000 Hz. The average of these values is 9.2 dB SPL. The ANSI (1969) threshold standard for speech is 20 dB SPL for the TDH 39 earphone. That is, 20 dB SPL = 0 dB HL. Thus, there is a calibration difference of about 10 dB between threshold of *detectibility* for pure tones and threshold of *intelligibility* for speech (SRT). Remember that the SRT should be about 10 dB poorer than the SAT. The SAT should require about the same SPL as pure tone thresholds across the mid frequency range. Therefore, the SRT and the pure tone threshold average (PTA) should agree closely with the use of audiometers whose calibration is that described above.

Relationship Between Speech and Pure Tone Thresholds in Flat Configurations

Numerous procedures have been proposed to relate pure tone and speech thresholds. One of the simplest is probably the best. Fletcher (1929) suggested that the average of the thresholds from 500 to 2000 Hz would provide a good estimate of sensitivity for speech. Carhart (1946) investigated several methods and also concluded that the average of thresholds at 500, 1000, and 2000 Hz was preferable. Actually both of these studies used the frequencies 512, 1024, and 2048 Hz since audiometers at that time were designed to produce those frequencies. Their conclusions persist, and it remains a common procedure to average thresholds at 500, 1000, and 2000 Hz to obtain one level which represents overall sensitivity for simple speech and with which the speech threshold is compared. For individuals with fairly flat audiograms (about the same sensitivity across frequency) speech threshold and pure tone threshold averages should agree closely.

Relationship Between Speech and Pure Tone Thresholds in Irregular Configurations

Fletcher (1950) observed that speech thresholds were likely to be better than three-frequency pure tone threshold averages in cases where there were substantial differences in sensitivity at the three frequencies. He proposed utilizing only the two best frequencies to obtain an average representing overall sensitivity for simple speech and with which to compare the speech threshold. He found this procedure gave better speech-pure tone threshold agreement. Fletcher's suggestion has become common clinical practice. If there is a difference greater than 15 dB between thresholds at the octave intervals, 500, 1000, and 2000 Hz, you should average the two best frequencies. When you record the result designate it as a "2 best frequency" average. Although justifiable in any irregular configuration, the use of Fletcher's proposal is most commonly associated with high frequency loss. In cases of precipitously dropping high frequency losses in which reliable speech thresholds can be obtained, you may find the speech threshold is closer to the threshold of the single best pure tone frequency, rather than even the two-frequency average.

Good to Poor Pure Tone-Speech Threshold Agreement

Carhart (1960) suggested that PTA-SRT agreement should be within 6 dB. The designations shown in Table 5.1 should apply to the PTA-SRT relationship. If good agreement exists, the speech threshold supports the pure tone results. If there is questionable agreement, try to find out what is causing the discrepancy. Retest to examine reliability of results. Poor agreement indicates that either speech or pure tone thresholds are not valid. Such results should not be reported until all efforts to correct them have been exhausted. If the results persist they

Table 5.1
Agreement Between Pure Tone Threshold Average and Speech Reception Threshold

For Thresholds Obtained in 2 dB Steps		For Thresholds Obtained in 5 dB Steps	
If PTA-SRT Agreement is	Agreement is	If PTA-SRT Agreement is	Agreement is
±6 dB	Good	±5 dB	Good
±12 dB	Questionable	±10 dB	Questionable
>±12 dB	Poor	>±10 dB	Poor

should be reported with a cautionary statement regarding the discrepancy and the failure of efforts to improve the relationship. If possible, the probable reason for the discrepancy should be mentioned.

Factors which Influence Speech-Pure Tone Threshold Relationship

Nonorganic (functional or feigned) hearing loss is known to result in poor SRT-PTA agreement. Ventry and Chaiklin (1965) reported that 70% of a group with functional loss gave speech reception thresholds at least 12 dB better than the PTA. Poor SRT-PTA agreement with speech thresholds better than pure tone averages should suggest the possibility of functional loss if the conditions described below do not apply.

SRT-PTA agreement is likely to deteriorate as the audiometric configuration moves more and more away from a flat loss with equal sensitivity at all frequencies. Even when the appropriate two-frequency average is used, the agreement may not be as good as that ordinarily seen in flat losses. Nevertheless, the agreement should be no poorer than in the "questionable" category to be minimally acceptable.

In speech threshold testing, demands on discrimination ability are minimized to reduce the effect of discrimination deficit on the threshold-finding process. Nevertheless, if discrimination ability is very poor, this variable may intervene. If the patient cannot readily repeat spondees at a suprathreshold level, it will be difficult to obtain a valid speech threshold. A special case is the individual with a sharply falling high frequency loss with sensitivity in the lower part of the speech range that is much better than in the high frequency part. You may find a range of many decibels across which the individual can repeat approximately 50% of the spondees. In these cases with discrimination problems, it is more meaningful to obtain a SAT rather than the conventional SRT.

MASKING

With some differences, the rules discussed in the previous chapter for masking during pure tone testing also apply to speech testing. Anticipating a minimum interaural attenuation for speech of 40 dB, you should mask during speech threshold testing when there is a difference of 40 dB or more between the speech threshold of the test ear and the bone conduction thresholds of the nontest ear. During pure tone testing when you looked at the nontest ear to evaluate the possibility of crossover, you needed to consider only the one frequency being tested. Now you must consider bone conduction sensitivity in the nontest ear across the range important for the audibility of speech. Several procedures are possible: If the bone conduction thresholds of the nontest ear are similar across frequency, the three frequency average (500, 1000, 2000 Hz) will be useful. If there is a difference between the test ear speech threshold and the bone conduction PTA of the nontest ear of 40 dB or more, masking is indicated.

Because of irregular configuration, a two-frequency average may be more representative of the nontest ear bone conduction sensitivity. Using the rules advocated for air conduction, average the two better thresholds of the frequencies, 500, 1000, and 2000 Hz. If there is a difference between the test ear speech threshold and the bone conduction two-frequency average of 40 dB or more, masking is indicated.

A more conservative approach is to look for the best bone conduction threshold across the frequency range, 500–4000 Hz. If there is a single frequency in which the bone conduction threshold is 40 dB or more better than the speech threshold, masking is indicated. Depending on circumstances, this conservative approach is probably the procedure of choice. Even though the probability of crossover is minimal it is better to mask when probably not necessary than to risk recording an invalid speech threshold.

Two masking problems present during pure tone audiometry persist in speech threshold testing: overmasking and central masking. Assuming a minimum of 40 dB and an expected value for interaural attenuation of about 50 dB, you should be alert for overmasking when the noise exceeds the pertinent bone conduction thresholds of the test ear by 40–50 dB or more. The methods for detecting and preventing overmasking during speech threshold testing are the same as those appropriate for pure tone testing, discussed in the previous chapter.

Central masking affecting spondee threshold has been demonstrated by Martin (1966). The magnitude was reported to be on the order of 5 dB. As is the case with pure tone testing, it is probably best to record masked speech thresholds even if the influence of central masking is suspected.

White noise is most commonly used for speech masking. A variation available on some audiometers is speech spectrum noise, sometimes called pink noise. It is generated by filtering white noise to approximate the long term spectrum of speech. Thus, its spectrum will show greatest energy in the range to 1000 Hz, with a gently sloping decrement in energy above 1000 Hz. Narrow band noise, of course, should not be used for masking the broad spectrum speech signal.

It is necessary to know the effectiveness of noise used to mask speech, just as is the case when masking pure tones. The same clinical calibration is appropriate. A column indicating the effectiveness of broad band noise for masking speech can be added to the masking table described in Chapter 4. Alternatively, a correction (*K*) factor for the masking noise can be determined. The procedure is similar to that for determining effective masking of pure tones. Direct the speech signal and noise to the same earphone. Set the noise attenuator to a reasonably high level, such as 60 dB. Determine the speech threshold in noise for a few reliable, normal hearing subjects. Compute the mean masked speech threshold. The difference between the resulting threshold and the masking noise dial setting can be used to construct a masking table or as a *K* factor. That is, if 60 dB of noise resulted in a speech threshold of 40 dB, a 50 dB setting can be expected to permit a 30 dB threshold, a 70 dB setting a 50 dB threshold, etc. In this example, the K factor is 20 dB. To utilize this factor, determine the desired effective masking, add to it the *K* factor, and set the masking dial at that level. You must remember that these generalizations apply only if linearity of the masking attenuator has been determined, the procedure for which is described in Chapter 2.

Either the Hood procedure or the formula method described in the previous chapter may be used. Using the Hood procedure, obtain a speech threshold in quiet on the poorer ear. Then shift the better ear threshold 10 dB with the appropriate masking. Re-establish the speech threshold. If there is no shift, introduce another 10 dB shift to the nontest ear. If the threshold is still unchanged over this 20 dB plateau, it may be recorded. However, if shifting the nontest ear results in a similar shift of obtained threshold, continue the procedure until a 20 dB plateau does result, or the maximum audiometer output is reached.

A more expeditious masking procedure for speech threshold audiometry is to estimate minimum and maximum masking levels, as explained in the previous chapter. Then deliver a masking level between these two values to the nontest ear while obtaining speech threshold. If the resulting threshold should not agree with the pure tone results, whenever they are obtained, then masking inadequacy should be one of the possibilities considered to explain the discrepancy. A final precaution: just as with pure tone audiometry, be alert for the presence of an air-bone gap in the nontest ear which will increase the probability that masking will be needed. Also remember that an air-bone gap in either or both ears may increase the danger of overmasking.

SPECIAL PROCEDURES IN OBTAINING SPEECH THRESHOLDS

Various attributes of the patient may preclude use of the standard procedure. Age is an example. Very young or aged patients may not respond well to the standard procedure. Appendix C gives a list of spondees which are more likely to be within the vocabulary of children. Patients with language or speech problems also may require special procedures. If the patient cannot respond verbally but can point to pictures or objects representing spondee words, a valid speech threshold can be obtained. The spondees in Appendix C can readily be represented by pictures. To reduce demands on memory span you probably should use no more than six pictures from which the patient must select by pointing. This small number may move the SRT slightly toward the threshold of detectibility.

A less formal procedure involves asking the patient to point to body or clothing parts. This method is good with young children who have not yet learned spondee words and who cannot or will not speak. It may also be useful with older aphasics. Find three or four spatially separated items which the patient can point to on request (for example, "hair," "mouth," and "shoes"). While these items do not meet good criteria for threshold material, their use may permit establishment of a minimum response level. Finally, if a threshold of intelligibility of any sort cannot be obtained, you may be able to establish thresholds of detectibility for speech. Remember this threshold is expected to be 8–10 dB better than the speech reception threshold would be if obtainable. Remember, too, that speech thresholds represent only overall sensitivity and are not very sensitive to audiometric configuration, such as high frequency loss. When speech thresholds are used as the only evidence of sensitivity, a high frequency loss cannot be ruled out.

Bone conduction speech thresholds may be useful estimates of cochlear reserve when pure tone thresholds cannot be obtained or for confirming bone conduction pure tone results. They serve only as overall estimates and are subject to the restrictions mentioned in the above paragraph. Masking is often necessary to isolate response to the test ear. Some audiometers are calibrated for bone conducted speech. Most are not. Biologic recalibration is possible. The simplest procedure may be to insert the bone conduction plug into one of the earphone jacks. Direct the speech signal through that circuit (remember to set your output selector for the appropriate air conduction output: that is, where your bone vibrator is plugged in). Obtain speech thresholds on a few normal subjects. You will probably find the average attenuator setting required for threshold is about 40 dB. This attenuator setting becomes 0 dB HL for purposes of bone conduction speech threshold testing.

SUMMARY

Speech threshold testing is a direct measure of overall sensitivity for speech. It serves as the basis for the presentation level for other auditory tests. It provides a comparative measure for confirming pure tone thresholds.

The most commonly used speech threshold is the threshold of intelligibility, usually called the speech reception threshold (SRT). It represents the lowest level in decibels at which 50% of the speech test material can be identified. An alternative is the threshold of detectibility, or speech awareness threshold (SAT). This threshold is the lowest level at which speech is detectable 50% of the time. SAT is expected to be 8–10 dB better than SRT.

The most commonly used words for SRT testing are spondees, two syllable words spoken with equal stress on each syllable. Lists appropriate for adults or children are included in the appendices. Thresholds may be obtained using recorded material or by monitored live voice. Live voice is more flexible, and careful measurement by an experienced clinician results in thresholds as reliable as those obtained with recordings.

During testing, the input signal should be adjusted so that the needle on the VU meter of the audiometer peaks at zero for each syllable. The patient should be familiarized with the words prior to testing and unintelligible words should be discarded. The level at which approximately 50% of the spondees can be identified represents the SRT.

If the pure tone audiogram is fairly flat, good agreement can be expected between the SRT and the PTA for the frequencies 500, 1000, and 2000 Hz. If the audiogram is irregular, averaging of the best two thresholds in the range 500–2000 Hz should result in better SRT-PTA agreement. If agreement is not good, efforts should be made to find the reason and reduce the discrepancy. Poor SRT-PTA relationship may be associated with functional hearing loss or extremely poor auditory discrimination ability. In the latter case, the SAT may be a more useful measure of sensitivity for speech.

Masking is necessary in speech threshold testing if the danger of crossover hearing exists. Rules and procedures are similar to those governing pure tone threshold audiometry. The major difference is that a range of sensitivity across the bone conduction thresholds of the nontest ear determines the need for masking rather than a single frequency, as is the case when testing an individual pure tone.

Formal procedures for establishing speech thresholds should be followed if possible. If not, modification of the usual methods may be useful to estimate minimum response levels. Bone conduction speech audiometry is a special modification which gives information about sensorineural levels.

STUDY QUESTIONS

1. What are the purposes of obtaining speech thresholds? What are the shortcomings of using the speech threshold as the *only* measure of hearing sensitivity?

2. Review the instrumentation for speech audiometry. How do you calibrate the input for (a) live voice testing? (b) recorded testing?
3. What are the requirements of good material for speech threshold testing?
4. What are the possible advantages of obtaining speech thresholds prior to pure tone threshold testing?
5. What are the methods for obtaining speech thresholds in (a) 2 dB steps? (b) 5 dB steps? What differences are expected between thresholds obtained with the two procedures?
6. What are the relationships between pure tone threshold averages (PTA) and speech reception threshold (SRT) that constitute good, questionable, and poor agreement? What are some factors which influence PTA-SRT agreement? How can adverse influences be minimized?
7. What are the rules for masking when establishing speech thresholds? How do the rules differ from those for masking in pure tone testing?

APPENDIX A

Children's Threshold Test (Keaster, 1947)

1. Put the *rabbit* on the floor.
2. Point to the *boat.*
3. Give the *pig* to mother.
4. Show the *bird* to the lady.
5. Put the *baby* on the floor.
6. Put the *spoon* on the window sill.
7. Point to the *car.*
8. *Show the bed* to mother.
9. Put the *cat* on the stool.
10. Give the lady the *ball.*
11. Point to the *house.*
12. Put the *shoe* on the window sill.
13. Put the *chair* on the floor.
14. Give mother the *dog.*
15. Point to the *cow.*
16. Show the lady the *squirrel.*
17. Put the *coat* on the chair.
18. Give the *cow* to the lady.
19. Point to the *train.*
20. Put the *knife* on the table.
21. Show mother the *fish.*
22. Point to the *airplane.*
23. Give the *chicken* to the lady.
24. Show the *apple* to mother.
25. *Put the horse* on the floor.

APPENDIX B

The CID Spondees (Hirsh *et al.*, 1952)

Airplane*
Armchair*
Baseball
Birthday*
Cowboy
Daybreak
Doormat
Drawbridge
Duckpond
Eardrum*
Farewell*
Grandson
Greyhound
Hardware*
Headlight
Horseshoe
Hotdog
Hothouse
Iceberg*
Inkwell
Mousetrap*
Mushroom
Northwest*
Oatmeal

Padlock	Schoolboy	Toothbrush
Pancake	Sidewalk*	Whitewash*
Playground*	Stairway*	Woodwork
Railroad*	Sunset*	Workshop

* Words indicated by Olsen and Matkin (1979) as most commonly determined to be heterogeneous for intelligibility.

APPENDIX C

Children's Spondee List

Airplane	Firetruck	Railroad
Baseball	Hotdog	Rainbow
Bathtub	Ice cream	Sailboat
Birthday	Pancake	Snowman
Cowboy	Popcorn	Toothbrush

CHAPTER 6 Speech Discrimination Testing

Some procedures in speech audiometry are common to both threshold testing and discrimination testing. For example, the instrumentation discussed in the preceding chapter will not be repeated here. Also, the use of the VU meter for input calibration will not be discussed again, except in those aspects unique to discrimination testing. You may want to review the instrumentation discussed in the preceding chapter before you read further. Also, you should remember that the speech threshold is related to speech discrimination ability in an important way: the sensation level (decibels above threshold) at which speech is presented is an important determinan of intelligibility.

PURPOSES

Speech discrimination ability is defined as the ability to differentiate speech sounds. The purpose of speech discrimination testing is to measure how well the listener can understand speech, as a function of the ability to differentiate sounds, under optimum circumstances. The speech discrimination score is intended to be a measure of the clarity with which a person hears speech. A common clinical measure involves presentation of 50 monosyllabic words to either ear, with the discrimination score representing the percentage of words correctly identified.

Diagnostic Uses of Speech Discrimination Testing

Before the development of some currently used diagnostic tests, speech discrimination scores were especially relied upon to help determine type of loss (Thurlow *et al.*, 1949). Patients with conductive loss were expected to have essentially normal discrimination scores once the presentation level became high enough to overcome the effects of the conductive blockage. Patients with sensorineural disorder were expected to have discrimination scores reduced in proportion to the magnitude of sensitivity loss. Thus, discrimination scores contributed to differentiation of conductive and sensorineural disorder. More sensitive differentiation was also expected. Shambaugh (1959) pointed out that in Meniere's disease discrimination scores are disproportionately reduced relative to the pure tone audiogram. Moreover, in cases of acoustic tumor, an even greater reduction in discrimination scores was expected. Schuknecht (1955) advocated discrimination testing to classify the pattern and problems of elderly hearing impaired persons.

The problem with diagnostic use of speech discrimination tests lies in the overlap in scores which may exist between types of hearing loss or pathologies. In part, this problem is related to inappropriate test selection (Carhart, 1965). With an easy discrimination test, patients with small sensorineural losses may score within normal limits. Conventional discrimination tests are usually not sensitive to disorders of the central auditory nervous system. Extensive damage to the brain can coexist with normal sensitivity and normal discrimination ability for conventional tests (Hodgson, 1967). The shortcomings of conventional speech tests for diagnostic purposes led to the development of many specialized speech tests beyond the scope of this book.

Development of other tests have minimized the use of conventional discrimination tests for diagnostic purposes. Today, conventional speech discrimination testing has limited diagnostic application. Nevertheless, discrepancies between audiometric indicators of type of loss and the discrimination score, such as poor scores when pure tone audiometry indicates conductive loss, indicate the need for retesting or a search for other explanations of the discrepancy.

Speech Discrimination Scores as a Measure of Handicap

If an individual can hear speech but cannot differentiate sounds well enough to understand what is said, hearing is of very limited value. An important use of speech discrimination test results is for predicting how well an individual should understand speech and the handicap that is to be expected in different situations. Many factors contribute to a hearing handicap in addition to speech discrimination ability. The testing of ability to differentiate sounds in the clinical evaluation is quite unlike many listening conditions. For these reasons the predictive ability of speech discrimination tests is only general and is subject to error. Nevertheless, used intelligently and with an awareness of their limitations, speech discrimination scores contribute to prediction of auditory handicap.

Predictor of Benefit from Amplification

Speech testing can provide information about the need for amplification and the benefit which may be expected. In general, the poorer the speech threshold the greater the need for amplification. The better the discrimination score the greater the benefit which can be expected from amplification.

Speech discrimination has played a varied role in the actual clinical process of hearing aid assessment and selection. Special speech testing procedures to replace or supplement conventional speech tests have been developed. This aspect of speech audiometry is beyond the scope of this book. If you are interested in more information about the role of speech audiometry in hearing aid selection, see Hodgson (1977).

HISTORY

Research related to the testing of telephone equipment provided basic concepts and some materials for speech testing (Fletcher, 1929 and 1953). French and Steinberg (1947) developed and evaluated the concept of the Performance-Intensity (PI) function: a measure of how intelligibility of speech grows with increase in the presentation level. They called it the articulation function because they were concerned about how well their communication equipment could "articulate" under different conditions. This important concept, the PI function, is discussed below.

During World War II researchers continued the study of communication equipment. They developed speech material for intelligibility testing which was the forerunner of tests in clinical use today. Much of this work was done at the Psycho-Acoustic Laboratory at Harvard University (Egan, 1948). Tests developed there utilized the concept called phonetic balancing: phonetic composition similar to that of the English language. That is, commonly occurring speech sounds were used often in the test while sounds which occur less often also occurred less often in the test. The name for commonly used discrimination test material, Phonetically Balanced (PB) lists, is derived from this concept. Subsequently, many revisions, refinements, and new developments occurred. Tests which have clinical utility are discussed below, in the section labeled Discrimination Test Materials.

PERFORMANCE-INTENSITY FUNCTION

The Performance-Intensity (PI) function shows how intelligibility grows as the presentation level of speech is increased above threshold. The function differs depending on the type of speech material used for speech discrimination testing (Hirsh *et al.*, 1954) and on the hearing characteristics of the listener being evaluated (Carhart, 1951). Figure 6.1 shows PI functions of various types of speech material for a group of normal hearing listeners. Notice that easy words (spondees) become audible at a lower presentation level than others. Notice, too, that the

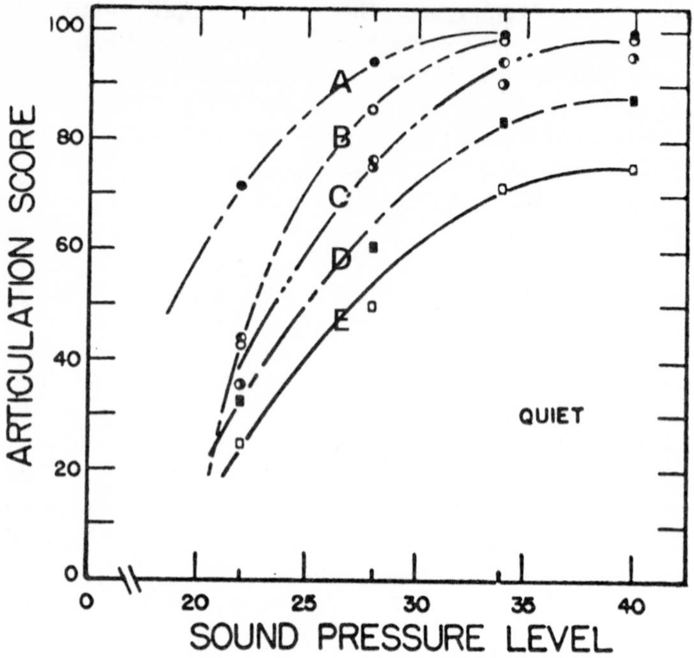

Fig. 6.1. Performance-intensity functions (articulation functions). *A*, spondees; *B*, polysyllables (words of more than two syllables); *C*, two syllable words spoken with unequal stress; trochees (stress on first syllable), and iambs (stress on second syllable); *D*, monosyllables; *E*, nonsense syllables. (Reprinted by permission from: Hirsh, I., Reynolds, E., and Joseph, M.: *J. Acoust. Soc. Am. 26*:530–538, 1954.)

slope of the function varies for the different types of material as intensity grows. Because spondees are nearly equivalent in intelligibility, once they begin to be audible intelligibility grows quickly to 100% with only a small additional increase in intensity. The result is a very steep function. Other material, such as monosyllables, varies in intelligibility and the slope is not as steep. PI functions indicate that connected speech is easiest of all. The redundancy resulting from meaning clues and rules of the language makes it possible for listeners to identify connected speech correctly at a lower presentation level.

Figure 6.2 shows PI functions for different listeners. One curve is for a normal hearing person, and you can see that speech becomes 100% intelligible as intensity increases. Of course 100% intelligibility may not result even with a normal listener, depending on the difficulty of the material. However, for familiar monosyllabic words, 100% intelligibility will occur about 25 dB above the speech threshold of a normal hearing listener (Carhart, 1951). Notice that the PI function of the listener with conductive loss is shifted to the right. That is, speech does not become audible until the presentation level is increased sufficiently to overcome the effects of the conductive blockage. Once speech begins to be audible, however, the PI function is quite normal, and 100% intelligibility results. This normal function, different only in that it is shifted to the right, reflects the reduced sensitivity but normal discrimination ability of the individual with conductive hearing loss. PI functions of two persons with sensorineural loss are shown. The first represents a flat, overall sensorineural loss. The PI function differs from normal in two ways. First, it is shifted to the right, representing the loss of sensitivity. As with the conductive loss, presentation level must be increased over normal before the test words become audible. Second, because of the reduction in discrimination ability associated with sensorineural loss, maximum intelligibility is less than 100%, even at the most favorable presentation level. The score obtained at the most favorable level is often called "PB-max" (Carhart, 1952)—maximum intelligibility of PB lists as a function of presentation level. The next curve in Figure 6.2 represents a high frequency sensorineural loss, with normal hearing sensitivity across part of the speech range. Because of the good low frequency sensitivity, speech starts to be audible at normal presentation levels. That is, there is no overall loss for speech. Therefore, the function is not shifted to the right. However, because of the sensorineural nature of the loss and the resulting audiometric configuration, intelligibility never reaches 100% as intensity increases.

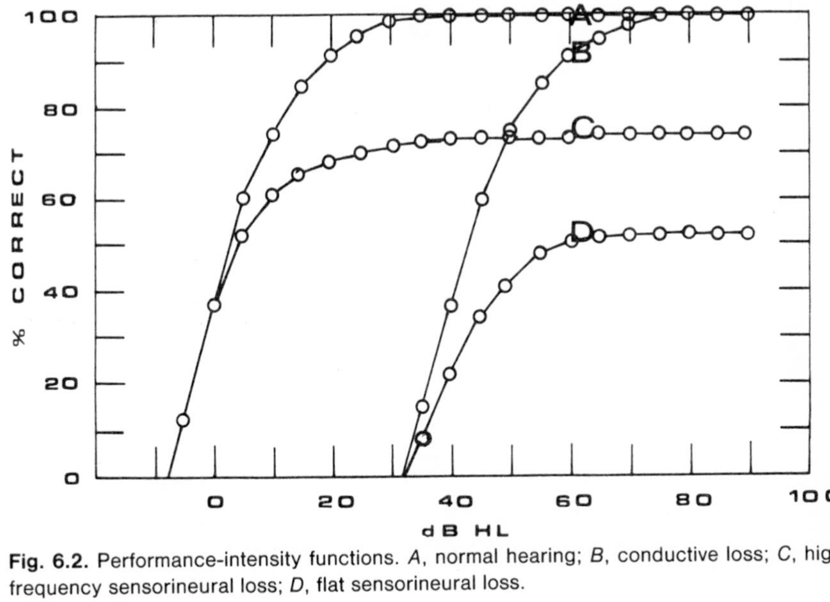

Fig. 6.2. Performance-intensity functions. *A*, normal hearing; *B*, conductive loss; *C*, high frequency sensorineural loss; *D*, flat sensorineural loss.

Because of the time required to establish complete PI functions, this sort of testing is ordinarily not done clinically. There are exceptions. As discussed later, presentation level may be especially critical in some situations and for some patients. In these cases, at least partial PI functions may be needed. Also, some special tests developed for diagnostic purposes utilize the PI function. Usually, however, the clinician strives to establish two values relative to the PI function. They are, first, the level at which speech becomes 50% audible—the speech threshold, and second, the discrimination score which is representative of maximum intelligibility. These two values give most, though not all, information present in the PI function. They tell how intense speech must be for audibility, and how well the patient can understand speech once it is presented at an optimum level. A problem may have occurred to you; it is sometimes difficult to know if discrimination testing has been done at the level eliciting maximum intelligibility. Selection of optimum presentation level is discussed later in this chapter.

DISCRIMINATION TEST MATERIALS

Egan (1948) described the following criteria used in developing the first PB lists: (1) monosyllabic words, (2) equal average difficulty of lists, (3) equal range of difficulty of words within each list, (4) equal phonetic composition of each list, (5) a composition representative of English speech (phonetic balance), and (6) words in common usage. Carhart (1965) added that materials for discrimination testing, unlike speech threshold test materials, should be made up of relatively nonredundant items. Otherwise the excessive clues may make the test too easy and obscure discrimination problems. Carhart also cautioned that the test material must be suitable to the linguistic background of the patient. If not, the words become nonsense items for the patient, increasing their difficulty and reducing the discrimination score. Carhart felt that phonetic balance was of secondary importance, as long as there was only moderate divergence. He cited as evidence the fact that the original PB lists were of approximately equal intelligibility in spite of some deviation in phonetic balance. To meet these criteria, Carhart recommended lists of monosyllabic words. He felt that monosyllables, less predictable than connected speech or spondees, would require patients to identify individual speech elements independently, assessing discrimination skills sensitively. He felt they were preferable to nonsense syllables, which are confusing to patients and difficult to score. Monosyllabic word lists have emerged as the most popular discrimination test material. However, some individuals have felt that monosyllabic words are so different from regular speech that it is difficult to generalize from discrimination scores obtained with monosyllabic word lists about how the patient will perform when listening to everyday speech (Jerger *et al.*, 1968). Therefore, sentence tests of speech intelligibility have been developed and some of them are reviewed below.

Open Versus Closed Set Tests

Open set tests are those in which the patient's response is not limited by the structure of the test. That is, on hearing the test item, the patient is free to make any response. The usual pattern for open set tests is to ask the patient to say or write the test word. Closed set tests, on the other hand, restrict the patient to one of a set number of possible responses. These are usually multiple choice tests in which the patient looks at a list of possible answers while listening to the test item and designates the correct selection.

Closed set tests have this advantage: they require neither a spoken nor written response. Rather the patient responds by pointing to a word or a picture, or by circling a word on a multiple choice list. Therefore, closed set tests are useful for individuals who cannot speak or write well enough to perform with open set tests. The use of pictures rather than printed words adapts the test to those who cannot read. However, Pollack and associates (1959) reported that closed set tests decrease in intelligibility as the number of possible responses increase. Related attributes in closed set tests can probably be interpreted as detrimental under most circumstances. First, the reduced number of responses from which the subject must choose makes the test easier. Hodgson (1973) reported an improvement of 10% in the scores of normal hearing listeners responding to a closed set test over those who listened to the same test in an open set condition. Second, closed set tests are less common in clinical use than are open set tests.

Open Set Discrete Word Tests

Harvard PAL PB-50 Word Lists. These lists are usually identified as the PB-50 lists. They are sometimes called the NDRC lists, having been developed under a Naval Defense Research Contract. Twenty lists, each consisting of 50 monosyllabic words, were developed (Egan, 1948). These lists appear in Appendix A. The PB-50 lists were used clinically in Veterans Hospitals during and after World War II. Their use continues to date. Egan reported that the range of difficulty is about the same in each list and that each list has nearly the same average difficulty. Further, the lists have nearly the same phonetic composition, and the phonetic composition is quite similar to that of the English language.

Rush Hughes Recording of the PB-50 Lists. Eight of the PB-50 lists were recorded at the Central Institute for the Deaf and made available commercially on phonograph discs.[1,2] The lists were modified slightly, more familiar words replacing a few of the most difficult words, as indicated in Appendix D. A number of factors made these recordings more difficult than anticipated. They include the lack of familiarity of some of the remaining words, the style of the speaker, Rush Hughes, and some recording variables. Because subjects with normal hearing did not routinely score 100% on this test, it was considered unduly difficult for routine clinical use.

Of the PB-50 lists recorded by Rush Hughes, Eldert and Davis (1951) determined that list 8 was more difficult and lists 11 and 12 easier than the others. The remaining lists—5, 6, 7, 9, and 10—were judged to be of approximately equivalent difficulty.

The Rush Hughes recording is not now in routine clinical use as a standard test of auditory discrimination ability. Because of expectations for discrimination performance developed from the use of easier tests, a score obtained with the Rush Hughes recording and interpreted in the usual way will overestimate the patient's discrimination deficit. However, it has been determined that the Rush Hughes recording is sensitive to *central* auditory disorders (Goetzinger and Angell, 1965).

The W-22 Recording.[1,2] Concerned with the difficulty of the Rush Hughes version, Hirsh *et al.* (1952), revised and re-recorded the PB-50 lists. The new recording was called CID Auditory Test W-22. Their goals were to improve the phonetic balance and to eliminate rare words. They selected 200 words, only 120 of which appeared in the PB-50 lists. The four lists were recorded in six different scramblings. Therefore, all the words on list 1 are different from the words on list 2 but the same words appear on lists 1A and 1B, recorded in different order. The W22 lists appear in Appendix B.

Use of the W-22 recording is likely to result in a considerably higher discrimination score than if the Rush Hughes recording is used. Just as the Rush Hughes recording had been criticized as too difficult, concern arose that the W-22 recording was too easy, that it failed to differentiate pathologies or to sensitively measure the discrimination ability of patients with mild hearing loss. Carhart (1965) commented that this problem was more the fault of the clinician who uncritically selected an inappropriate test for a given patient than of the tests themselves. Of the recorded tests available today, the W-22 is probably the most widely used.

Northwestern University (NU) Auditory Test No. 6. Lehiste and Peterson (1959) developed new lists composed entirely of common

[1] Available from Technisonic Studios, Inc., 1201 S. Brentwood Blvd., Richmond Heights, MO 63317 (phonograph disc).

[2] Available from Auditec of St. Louis, 330 Selma Ave., St. Louis, MO 63119 (audiotapes).

words with an initial consonant, a vowel nucleus and a final consonant. Tillman *et al.* (1963) developed NU Auditory Test No. 4 primarily using words from the Lehiste and Peterson lists. This test, consisting of two lists, was revised and expanded by Tillman and Carhart (1966). The new test was called NU Auditory Test No. 6. It consists of four lists of 50 consonant-nucleus-consonant (CNC) words each. The authors reported that the linear part of the NU 6 test has a slope of about 5.6%/dB for normals and about 3.4%/dB for subjects with sensorineural loss. Tillman and Carhart established high test-retest reliability and good interlist equivalence. The NU 6 lists appear in Appendix C.

A recording of the NU 6 lists is available from Auditec.[2] Orchik and associates (1979) compared the Auditec recordings of the W-22 and NU 6 lists. The scores of subjects with sensorineural loss were consistently better for the W-22 recording. Differences of 10% or more were obtained from 14 of the 30 subjects. The authors concluded that these versions of the two tests should not be used interchangeably with individuals who have sensorineural loss.

Rintelmann *et al.* (1974*a*) recorded and evaluated their own version of the NU 6 test.[3] They found their recording to be a little more difficult than the original recorded version of Tillman and Carhart. They reported good test-retest reliability for both normal and sensorineural subjects. The lists were essentially equal in difficulty, although their recording of list 4 appeared to be a little easier than the others (Rintelmann *et al.* 1974; Rintelmann and Schumaier, 1974).

Rintelmann and associates (1974*b*) evaluated four randomizations of the words on each of the NU 6 lists. They found that the PI function did not change because of the difference in word order. They also found that increasing the number of forms of each list from one to four did not increase the variability within the lists.

An, audio tape recorded version of the NU 6 is also available from Auditec.[2] Characteristics of this recorded version were examined by Wilson *et al.* (1976). They established good interlist equivalence. They found the Auditec version more difficult than the recording originally used by Tillman and Carhart. Relative to the original, the Auditec PI function was shifted to the right an average of 5.2 dB for normals and 4.9 dB for subjects with sensorineural loss. These findings reinforce the admonition of Kreul *et al.* (1969) that different recorded versions of the same test may differ significantly, depending on the talker and recording conditions.

PB-Kindergarten (PB-K) Lists. Haskins (1949) developed PB lists composed of words likely to be within the vocabulary of young children.

---

[3] Available from Gordon N. Stowe & Associates, 3217 Doolittle Dr., Northbrook, IL 60062.

Three of the lists appear in Appendix D. An audio tape recording of these lists, along with recorded spondees suitable for threshold testing of children, is available from Auditec.[2]

Open Set Sentence Tests

Open set sentence tests are not in common clinical use. Sentences tend to be undesirably easy since the redundancy supplied by semantic and syntactic clues may permit the patient to supply a key word even if the word was not heard. Conversely, auditory memory or confusion regarding the meaning of a sentence may tend to reduce discrimination scores derived from sentence tests. As mentioned in the previous chapter, sentences used for discrimination testing were developed by the Bell Telephone Laboratories (Fletcher, 1929). Other sentence tests suitable for open set use include the PAL Auditory Test No. 12 (Hudgins *et al.*, 1947), and the CID Everyday Speech Sentences (Davis, 1978, pp. 536–538).

Closed Set Discrete Word Tests

Modified Rhyme Test. House *et al.*, (1965) adapted Fairbanks' Rhyme Test (1958) for use as a multiple choice discrimination test. As modified, the test consists of six lists of 50 monosyllabic words (see Appendix E). As you can see, most of the words in each row vary only in the initial or final consonant. The patient listens to the test word and circles on the form the word as heard. House *et al.* evaluated the test with normal hearing listeners at various signal-to-noise ratios. They found no statistically significant differences between the lists and concluded that the test was stable, required little or no training of listeners before use, and lent itself readily to mechanized administration and scoring.

Kreul *et al.* (1968) reported efforts to adapt the Modified Rhyme Test for clinical use. Administering the test at three different signal-to-noise ratios, they felt it capable of ranking patients on the basis of their everyday listening abilities. However, Gengel (1973) reported considerable variability in Modified Rhyme Test scores of subjects with moderate to severe sensorineural loss. The variability of subjects' scores was about equal either when the same list was repeated four times or when scores of all four lists were considered. The range of scores for a different subject for four tests was as little as 2% and as much as 34%. To minimize the effects of variability, Gengel recommended use of practice words to familiarize the subject with the procedure and basing the discrimination score on results from two or three lists rather than from a single list.

The WIPI Test. For young children or others who have a restricted receptive vocabulary and cannot read, discrimination ability may be

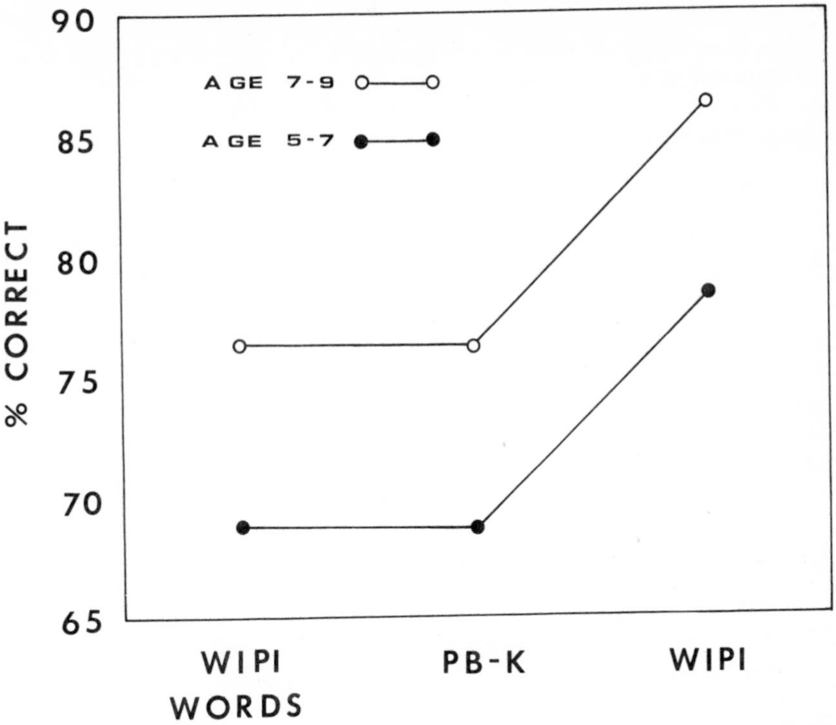

Fig. 6.3. Relationships between intelligibility of WIPI words, PB-K words, and the WIPI test for normal hearing children in two age groups ($n = 12$ in each age group). To reduce intelligibility, words were passed through a low-pass filter (1560 Hz) which had a rejection rate of 39 dB per octave. (Data from Hodgson, W., 1973.)

estimated through use of a picture discrimination test. In this format, the patient listens for the test word while looking at a number of pictures, one of which represents the test word. The child points to the picture of the test word. A commonly used picture discrimination test is the Word Identification Picture Index, or WIPI[4] test (Ross and Lerman, 1970). The WIPI consists of four lists of 25 monosyllabic words. The test manual contains 25 plates plus a practice plate. On each plate are six pictures. Only four pictures per plate are ever used as test words. On administering the WIPI to 61 hearing impaired children between the ages of 4 years 7 months and 13 years 9 months (mean, 10 years 2 months), the authors concluded the test-retest reliability and equivalence of the four lists were high.

When interpreting WIPI results, remember the effects of a closed set test. Figure 6.3 shows the relationship between the WIPI words used as

[4] Available from Stanwix House, Inc., 3020 Chartiers Ave., Pittsburgh, PA 15204.

an open set and as a closed set test for normal hearing children. In the open set condition subjects repeated the WIPI words as they heard them, without seeing the WIPI pictures. The closed set response required the usual picture identification task. Subjects also repeated the words of a PB-K list administered in the conventional open set fashion. While there was no difference in the intelligibility of the WIPI and the PB-K words, use of the WIPI as a closed set test improved the discrimination scores by about 10%. Whenever the WIPI is used in discrimination testing, its use should be identified on the Audiologic Record so that those who see the test results can interpret them accordingly.

An Adaptive Speech Discrimination Test for Children. Katz and Elliott (1978) and Elliott *et al.* (1979) reported the development of a children's speech discrimination test which used an adaptive procedure. That is, instead of obtaining scores in percentages, presentation level was varied when testing in quiet or in the presence of a fixed level of noise to achieve 71% correct response. Stimuli (monosyllabic nouns) were within the receptive vocabulary of 3-year-old inner city children.

Subjects responded by pointing to one of four pictures after hearing the stimulus word. In another condition, subjects repeated the test word (an open set response).

The authors concluded that children at least as young as age 5 could perform the test successfully when an adaptive test was used. They found that performance of normal hearing children with learning problems was poorer than that of children progressing normally in school.

The SERT. The Sound Effects Recognition Test (SERT) was developed to estimate gross discrimination ability of children not capable of differentiating verbal stimuli (Finitzo-Hieber *et al.*). The test consists of familiar environmental sounds recorded on audiotape. There are three equivalent subtests, each containing 10 sounds. The listener responds by pointing to one of four pictures after hearing each sound. The test has been used with school age children who have very limited verbal language because of profound hearing loss and with preschoolers. The authors report successful use of the SERT in hearing evaluations and hearing aid evaluations. The test is available from Auditec.[2]

Closed Set Sentence Tests

The PAL Auditory Test No. 8. The PAL 8 (Karlin *et al.*, 1944) is an interesting example of a closed set sentence test. The subject looks at a multiple choice answer sheet while listening to the test sentence. On hearing the sentence, the subject circles the correct answer from a choice of four. The developers tried to reduce the effects of redundancy and require the subject to hear as much of the sentence as possible to answer correctly. All of the possible answers have some relation to the test sentence. An example is, "The thing without any legs is . . . " and the words from which the answer must be chosen are, "centipede," "fish" "man," and "dog." Nevertheless, Jirsa and Hodgson (1970) found the PAL 8 sentences considerably easier than the W-22 or NU 6 word lists when all tests were presented under the same conditions.

The SSI Test. Speaks and Jerger (1965) and Jerger and associates (1968) reported development of the SSI (Synthetic Sentence Identification) Test. They felt that the changing pattern of speech over time is an important element of auditory discrimination ability which can be assessed by sentences but not by discrete words. Syntactical clues, which may make sentence tests too easy, are reduced in the SSI. The test consists of lists of 10 sentences which follow a third-order approximation to the rules of English. That is, in preparing the sentences, selection of a given word from the pool of possible words was permitted only if that word made good sense in conjunction with the two previous words. For examples see Appendix F. In responding to the SSI, the patient listens while looking at the 10 sentences constituting a list and selects the test sentence on hearing it. To make the procedure more difficult, a competing message is incorporated under various conditions, depending on the purpose of the test. The competing message consists of a single speaker reading prose. In addition to conventional discrimination testing, various applications of the SSI have been developed which are beyond the scope of this book. The interested reader should consult these sources: for the SSI and hearing aid evaluation refer to Jerger and Hayes (1976); for use of the SSI in testing central auditory nervous system function see Jerger and Jerger (1975).

Foreign Language Tests

If there is extensive demand for evaluation of individuals who do not speak English, a clinician with fluency in the involved language should be available. For occasional use it may be possible to use a recorded closed set test even though the clinician does not speak the language involved. The patient should respond by circling the correct word on a printed response form or by pointing to the correct picture while the clinician refers to an answer sheet printed in English. The clinician who does not have command of the language involved should not attempt to score verbal responses. As always, you should indicate on the Audiologic Record the test procedure used to elicit the discrimination score.

TEST PROCEDURES

Presentation Level

As mentioned earlier, the goal of discrimination testing in which only one test list is delivered (as opposed to establishing a PI curve) is to find the patient's maximum discrimination score, or PB-max. To achieve PB-max, it is necessary to determine the presentation level which affords optimum intelligibility, a complex problem.

There is no one sensation level (SL: dB above threshold) which will afford maximum intelligibility for all patients. Several factors contribute to the SL needed for PB-max, notably the difficulty of the material and the differential effects of the hearing loss. The configuration of the audiogram also may be a factor, and patients with high frequency hearing loss may benefit from an increased presentation level. In sensory losses with loudness recruitment, however, tolerance problems commonly limit the SL at which discrimination testing is done. In severe losses, maximum audiometer output limitations may intervene. In some cases of conductive loss, problems associated with masking must be considered when the presentation level is selected. Some individuals exhibit rollover in the articulation function—after PB-max is reached, further increase of the presentation level causes a decrease in the discrimination score. This behavior contrasts with that of most patients, in which there is a plateau in the PI function after PB-max is reached. All of these factors are considered in the following discussion of presentation level.

Difficulty of Test Material. Carhart (1965) noted that normal listeners will approximate PB-max for the W-22 recording at about 25 dB SL. For the more difficult Rush Hughes recording, a sensation level of 40 dB is required for PB-max. Carhart estimated that most talkers when using live voice will approximate the results of the W-22 recording. This assumes a trained and careful talker who follows the rules of speech audiometry.

Developers of the NU 4 discrimination test (Tillman *et al.*, 1963) found their normal subjects reached PB-max at 24 dB SL. In the expanded version (NU 6), Tillman and Carhart (1966) reported PB-max for normals at 32 dB SL. In each study the authors reported an increase in intelligibility of about 6% per dB along the linear part of the PI function. The function was linear to an SL of about 9 dB, at which level the discrimination score was about 80%. From there, as the presentation level increased, there was a progressive decrement in intelligibility improvement until the maximum score was reached. With their own recording of the NU 6. Rintelmann and associates (1974) reported PB-max for normals at about 32 dB SL. Beattie *et al.* (1977) studied the Auditec recording of the W-22 lists and the NU 6. PI functions of the two tests were similar and 95% intelligibility for normals was obtained at 32 dB SL. Wilson *et al.* (1976) also found PB-max for the Auditec recording of the NU 6 at 32 dB SL using normal subjects. It should be noted that the studies cited above established PI functions by presenting PB lists at increasing presentation levels in 5–8 dB steps. Ordinarily the next to highest presentation level resulted in scores very close to PB-max, and it seems probable that maximum intelligibility for normals would have occurred at a level a little lower than these studies suggest.

It is clear that, for commonly used clinical tests, maximum intelligibility for normals occurs by a presentation level of around 30 dB SL. Presentation at a 40 dB sensation level is comfortable for normal listeners and will assure adequate intensity for PB-max. Therefore, 40 dB SL is a commonly used presentation level.

Effects of Hearing Loss. Tillman and associates (1963) established PI functions on normals and subjects with conductive loss. They found them highly similar, with equal slope and PB-max occurring at the same SL. They concluded that the performance of subjects with conductive loss duplicated very closely that of normals. Clinically, a presentation of 40 dB SL will ordinarily be comfortable for an individual with conductive loss and will assure adequate intensity for maximum intelligibility. If, because of the conductive nature of the disorder, overmasking becomes a problem, the presentation level could be reduced by as much as 10 dB without much concern.

The presentation level required for PB-max with patients who have sensorineural loss is clearly different. To illustrate, Tillman and Carhart (1966) reported a slope of 5.6%/dB for the linear part of the PI function of normals but only 3.4%/dB for sensorineural subjects. PB-max occurred by at least 32 dB SL for the normals, but not until about 40 dB SL for the sensorineural subjects.

Certain problems prevent use of 40 dB SL as a universal presentation level for discrimination testing. If the loss is sufficiently severe, maximum output limitations of the audiometer will prevent an SL of 40 dB. At any rate, most patients with sensory loss will find 40 dB SL uncomfortably loud. Many will complain about the loudness of the signal at levels considerably less than 40 dB SL. On the other hand, patients with high frequency sensorineural loss and normal hearing across the lower part of the speech range may benefit from a presentation level greater than 40 dB SL. These individuals may not hear the important higher frequencies of speech until an SL greater than 40 dB.

Aside from the problem of tolerance, another consideration prevents the uniform application of a high presentation level in sensorineural loss. In some patients, after PB-max is reached, additional increase in presentation level will result in a decrease in discrimination scores. This rollover in the PI function has been associated with retrocochlear disorder (Jerger and Jerger, 1967 and 1974). The phenomenon is not limited to active VIIIth nerve disorder, such as acoustic tumor. Schuknecht (1955) demonstrated degenerative changes in the auditory nerve of elderly individuals. Gang (1976) reported rollover in the PI function of some elderly subjects, apparently associated with retrocochlear changes.

Problems with tolerance and individual differences in loudness preference led to the practice of conducting discrimination testing at a comfortably loud listening level, or Most Comfortable Loudness (MCL). The rationale is appealing to test discrimination ability at the loudness level which the patient prefers. However, Posner and Ventry (1977) found that MCL was not likely to result in PB-max for subjects with sensorineural loss. Their subjects chose a mean 14.6 dB SL as MCL. At this presentation level, average discrimination score was 61.4%. PI functions established PB-max of 82.4%, which occurred at a mean SL of 37.2 dB. Lezak (1963) found that maximum scores were obtained when the test was administered at the *upper limits* of the range which subjects reported to be comfortable.

The complexities of this problem indicate that you cannot be sure you have determined PB-max if you test discrimination at only one presentation level unless the score approximates 100%. The only way you can be sure otherwise is to test at enough presentation levels to explore the upper part of the PI function. Desirable as this procedure is, time limitations may prevent its application. If so, consider all the variables discussed above to pick a level that is feasible and most likely to measure PB-max. In most cases, this level is at the upper range of the comfortable loudness noted by the patient. It is preferable for the presentation to be at least 25 dB SL and as close to 40 dB SL as the patient finds comfortable. If you find the resulting discrimination score at odds with other audiometric data, perform discrimination testing at more than one presentation level in spite of the demands of time. Remembering that a reduced score may result from a presentation level either too low or too high, a sensible clinical procedure would be to obtain additional scores at 5 or 6 dB above and below the presentation level which resulted in the suspect score.

If the patient has nearly normal sensitivity or a fairly flat audiometric configuration, an MCL greater than 40 dB SL may result. In these cases, there is probably no need to exceed a presentation level of 40 dB SL. To do so would necessitate masking which otherwise may be unnecessary.

Discrimination Testing for Special Purposes. In the preceding discussion of conventional discrimination testing, the goal was to ascertain how well the listener could differentiate sounds at optimum intensity under the best of listening circumstances. Discrimination testing can also be conducted for other purposes. For example, testing in noise may give a more realistic estimate of how well an individual performs under adverse listening conditions. As another example, aided discrimination testing is conducted at reduced presentation levels to determine how well a person can function when listening to speech at a level which would be handicapping unaided. Under this circumstance, the hearing aid supplies the required amplification.

Monitored Live Voice Versus Recorded Testing

Beattie and co-workers (1977) showed that different experienced examiners can obtain the same speech thresholds from subjects using monitored live voice procedures, and that the thresholds so obtained do not differ from thresholds obtained with recorded material. No such interexaminer reliability has been reported with the use of monitored live voice for discrimination testing. This shortcoming has led to advocacy of recorded tests for all discrimination evaluation. However, Carhart (1965) noted that the individual speaker's characteristics are built into recorded tests and that two recorded versions, even of the same test material, may also yield significantly different results. To illustrate, recall that Wilson *et al.* (1976) found the Auditec recording of the NU 6 test to be more difficult than the original recording of that test. Therefore, if discrimination scores obtained via recording are really to be interchangeable from clinic to clinic, one standardized recording must be universally used. Such is not the case and perhaps should not be. Carhart (1965) reminds us that appropriate test selection is an important clinical prerogative, depending on the client's receptive language level, expressive ability, and the level of difficulty necessary to achieve a sensitive measure of auditory discrimination ability.

Recorded tests are inflexible. Their use with the very young or old may be difficult. These patients may require more time for response than that allotted on recordings. They may require intermittent reinstruction, reinforcement, or questioning. These procedures, while not impossible during a recorded test, are difficult. The routine use of recorded tests takes more time than their live voice counterparts would ordinarily require. That is, more time is allotted for response on recorded tests than most patients require. Coupled with the time required for preparing and calibrating the recorded presentation, this restraint tends to make recorded tests unpopular.

It is probably safe to generalize that experienced clinicians can obtain test results using monitored live voice that agree as well as two recorded versions of the same test. However, this skill is not automatic; it requires practice to achieve and care to maintain. For example, we have a natural tendency to speak more carefully as we observe our listeners having more difficulty in following what is said. Unchecked, this tendency may result in very good scores from individuals who have very poor discrimination ability. To use monitored live voice testing effectively you must work to achieve a standard, unvarying presentation. The time you allot for response may vary, depending on the patient's needs. But the presentation of each test word must always be the same from patient to patient. In this fashion you can develop a concept of how patients with problems of varying magnitude respond to your testing and learn to use your testing in a dependable way. Even so, you must remember the ultimate limitation of monitored live voice testing. Results so obtained cannot be uncritically compared with the test results of other speakers.

Half List Versus Full List Testing

Egan (1948) reported that in the original development of PB lists, lists of 50 words were made up because it was not possible to satisfy the developers' criteria with 25 word lists. The time required for testing with full lists, particularly in situations where several discrimination tests were necessary at one time, led people to wonder if the same results could be achieved with half lists. That is, if 25 rather than 50 words could make up a test, each word counting 4% instead of 2%. Half list usage modifies the phonetic balance of the full list, but Carhart (1965) reported that moderate differences in phonetic balance produce no important change in discrimination scores.

Variability in test scores is the biggest problem with using half lists. In the measurement of any behavior that is not stable, variability increases as the number of measures decrease. As variability increases, the probability of a measure being truly representative of the individual's performance decreases. Obviously reliability of a test is important. Obviously time constraints in a clinical setting are important. How to solve the dilemma?

Research regarding the advisability of half list versus full list usage has often been based on part-whole correlation and on group rather than individual differences between half and whole list scores. On the whole, it has not been particularly illuminating and has not answered the clinical question.

Egan (1948) pointed out that the distribution of difficulty of words in the PB lists in most cases follows a bell-shaped curve. For this reason discrimination tests are not uniformly sensitive over the entire range of possible scores. Near the two ends of the range, 0 and 100%, variability is minimized, with greatest variability in patients who score near the middle of the range. Therefore, it makes sense to use half lists with those patients in whom lowest variability can be expected, those whose performance falls at either end of the range. For those in between, you should strive to reduce the invalidating effects of variability by the common expedient of increasing the number of test items.

Beattie *et al.* (1978) found that in individuals with sensorineural loss, half list testing was an effective screening procedure to determine advisability of full list testing. They found that 95% of the subjects who missed three words or less on the half lists had 4% or less variability between the half list and the whole list score. However, subjects who missed 10–19 words on the half lists had half-full list agreement within 8%, only 83% of the time, and the disagreement ranged as high as 14%.

Here is a clinical rule of thumb based on the data and reasoning discussed above: use full lists for patients whose half list score is poorer than 88% but better than 12%. If a full list results in great variability between the halves, a more careful assessment is called for. Administer a second full list and take an average. Two precautions: First, reliance on half list testing under any circumstances calls for care in controlling the other variables which may influence discrimination testing, such as standard presentation and adequate presentation level. Second, whenever discrimination scores based on half list testing are at odds with expected results based on other audiometric data and observation of performance, administer additional testing to gather more information.

Carhart (1965), studying the W-22 scores of 170 hearing impaired subjects, noted that 60% scored 90% or better. For this group, auditory discrimination was good enough to identify almost all of the words on the test. Rose (1974) ranked the words from the W-22 list in order of difficulty. He then devised a procedure to reduce administration even further than half lists, still retaining full list capability when the initial screening procedure indicates the need for it. His screening procedure is to administer the 10 most difficult words first. If the patient does not meet a screening criterion, such as 80 or 90% correct, the half list or full list is administered. However, if the patient gets eight or nine of the most difficult words correct, discrimination is judged good enough to obviate additional testing. See Appendix G for the ranking of the difficulty of the W-22 words.

Methods for Administering Discrimination Tests

Prior to the test, be sure the seating arrangement permits you to see and hear the patient well. That is, with the patient seated in the examination room, you must be able to see clearly from the control room. The patient's voice must be clearly audible via the talkback system. When using live voice, be sure the patient cannot see you, to avoid the possibility of affording visual clues. A seating arrangement which permits you to see the patient in profile is useful. Ask the patient not to watch you, if necessary.

Input calibration is an important preliminary to discrimination testing. This procedure assures you, if the audiometer is working properly, that the level shown on the hearing loss dial is the actual presentation level at which the test was administered. The procedure differs for recorded and monitored live voice testing.

Recorded tests will incorporate a 1000 Hz tone to facilitate input calibration. With that tone fed into the speech audiometer, adjust the input gain control until the VU meter needle rests at zero. Occasionally a recorded test may have instructions to set the VU meter at some level other than zero but this exception should be rare, for the calibration tone should be recorded at the same level as the speech material.

To prepare for live voice testing, speak into the microphone while monitoring the VU meter and adjusting the input gain control. You will be using a carrier phrase. The most common is probably, "Say the word . . . ," although the carrier phrase on the W-22 recording is "You will say. . . . " Egan (1948) includes in his justification of carrier phrases these purposes: (1) to prepare the listener for the advent of the test item and thereby reduce variability due to inattention and distraction, and (2) to permit the speaker to modulate the voice so that the level is even from presentation to presentation. You should speak each carrier phrase and adjust the input gain so that the VU meter peaks at zero on the final word of the carrier phrase. Do not attempt to peak the meter at zero for each word of the PB list. Each word has intrinsic differences in power, depending on its vowel. If you peak the meter at zero for each carrier phrase and speak each test word with equal effort, you will retain something of the natural variability intrinsic in the test words. You should practice for a consistent and standard presentation. Listen to a recording of PB lists, such as the W-22 recording or one of the commercially available recordings of NU 6. Before actually doing live voice testing in the clinic you must achieve a standard presentation with results similar to those obtained by recorded tests, such as the W-22.

When you are ready to begin the test, place the headset on the patient. Be sure that the earphone diaphragm is directly over each ear canal and that the placement is comfortable. Double check: right phone on right ear, left phone on left.

Instruct the patient. I think we tend to over-instruct patients, taking unnecessary time and sometimes creating confusion. For live voice testing it is probably necessary to say no more than, "Listen carefully and do the best you can. Would you say the word . . . " When using a recorded test, you should explain to the patient that the test is recorded and that the patient will be asked to repeat one syllable words. Caution the patient not to consider each reply too long, in order to be ready for the next recorded item. Be alert to stop the recording, however, if the patient does need more time to reply than afforded by the record.

It is probably more common to request a spoken rather than a written response. There is some concern about error in scoring spoken responses. Merrell and Atkinson (1965) reported that judges on the average disagreed by 5.92% between a subject's written and spoken responses when the judges listened to tape recorded responses. Variability of scores from 25 judges was as high as 21% for a given list. However,

Norton and Hodgson (1973) reported better interjudge agreement when the judges could both hear and see subjects. They found that two experienced listeners judging responses consisting of 100 monosyllabic words spoken by 40 subjects disagreed by 0% in 27 of the cases, by 1% in 10 of the cases, and by 2% in 3 of the cases. Provision should be made in your training program for someone to score responses along with you from time to time, to assess the accuracy of your scoring. Certainly the use of spoken responses places a heavier responsibility on the audiologist, and the following conditions should be obtained: The audiologist must be able to see and hear the patient clearly and to watch and listen carefully. A talkback system with good fidelity is required. The patient must have intelligible speech. The hearing of the audiologist must be normal. The audiologist must be alert to ask the patient to repeat, spell, or define unclear responses.

If the above conditions cannot be met, alternatives to spoken responses, such as written responses, should be utilized. When scoring written responses, be alert for homonyms: for the test word, "ail," "ale" is also acceptable. If the patient cannot write well, special procedures are available, and some of these are discussed on the following pages. If circumstances require that you utilize spoken responses when all the criteria described above are not met, you should note these qualifications on the Audiologic Record.

As you score discrimination responses, you must have a printed list of the discrimination test in front of you to read the words in live voice testing and to score the patient's response in either MLV or recorded testing. Some audiologists write the patient's response phonetically on the printed list to permit later analysis of the kind of errors made by the patient. Such qualitative analysis may give helpful information in addition to the percentage score. A pattern of discrimination errors which involves only difficult-to-differentiate consonants is less handicapping than one in which vowel errors are also involved.

You will learn to expect representative patterns of error depending on the hearing loss; marked deviation from the expected pattern may have diagnostic significance. Discrimination ability much poorer than the audiogram would suggest should alert you to the possibility of a retrocochlear problem. An atypical response pattern may indicate the need to explore for nonorganic loss. Campbell (1965) developed an index to alert the clinician to the probability of invalid responses. The index is based on responses which, in valid assessment, (1) rarely occur, (2) lack phonetic resemblence to the test word, and (3) involve an easy, seldom missed, test word. A fourth element of the index consists of failure to guess despite instructions to do so if necessary.

Having completed the discrimination test on either ear, you should record the scores and the presentation level at which testing was done.

Remember that each correct response contributes 2% to the score if a complete list is used. Each correct response is worth 4% if a half list is used.

In summary, here is a step-by-step procedure for administering the discrimination test:

1. Utilize a seating arrangement which prevents the patient from watching you but permits you to see the patient's face, at least in profile.
2. Instruct the patient to respond appropriately. Position the earphones correctly.
3. Adjust the input gain control so that the VU meter peaks at zero for the calibration tone of a recorded test or the final word of the carrier phrase in live voice testing.
4. Select appropriate presentation levels. The goal is a level high enough for maximum discrimination score without discomfort. This level will probably approximate the upper limit of the range of comfortable loudness. It is preferable for the presentation to be at least 25 dB SL and as close to 40 dB SL as is comfortable. Be alert to the possibility of crossover and the need for masking. Masking during discrimination testing is discussed in the next section.
5. Test each ear. Testing may be discontinued after the first half list if the discrimination score is very good or very poor. It is advisable to use a full list if the score is poorer than 88% but better than 28%.
6. If the score appears incongruent with the pure tone audiogram, you may want to administer retests. Perhaps exploring different presentation levels will resolve the incongruity.

MASKING

Because discrimination testing is a suprathreshold procedure, masking is often necessary. The basic rule is similar to that for threshold testing. Masking is needed when there is a difference of more than 40 dB between the bone conduction thresholds of the nontest ear and the presentation level to the test ear. You probably noticed that in tests for establishment of threshold, I have advised masking when the difference is *40 dB or greater*. Now, for suprathreshold testing, the statement is changed to "greater than 40 dB." It is common practice to administer discrimination tests in bilaterally equal losses at 40 dB SL without masking. This procedure may be justifiable in *suprathreshold* testing since (1) actual instances of interaural attenuation for speech as little as 40 dB are probably rare, and (2) when they do occur, effective crossover at 0 dB SL would contribute relatively little to the discrimination score.

In threshold testing, on the other hand, crossover at 0 dB SL would result in an invalidating response.

A broad band signal should be used for masking, either white noise or pink noise. The noise should be calibrated for effective masking, as explained in Chapter 5 (Speech Threshold Testing).

A conservative approach is to select the best bone conduction threshold of the nontest ear for the frequencies 500–4000 Hz as the representative threshold. If there is more than 40 dB difference between that threshold and the presentation level, introduce enough effective masking to reduce the difference to less than 40 dB. Remember that any air-bone gap in the nontest ear will reduce the effectiveness of the masking. Introduce additional masking to compensate for the air-bone gap, thereby shifting the bone conduction thresholds to the desired level. In cases of conductive loss, be alert for the possibility of overmasking. You should estimate minimum and maximum masking levels, as described in Chapter 4 (Masking).

SPECIAL PROCEDURES

Conventional procedures are not feasible with some individuals because of age, intelligence, language ability, or other reasons. In such cases, special procedures will sometimes permit estimation of discrimination ability.

Congenital hearing loss usually is associated with reduced language ability. Word familiarity plays an important role in intelligibility. Therefore, language retardation will reduce discrimination scores. Patients should be tested with words which are within their vocabulary.

To minimize the effect of language on the discrimination score, Matkin (1977) recommended selecting the discrimination test on the basis of established or estimated Receptive Vocabulary Age (RVA). Information regarding RVA may be obtained by questioning parents and teachers or through use of appropriate materials, such as the Peabody Picture Vocabulary Test. Matkin recommended the following guide: Adult word lists should be used if the RVA is 12 years or greater. The PB-K lists are appropriate if the RVA is between 6 and 12. If the RVA is 4 to 6, the WIPI test is recommended. If the RVA is less than 4 years, selected words known by the child may be used. For example, if 10 pictures or objects can be found for which the child knows the name, an estimate can be obtained by determining how many of the 10 the patient can identify on hearing the words presented. In this case, discrimination scores can be recorded as the number correct out of 10, rather than in percentages. Always describe the informal procedure which was used so that those who see the test results later can interpret them meaningfully. For children who cannot differentiate verbal stimuli, the SERT may provide a gross estimate of discrimination ability.

RELATIONSHIPS BETWEEN PURE TONE THRESHOLDS AND SPEECH DISCRIMINATION SCORES

A number of limitations reduce our ability to predict discrimination scores from observation of the pure tone audiogram. One limitation is the lack of a universal standard test. Another is receptive language level, which affects discrimination scores. Furthermore, various causes of hearing loss affect discrimination ability in a fashion which is not always predictable. In spite of these influences, which should be minimized as much as possible by good clinical practice, useful generalizations can be drawn from discrimination testing. The relationships discussed below apply to hearing losses acquired after the acquisition of language and speech. It is assumed additionally that discrimination scores were obtained from a test similar to the W-22 recording.

In cases of conductive loss, discrimination scores should be between 90 and 100%. This is the approximate range which would be expected with normal hearing sensitivity. Once the presentation level is sufficient to compensate for the conductive blockage, performance should be normal. Accurate discrimination testing is particularly important in cases with conductive components, such as in otosclerosis, when surgery may be contemplated. Unimpaired discrimination ability indicates good potential for improvement in auditory function if surgery is feasible to improve auditory sensitivity.

The relationship between magnitude of loss and discrimination scores in sensorineural loss is more difficult to predict. Configuration, site of lesion, and etiology are contributing factors.

In general, individuals with auditory nerve lesions will produce lower discrimination scores than those with cochlear disorders. However there is considerable overlap in performance between the two groups and the dramatic deterioration of discrimination ability associated with such retrocochlear disorders as acoustic tumor does not always occur. Cochlear disorders are associated with variable influence on discrimination ability. Historically patients with Meniere's disease, a labyrinthine disorder, have been expected to exhibit poorer discrimination ability than those with other cochlear etiologies. Other disorders associated with inordinately poor discrimination ability in relation to the pure tone audiogram are discussed below in the section under phonemic regression.

The limitations discussed above should make it obvious that it is precarious to comment on the expected relationship between magnitude of sensorineural loss and auditory discrimination scores. Keep these

Table 6.1
Auditory Discrimination Scores of Patients With Acquired Sensorineural Loss[a]

Sensitivity (dB re: ANSI. 1969 Norm)	Age in Years	Number of Ears	Mean % Score
Normal	Under 65	175	97.31
(0–10 dB)	Over 65	5	96.40
Borderline	Under 65	75	97.07
Normal (11–25 dB)	Over 65	15	94.67
Mild loss	Under 65	55	88.36
(26–45 dB)	Over 65	57	83.12
Moderate loss	Under 65	12	63.83
(46–65 dB)	Over 65	24	66.33
Severe loss	Under 65	2	26.00
(66–85 dB)	Over 65	4	26.50
Profound loss	Under 65	2	2.00
(86 + dB)			

[a] Slope of audiometric configuration was no more than 15 dB per octave from 500–2000 Hz. Patients had interweaving air and bone conduction thresholds. Tympanograms, if obtained, were normal.

limitations and the numerous exceptions which can be expected in mind.

On the average, discrimination scores decrease as the magnitude of sensorineural loss increases. The relationship between discrimination scores and sensitivity in patients with relatively flat sensorineural loss is shown in Table 6.1.

The effect of high frequency loss on discrimination ability in patients with normal sensitivity across part of the audiogram and a sharply falling loss has been estimated by administering discrimination tests to normals with the speech filtered to simulate high frequency losses of varying degree. Table 6.2 summarizes the discrimination scores which may be expected from individuals with varying degrees of high frequency sensorineural loss.

The term *phonemic regression* was coined by Gaeth (1948) to describe certain auditory characteristics in elderly individuals. They include a mild or moderate sensorineural loss with auditory discrimination scores which are disproportionately poor. Gaeth determined that this condition does not exist in all individuals with presbycusis, or hearing loss associated with aging. Table 6.1, showing scores of patients above and below age 65, does not reveal scores consistently poorer for the older group. Some presbycusics exhibit quite good discrimination scores.

Table 6.2
Expected Relationships Between Discrimination Scores and Pure Tone Configurations in a Sharply Falling Sensorineural Loss[a]

If Sensitivity is Normal Between	Expect % Discrimination Score to Be
125 and 4000 Hz	96 to 100
125 and 3000 Hz	90 to 94
125 and 2000 Hz	84 to 88
125 and 1000 Hz	64 to 82
125 and 500 Hz	40 to 62
125 and 250 Hz	22 to 38
Up to 125 Hz	0 to 20

[a] Based on data from French and Steinberg (1947); Hirsh *et al.* (1952); Carhart (1960); Giolas and Epstein (1963); and clinical experience.

Other etiologies already mentioned may cause unduly low discrimination scores—acoustic tumor and Meniere's disease.

Even if presbycusis and phonemic regression appear a likely reason for an unusually reduced discrimination score, you should explore for the possibility of better performance. The patient may be insufficiently motivated or may not understand the instructions or purpose of the test. It is also possible that retesting, at more appropriate presentation levels, may improve performance.

SUMMARY

The purpose of discrimination testing is to establish how well an individual can differentiate speech sounds when speech is presented at an optimum listening level. This information provides an estimate of auditory handicap and the ability to benefit from amplification. Many discrimination tests have been developed. The most commonly used are lists of monosyllabic words to which the patient responds by repeating the test word.

The difficulty of the test material and its appropriateness to the RVA of the patient must be taken into account when administering and interpreting discrimination tests. The presentation level is also an important variable and in some instances retesting at various presentation levels is indicated to be sure that the maximum intelligibility score is elicited.

Recorded tests of discrimination ability are available. Much discrimination testing is done by monitored live voice. The clinician must learn a carefully monitored and standard presentation for live voice testing. Even so, you must realize that speaker differences reduce the confidence with which you can compare results obtained by different talkers. These differences also apply to recorded versions of the same test which utilize different talkers.

There is, in general, a predictable relationship between discrimination scores and type, magnitude, and configuration of hearing loss. This relationship is affected by the lack of a standardized discrimination test, by receptive language levels, and etiology of hearing loss.

STUDY QUESTIONS

1. What are the purposes of speech discrimination testing? How well are the purposes realized with our current tests?
2. Instead of a complete performance-intensity (PI) function what two points of the function are usually established? Under what circumstances should discrimination ability be tested at more than one presentation level?
3. What are the influences on intelligibility of the following factors: (a) word length? (b) word familiarity? (c) open versus closed set tests? (d) receptive vocabulary? (e) presentation level? (f) sensorineural loss?
4. Under what circumstances should you administer to each ear (a) less than a full PB list? (b) a full PB list? (c) more than one full PB list?
5. What are the rules for masking when establishing speech discrimination scores? How do the rules differ from masking during speech threshold testing?
6. Consider the need for masking during speech discrimination testing in the following cases. In each instance the patient has a bilaterally equal 30-dB hearing loss. Presentation level for testing is 40 dB SL (70 dB HL). Common procedure requires that the bone conduction thresholds of the nontest ear be shifted to within 40 dB or less of the presentation level to the test ear. *Remember*: if the 30dB loss in the *masked* ear is *conductive*, 30 dB of masking will be dissipated by the conductive disorder. Recording the examples given below on an audiogram form may be helpful as you solve the problems.
   (a) If the 30-dB loss is *bilaterally sensorineural*, how much effective mask is required? Is overmasking probable?
   (b) If the 30-dB loss is *sensorineural* on the *test ear* and *conductive* on the *nontest ear*, how much effective masking is required? Is overmasking probable?
   (c) If the 30-dB loss is *bilaterally conductive*, how much effective masking is required? Is overmasking probable?
7. Review the expected relationship between magnitude of hearing loss and auditory discrimination scores. What factors influence the relationship? How can adverse influences be minimized?

APPENDIX A

PB-50 Word Lists (Egan, 1948)

The PAL-50 (NDRC) PB lists appear below. The words are in alphabetical order and should be randomized before clinical use. Lists 5 to 12 were used, with slight modification, for the Rush Hughes recording. On these lists, words followed by an asterisk (*) are omitted from the Rush Hughes recording. The replacement words are given at the end of each list.

PB-50 List 1

are	death	fuss	not	rub
bad	deed	grove	pan	slip
bar	dike	heap	pants	smile
bask	dish	hid	pest	strife
box	end	hive	pile	such
cane	feast	hunt	plush	then
cleanse	fern	is	rag	there
clove	folk	mange	rat	toe
crash	ford	no	ride	use (yews)
creed	fraud	nook	rise	wheat

PB-50 List 2

awe	dab	hock	perk	start
bait	earl	job	pick	suck
bean	else	log	pit	tan
blush	fate	moose	quart	tang
bought	five	mute	rap	them
bounce	frog	nab	rib	trash
bud	gill	need	scythe	vamp
charge	gloss	niece	shoe	vast
cloud	hire	nut	sludge	ways
corpse	hit	our	snuff	wish

PB-50 List 3

ache	crime	hurl	please	take
air	deck	jam	pulse	thrash
bald	dig	law	rate	toil
barb	dill	leave	rouse	trip
bead	drop	lush	shout	turf
cape	fame	muck	sit	vow
cast	far	neck	size	wedge
check	fig	nest	sob	wharf
class	flush	oak	sped	who
crave	gnaw	path	stag	why

PB-50 List 4				
bath	dodge	hot	pert	shed
beast	dupe	how	pinch	shin
bee	earn	kite	pod	sketch
blonde	eel	merge	race	slap
budge	fin	move	rack	sour
bus	float	neat	rave	starve
bush	frown	new	raw	strap
cloak	hatch	oils	rut	test
course	heed	or	sage	tick
court	hiss	peck	scab	touch

PB-50 List 5				
add	flap	love	rind (rīnd)	thud
bathe	gape*	mast	rode	trade
beck	good	nose	roe	true
black	greek	odds	scare	tug
bronze	grudge	owls	shine	vase (vace)
browse*	high	pass	shove	watch
cheat	hill	pipe	sick	wink
choose	inch	puff	sly	wrath
curse	kid	punt	solve	yawn
feed	lend	rear	thick	zone

* Rush Hughes: bake, drive

PB-50 List 6				
as	deep	gap	prig*	shank
badge	eat	grope	prime	slouch
best	eyes	hitch	pun	sup
bog*	fall	hull	pus	thigh
chart	fee	jag	raise	thus
cloth	flick	kept	ray	tongue
clothes	flop	leg	reap	wait
cob	forge	mash	rooms	wasp
crib	fowl	nigh	rough	wife
dad	gage	ode	scan	writ*

* Rush Hughes: beg, match, plug

PB-50 List 7				
act	dope	jug	pounce	siege
aim	dose	knit	quiz	sin
am	dwarf	mote*	raid	sledge
but	fake	mud	range	sniff
by	fling	nine	rash	south
chop	fort	off	rich	though
coast	gasp	pent	roar	whiff*
comes	grade	phase*	sag	wire
cook	gun	pig	scout	woe
cut	him	plod	shaft	woo

* Rush Hughes: meet, shave, whip

PB-50 List 8				
ask	cod	forth	look	shack
bid	crack	freak	night	slide
bind	day	frock	pint	spice
bolt	deuce	front	queen	this
bored	dumb	guess	rest	thread
calf	each	hum	rhyme	till
catch	ease	jell	rod	us
chant	fad	kill	roll	wheeze*
chew	flip	left	rope	wig
clod	food	lick	rot	yeast

* Rush Hughes: horse

PB-50 List 9				
arch	crowd	grace	odd	than
beef	cud*	hoof	pact*	thank
birth	ditch	ice	phone	throne
bit	flag	itch	reed	toad
boost	fluff*	key	root	troop
carve	foe	lit	rude	weak
chess	fume	mass	sip	wild
chest	fuse	nerve	smart	wipe
clown	gate	noose	spud	with
club	give	nuts	ten	year

* Rush Hughes: skill, tax, tub

PB-50 List 10				
ail	cue	gull	pink	staff
back	daub*	hat	plus	tag
bash*	ears	hurt	put	those
bob	earth	jay	rape*	thug
bug	etch*	lap	real	tree
champ	fir	line	rip	valve
chance	flaunt	maze	rush	void*
clothe	flight	mope*	scrub	wade
cord	force	nudge	slug	wake
cow	goose	page	snipe	youth

* Rush Hughes: died, dust, gold, lock, rake, spin

PB-50 List 11				
arc	doubt	jab	pond	shot
arm	drake	jaunt*	probe	sign
beam	dull	kit	prod	snow
bliss	feel	lag	punk	sprig*
chunk	fine	latch	purse	spy
clash	frisk*	loss	reef	stiff
code	fudge	low	rice	tab
crutch	goat	most	risk	urge
cry	have	mouth	sap	wave
dip	hog	net	shop	wood

* Rush Hughes: door, fist, skin

PB-50 List 12				
and	cling	frill	lash	rove
ass*	clutch	gnash	laugh	set
ball	depth	greet	ledge	shut
bluff	dime	hear	loose	sky
cad	done	hug	out	sod
cave	fed	hunch	park	throb
chafe*	flog*	jaw	priest	tile
chair	flood	jazz	reek*	vine
chap	foot	jolt	ripe	wage
chink	fought	knife	romp	wove

* Rush Hughes: glass, make, speed, teeth

PB-50 List 13

bat	few	jig	nip	sled
beau	fill	made	ought	smash
change	fold	mood	owe	smooth
climb	for	mop	patch	soap
corn	gem	moth	pelt	stead
curb	grape	muff	plead	taint
deaf	grave	mush	price	tap
dog	hack	my	pug	thin
elk	hate	nag	scuff	tip
elm	hook	nice	side	wean

PB-50 List 14

at	dead	isle	prude	stuff
barn	douse	kick	purge	tell
bust	dung	lathe	quack	tent
car	fife	life	rid	thy
clip	foam	me	shook	tray
coax	grate	muss	shrug	vague
curve	group	news	sing	vote
cute	heat	nick	slab	wag
darn	howl	nod	smite	waif
dash	hunk	oft	soil	wrist

PB-50 List 15

bell	fact	less	pup	teach
blind	flame	may	quick	that
boss	fleet	mesh	scow	time
cheap	gash	mitt	sense	tinge
cost	glove	mode	shade	tweed
cuff	golf	morn	shrub	vile
dive	hedge	naught	sir	weave
dove (duv)	hole	ninth	slash	wed
edge	jade	oath	so	wide
elf	kiss	own	tack	wreck

PB-50 List 16

aid	droop	kind	pump	stress
barge	dub	knee	rock	suit
book	fifth	lay	rogue	thou
cheese	fright	leash	rug	three

(con't)

cliff	gab	louse	rye	thresh
closed	gas	map	sang	tire
crews	had	nap	sheep	ton
dame	hash	next	sheik	tuck
din	hose	part	soar	turn
drape	ink	pitch	stab	wield

PB-50 List 17

all	crush	hence	past	sell
apt	dart	hood	pearl	ship
bet	dine	if	peg	shock
big	falls	last	plow	stride
booth	feet	ma	press	tube
brace	fell	mist	rage	vice
braid	fit	myth	reach	weep
buck	form	ox	ridge	weird
case	fresh	paid	roam	wine
clew	gum	pare	scratch	you

PB-50 List 18

aims	chip	flare	hush	sack
art	claw	fool	lime	sash
axe	claws	freeze	lip	share
bale	crab	got	loud	sieve
bless	cub	grab	lunge	thaw
camp	debt	gray	lynch	thine
cat	dice	grew	note	thorn
chaff	dot	gush	ouch	trod
chain	fade	hide	rob	waste
chill	fat	his	rose	weed

PB-50 List 19

age	chose (choz)	fond	notch	slid
bark	crude	gin	on	splash
bay	cup	god	paste	steed
bough	dough	gyp	perch	thief
buzz	drug	hike	raft	throat
cab	dune	hut	rote	up
cage	ebb	lad	rule	wheel
calve (cav)	fan	led	sat	white
cant	find	lose (looz)	shy	yes
chat	flank	lust	sill	yield

PB-50 List 20				
ace	duke	joke	retch	slush
base	eye	judge	robe	soak
beard	fair	lid	roost	souse
brass	fast	mow (mo)	rouge	theme
cart	flash	pack	rout (rowt)	through
click	gang	pad	salve	tilt
clog	get	pew	seed	walk
cork	gob	puss	sigh	wash
crate	hump	quip	skid	web
did	in	ramp	slice	wise

APPENDIX B

W-22 Words (Hirsh *et al.*, 1952)

W-22 word lists appear below in alphabetical order. They should be randomized before clinical use.

List 1				
ace	day	it	owl	toe
ache	deaf	jam	poor	true
an	earn (urn)	knees	ran	twins
as	east	law	see (sea)	yard
bathe	felt	low	she	up
bells	give	me	skin	us
carve	high	mew	stove	wet
chew	him	none (nun)	them	what
could	hunt	not (knot)	there (their)	wire
dad	isle (aisle)	or (oar)	thing	you (ewe)

List 2				
ail (ale)	dumb	ill	off	that
air (heir)	ease	jaw	one (won)	then
and	eat	key	own	thin
bin (been)	else	knee	pew	too (two, to)
by (buy)	flat	live (verb)	rooms	tree
cap	gave	move	send	way (weigh)
cars	ham	new (knew)	show	well
chest	hit	now	smart	with
die (dye)	hurt	oak	star	yore (your)
does	ice	odd	tare (tear)	young

List 3				
add (ad)	done (dun)	is	out	this
aim	dull	jar	owes	though
are	ears	king	pie	three
ate (eight)	end	knit	raw	tie
bill	farm	lie (lye)	say	use (yews)
book	glove	may	shove	we
camp	hand	nest	smooth	west
chair	have	no (know)	start	when
cute	he	oil	tan	wool
do	if	on	ten	year

List 4				
aid	clothes	his	ought (aught)	through
all (awl)	cook	in (inn)	our (hour)	tin
am	darn	jump	pale (pail)	toy
arm	dolls	leave	save	where
art	dust	men	shoe	who
at	ear	my	so (sew)	why
bee (be)	eyes (ayes)	near	stiff	will
bread (bred)	few	net	tea (tee)	wood (would)
can	go	nuts	then	yes
chin	hang	of	they	yet

APPENDIX C

NU 6 Words (Tillman and Carhart, 1966)

The Nu 6 word lists appear below in alphabetical order. They should be randomized before clinical use.

List 1				
bean*	gap	knock	pool	sure
boat	goose	laud	puff*	take
burn	hash*	limb	rag*	third
chalk	home	lot	raid*	tip*
choice	hurl*	love*	raise*	tough*
death*	jail	met	reach*	vine*
dime*	jar	mode*	sell*	week*
door	keen	moon	shout*	which
fall*	king	nag*	size*	whip
fat*	kite*	page	sub	yes*

List 2				
bite	far*	learn	pick*	south*
book*	gaze	live	pike	thought*
bought*	gin*	loaf	rain	ton*
calm	goal	lore	read*	tool
chair	hate*	match	room	turn*
chief	haze	merge*	rot*	voice
dab*	hush*	mill	said	wag*
dead*	juice	nice*	shack*	white*
deep*	keep	numb	shawl	witch
fail	keg	pad*	soap*	young

List 3				
bar*	dodge*	lid*	phone	soup
base*	five*	life*	pole	talk
beg	germ	luck	rat*	team
cab*	good*	mess	ring	tell*
cause	gun*	mop*	road*	thin*
chat*	half	mouse	rush*	void*
cheek	hire*	name	search	walk*
cool	hit*	note*	seize	when
date	jug*	pain	shall	wire*
ditch*	late	pearl*	sheep*	youth*

List 4				
back*	food	lean	peg*	such*
bath*	gas*	lease	perch*	tape
bone	get*	long	red*	thumb*
came	hall	lose	ripe*	time*
chain*	have*	make	rose*	tire*
check*	hole*	mob	rough*	vote*
dip*	join	mood*	sail	wash*
dog*	judge*	near	shirt	wheat*
doll	kick*	neat*	should	wife*
fit*	kill*	pass*	sour*	yearn

* Also in original PB-50 lists.

APPENDIX D

PB/K Word Lists (Haskins, 1949)

please	ways	are	pink	beef
great	five	teach	thank	few
sled	mouth	slice	take	use
pants	rag	is	cart	did
rat	put	tree	scab	hit
bad	fed	smile	lay	pond
pinch	fold	bath	class	hot
such	hunt	slip	me	own
bus	no	ride	dish	bead
need	box	end	neck	shop
laugh	ax	sing	crab	grew
falls	cage	all	peg	knee
paste	knife	bless	freeze	fresh
plow	turn	suit	race	tray
page	grab	splash	bud	cat
weed	rose	path	darn	on
gray	lip	feed	fair	camp
park	bee	next	sack	find
wait	bet	wreck	got	yes
fat	his	waste	as	loud
tire	those	vase	air	bush
seed	true	press	set	clown
purse	ache	fit	dad	cab
quick	black	bounce	ship	hurt
room	else	wide	case	pass
bug	nest	most	you	grade
that	jay	thick	may	blind
sell	raw	if	choose	drop
low	had	them	white	leave
rich	cost	sheep	frog	nuts

APPENDIX E

Modified Rhyme Test (House *et al*., 1965)

	Forms				
A	B	C	D	E	F
1. bat	bad	back	bass	ban	bath
2. bean	beach	beat	beam	bead	beak
3. bun	bus	but	buff	buck	bug
4. came	cape	cane	cake	cave	case
5. cut	cub	cuff	cup	cud	cuss
6. dig	dip	did	dim	dill	din
7. duck	dud	dung	dub	dug	dun
8. fill	fig	fin	fizz	fib	fit
9. hear	health	heal	heave	heat	heap
10. kick	king	kid	kit	kin	kill
11. late	lake	lay	lace	lane	lame
12. map	mat	math	man	mass	mad
13. page	pane	pace	pay	pale	pave
14. pass	pat	pack	pad	path	pan
15. peace	peas	peak	peal	peat	peach
16. pill	pick	pip	pig	pin	pit
17. pun	puff	pup	puck	pus	pub
18. rave	rake	race	rate	raze	ray
19. sake	sale	save	sane	safe	same
20. sad	sass	sag	sack	sap	sat
21. seep	seen	seethe	seed	seem	seek
22. sing	sit	sin	sip	sick	sill
23. sud	sum	sub	sun	sup	sung
24. tab	tan	tam	tang	tack	tap
25. teach	tear	tease	teal	team	teak
26. led	shed	red	bed	fed	wed
27. sold	told	hold	fold	gold	cold
28. dig	wig	big	rig	pig	fig
29. kick	lick	sick	pick	wick	tick
30. book	took	shook	cook	hook	look
31. hark	dark	mark	lark	park	bark
32. gale	male	tale	bale	sale	pale
33. peel	reel	feel	heel	keel	eel
34. will	hill	kill	till	fill	bill
35. foil	coil	boil	oil	toil	soil
36. fame	same	came	name	tame	game

37. ten	pen	den	hen	then	men
38. pin	sin	tin	win	din	fin
39. sun	nun	gun	fun	bun	run
40. rang	fang	gang	bang	sang	hang
41. tent	bent	went	dent	rent	sent
42. sip	rip	tip	dip	hip	lip
43. top	hop	pop	cop	mop	shop
44. meat	feat	heat	seat	beat	neat
45. kit	bit	fit	sit	wit	hit
46. hot	got	not	pot	lot	tot
47. nest	vest	west	test	best	rest
48. bust	just	rust	must	gust	dust
49. raw	paw	law	jaw	thaw	saw
50. way	may	say	gay	day	pay

APPENDIX F

Examples of Third-Order Approximation Synthetic Sentences (Jerger *et al.*, 1968)

1. Small boat with a picture has become
2. Built the government with the force almost
3. Forward march said the boy had a
4. Go change your car color is red
5. March around without a care in your
6. That neighbor who said business is better
7. Battle cry and be better than ever
8. Down by the time is real enough
9. Agree with him only to find out
10. Women view men with green paper should

APPENDIX G

W-22 Words Ranked from Most Difficult to Easiest (Rose, 1974)

List I		List II	
A	B	A	B
1. mew	1. bells	1. rooms	1. knee
2. bathe	2. deaf	2. thin	2. else
3. felt	3. chew	3. pew	3. bin
4. ache	4. ace	4. ease	4. ill
5. knees	5. owl	5. hit	5. cap
6. twins	6. an	6. tare	6. gave
7. thing	7. dad	7. that	7. send
8. stove	8. carve	8. off	8. cars
9. true	9. east	9. ail	9. key
10. skin	10. us	10. jaw	10. then
11. as	11. earn	11. flat	11. with
12. she	12. law	12. chest	12. does
13. or	13. poor	13. air	13. ham
14. it	14. day	14. smart	14. own
15. jam	15. him	15. oak	15. move
16. me	16. see	16. new	16. star
17. there	17. what	17. your	17. by
18. isle	18. tone	18. dumb	18. ice
19. them	19. high	19. die	19. odd
20. wet	20. give	20. way	20. live
21. could	21. ran	21. eat	21. now
22. toe	22. low	22. hurt	22. tree
23. not	23. hunt	23. one	23. too
24. up	24. wire	24. end	24. well
25. you	25. yard	25. show	25. young

List III		List IV	
A	B	A	B
1. wool	1. owes	1. dolls	1. few
2. dull	2. tan	2. net	2. nuts
3. he	3. nest	3. his	3. than
4. though	4. ears	4. all	4. pale
5. is	5. pie	5. tin	5. stiff
6. bill	6. say	6. ought	6. darn
7. cute	7. smooth	7. yes	7. ear
8. knit	8. farm	8. why	8. eyes
9. ten	9. king	9. chin	9. near
10. this	10. year	10. go	10. they
11. use	11. aim	11. hang	11. bee
12. ate	12. if	12. through	12. dust
13. oil	13. end	13. at	13. save
14. glove	14. west	14. shoe	14. tea
15. tie	15. camp	15. our	15. am
16. shove	16. raw	16. of	16. my
17. have	17. start	17. aid	17. can
18. done	18. three	18. who	18. art
19. hand	19. may	19. arm	19. in
20. jar	20. add	20. men	20. so
21. when	21. chair	21. leave	21. bread
22. lie	22. do	22. will	22. where
23. are	23. book	23. jump	23. yet
24. out	24. we	24. toy	24. cook
25. on	25. no	25. wood	25. clothes

CHAPTER 7 Basic Impedance Measurements

Different pathologies yield similar pure tone audiometric results but different mechanical states of the middle ear. It is important to have objective evidence to differentiate the causes of conductive disorders. Impedance measurement gives information about the nature of conductive hearing loss in situations where conventional audiometry only differentiates between conductive and sensorineural loss.

PURPOSE

The purpose of impedance measurement is to confirm and extend information gained via conventional audiometry by looking at the mechanical status and function of the middle ear in several ways. The tympanogram is one measure. Acoustic reflex measurement is another, giving confirmatory data about the status of the middle ear and also gleaning information about the sensorineural mechanism. In the following sections you will learn to identify tympanogram types and associate these types with the most common underlying conditions of the middle ear. You will also learn about acoustic reflex thresholds and the interpretation of reflex testing. The use of tympanometry in screening to differentiate normal and abnormal populations is also discussed.

Some impedance measures are beyond the scope of this text. For those areas not covered, references are given here to direct the interested reader. Basic Eustachian tube measurement is described in this chapter. Detailed assessment of Eustachian tube function is discussed by Bluestone (1975).

Basic impedance measurement gives some information about hearing sensitivity in those who cannot or will not make behavioral responses to conventional audiometry. There are additional techniques to estimate threshold sensitivity. These include the procedure of Niemeyer and Sesterhenn (1974) and the SPAR (Sensitivity Prediction by Acoustic Reflex) test (Jerger and associates, 1974a).

A simple procedure to detect loudness recruitment, based on the sensation level which elicits the acoustic reflex, is discussed in this chapter. Recruitment (abnormal growth of loudness) suggests a cochlear rather than retrocochlear disorder (Jerger and Harford, 1960). Tests measuring reflex decay to detect active VIIIth nerve disorder are described by Jerger and associates (1974b). The further use of acoustic reflex information to differentiate VIIIth nerve versus brainstem disorders is discussed by Jerger and Jerger (1977). Loss of function and recovery of the facial nerve can also be monitored by acoustic reflex testing (Jerger, 1970).

PRINCIPLES

Compatible with the basic nature of this discussion, a cursory explanation of principles related to impedance measurement is presented below. For a detailed explanation of impedance principles, the interested reader should refer to Berlin and Cullen (1975) or Feldman and Wilber (1976).

Impedance instruments are classified as either bridges or meters. The circuitry and operation of the two types differ, but the attributes measured are the same. In general, I have used the word meter to refer to impedance instruments in this chapter. The comments apply equally to impedance bridges.

In effect, the impedance meter gives information about middle ear functioning by measuring the sound pressure level in a probe tone introduced into the external ear canal which is reflected from the eardrum. We therefore learn how much energy is accepted by the middle ear. Since we know the characteristics of the normal middle ear in this respect, and of ears with various conductive disorders, inferences of diagnostic importance can be made from the impedance measurements.

Impedance means the acceptance or rejection of energy per unit of time. A system with low impedance readily accepts energy; a high impedance system does not. Several factors combine in a complex fashion to determine the impedance of a system: its mass, resistance, and stiffness. Of these, stiffness is the factor which is ordinarily utilized for measurement.

As the stiffness of a system increases, its ability to accept low frequency energy diminishes. Most impedance meters utilize a low frequency probe tone of approximately 220 Hz. Others also incorporate a higher frequency tone (such as 660 Hz) to gather additional information. Therefore, of the factors in the ear which determine its impedance, only stiffness affects the impedance meter in a material fashion. The reciprocal of stiffness, compliance, is a term in common clinical use for the measure accomplished with the impedance meter. A compliant system readily accepts low frequency energy while a stiff system does not.

As the field grew and new impedance instruments came on the market, terminology proliferated too. Although an ANSI standard is forthcoming, currently there is the tendency for instruments of each manufacturer to measure via a different impedance related concept and to express results in a different unit. Table 7.1 summarizes and explains some of the terminology currently used. Regardless of the terminology and units, each impedance instrument makes basically the same measure. Jerger (1975, p. 590) suggested that the clinician minimize attention on terminology and "concentrate on learning the intricate patterns of interaction among audiograms, tympanograms, and acoustic reflex thresholds."

The common measurement unit for compliance is the cubic centimeter (cm^3) of equivalent volume of air. A given value in this unit does not represent the actual volume of air being measured; rather it represents the volume of a hard walled cavity which has characteristics

Table 7.1
Summary of Impedance Terminolgy[b]

Term	Symbol	Concept	Clinical Importance
Impedance	Z	Total opposition to energy flow	Extremely limited: useful only when very high or very low
Admittance	Y	Total energy flow (reciprocal of Z)	See Z
Reactance	X	Opposition to energy flow due to storage	See Y
Susceptance	B	Energy flow associated with reactance (reciprocal of X)	See X
Resistance	R	Opposition to energy flow due to dissipation	HNSY[a]
Conductance	G	Energy flow associated with resistance (reciprocal of R)	HNSY[a]
Compliance	C	Reciprocal of stiffness: principal component of X at low frequencies	See Z
Tympanogram	T	Graph relating air pressure to either, Z,Y,X,B, or C	Great: second in importance only to AR
Acoustic reflex	AR	Contraction of stapedius muscle as detected by change in either Z,Y,X,B, or C	Very great: a powerful diagnostic tool

[a] *HNSY*, has not surfaced yet.
[b] From Jerger J.: *Arch. Otolaryngol., 101:* 589–590, 1975. (Copyright 1975, American Medical Association.)

similar to the ear being measured. A large volume of air is very compliant; a small volume of air has low compliance. Therefore, a middle ear system with high compliance will respond tympanometrically with a large cm^3 value and a stiff system will register a small cm^3 value.

INSTRUMENTATION

Without reference to the internal circuitry which mediates the measurement, a block diagram of an impedance meter is shown in Figure 7.1. As you can see, there is provision for a tube to be inserted into the ear canal. A closeup of an impedance headset is shown in Figure 7.2. The tube delivers a low frequency (usually 220 Hz) "probe tone." The typical level of the probe tone is approximately 90 dB SPL. One channel connects to a microphone which permits measurement of the SPL in the ear canal. If the ear under measure has high compliance, relatively little of the probe tone will be reflected from the eardrum. Conversely, in the case of a stiff system which does not readily accept the energy of the low frequency probe tone, a larger amount will be reflected. A meter of one type or another permits readout of the result in whatever units the particular impedance instrument uses. Additionally, the unit may include a graphic recorder which plots the results automatically.

Another channel is attached to an air pump, permitting change of air pressure in the ear canal. Of course, to maintain a variation in air pressure, an airtight seal must be obtained in the ear canal. This seal is

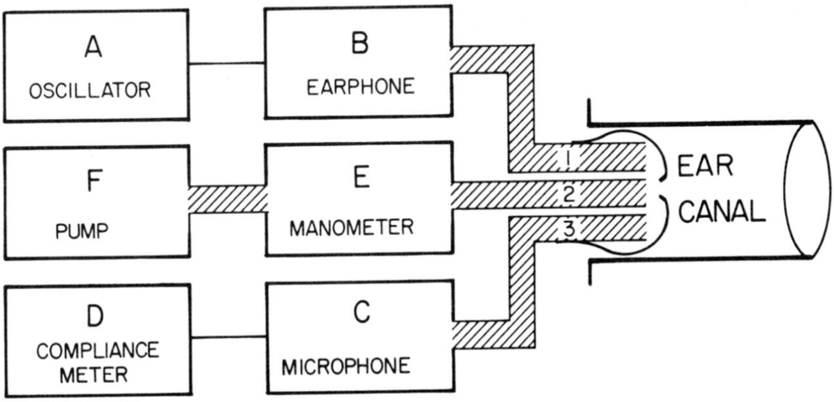

Fig. 7.1. Block diagram of an impedance instrument. The oscillator (*A*) and its earphone (*B*) send a low frequency probe tone into the ear canal via channel *1* of the probe tube. Channel *3* of the probe tube carries sound energy to the microphone (*C*) which enables the meter (*D*) to indicate compliance. Another channel (2) is connected to a manometer (*E*) which measures ear canal air pressure, regulated by a pump (*F*).

accomplished by a soft tip, available in various sizes, which fits over the probe tube and inserts snugly into the ear canal. A number of tips are shown in Figure 7.3. The pump functions to produce changes in air pressure in the sealed ear canal. This permits us to obtain the tympan-

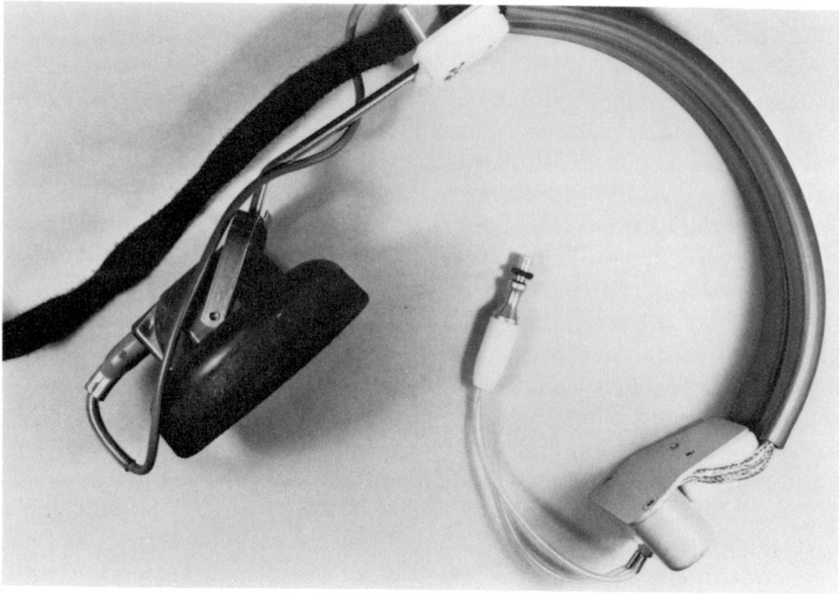

Fig. 7.2. Impedance meter headset. On one side there is a conventional audiometer earphone-cushion combination. On the other, a probe tube which is covered with a tip to promote an acoustic seal and inserted into the ear canal.

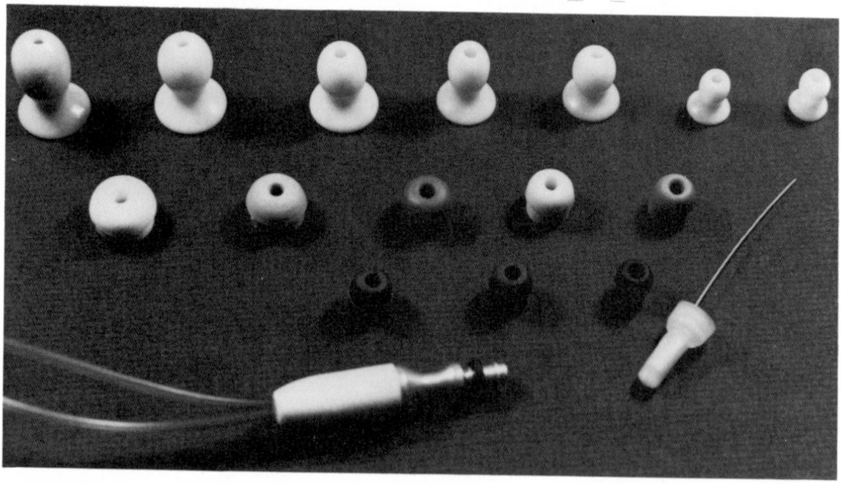

Fig. 7.3. Probe tips of various sizes, the probe tube, and probe tube cleaning wire.

ogram, a measure of middle ear compliance as a function of ear canal air pressure and also to determine, indirectly, the prevailing air pressure in the middle ear space.

THE BASIC IMPEDANCE BATTERY

The basic impedance battery consists of the tympanogram and acoustic reflex thresholds. Data from the tympanogram permit determination of the static (resting) compliance of the middle ear and a statement about the function of the Eustachian tube. Inspection of acoustic reflex test results permits inferences to support the presence of a conductive, sensory, or neural disorder. Each of these measures, and the interpretation, is discussed below.

The Tympanogram

The tympanogram indicates (1) the stiffness of the middle ear mechanism relative to normal and (2) Eustachian tube function, through a measure of the air pressure of the middle ear space. The tympanogram is a measure of middle ear compliance as a function of varying canal air pressure. The middle ear mechanism works best (has highest compliance) when air pressure is the same on either side of the eardrum. Therefore, the normal mechanism has highest compliance when the air pressure in the external canal is the same as that prevailing in the atmosphere (and, since the Eustachian tube function is normal, in the middle ear space).

To obtain a tympanogram, the middle ear mechanism is first made abnormally stiff by introducing a positive pressure into the ear canal. The unit in which this pressure is expressed is millimeters of water (mm H_2O). Conventionally, a pressure of 200 mm H_2O is introduced into the sealed ear canal for the first compliance measure. Then, the ear canal air pressure is reduced, crossing zero relative to the atmosphere and going into the negative range as far as −200 or even 300 or 400 mm H_2O. During this process, repeated compliance measures are taken from the impedance meter. Measurement is made at either 50 or 100 mm H_2O intervals if point-by-point measures are obtained or continuously if a graphic recording is made of compliance as air pressure changes. The ear canal air pressure at which the peak of compliance occurs, as well as the magnitude of that compliance, is also noted. Since the middle ear mechanism has highest compliance when air pressure is the same on either side of the eardrum, the ear canal pressure at which the peak of compliance occurs provides an indirect measure of the air pressure in the middle ear space. If the Eustachian tube is functioning well, the middle ear pressure should be quite similar to that of the atmosphere.

Test results obtained as described above are recorded on the tympanogram form. The air conduction threshold symbols are often used to record tympanometric results, a circle for the right ear and an X for the left ear. An Impedance Record is shown in Figure 7.4. On this particular form, ear canal air pressure in mm H_2O is displayed along the horizontal axis, from +200 mm H_2O to −400 mm H_2O. Compliance is displayed along the vertical axis, in cubic centimeters (cm^3) of equivalent volume of air. Impedance meters manufactured by various companies read out their results in units of various size, and there is no standard form for the vertical axis of the tympanogram. Therefore, the normal tympano-

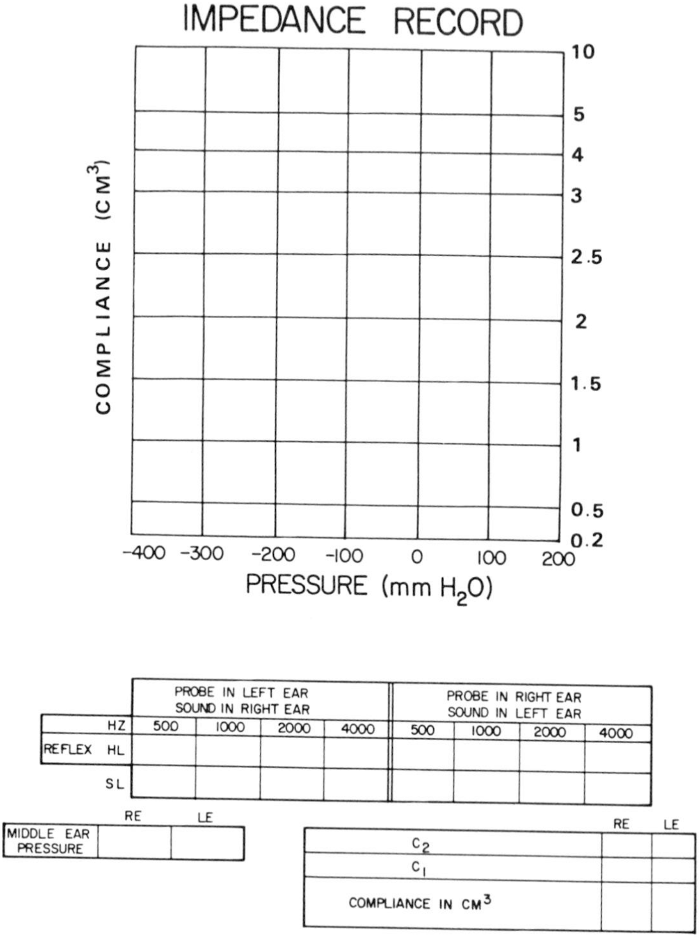

Fig. 7.4. Impedance Record. Because tympanograms usually fall into the range between 0.5 and 3.0 cm^3, relatively greater space is often devoted to this range in order to display more detail.

gram may vary considerably in its appearance, depending on the instrument with which it was obtained. Figure 7.5 shows tympanograms obtained on the same person with two different instruments. This lack of standardization means that you must interpret each tympanogram in terms that are compatible with the instrument on which it was obtained. In most cases in this text, I have used cm^3.

Static Compliance

On completion of the tympanogram, a simple computation permits determination of the static, or resting, compliance of the middle ear. Two values are involved in the computation: compliance obtained with +200 mm H_2O pressure in the ear canal and the compliance at its peak, or maximum compliance which occurred while obtaining the tympanogram.

The air in the ear canal contributes to compliance measures. With the canal pressure at +200 mm H_2O the eardrum is "locked" and the compliance measure obtained at that time approximates the equivalent volume of the ear canal alone. For purposes of determining static compliance this measure is called C_1. Recall that the second measure (C_2) is the peak or maximum compliance, obtained by changing ear canal air pressure until the middle ear is most compliant. C_2 approximates the equivalent volume of the canal *and* the middle ear. With

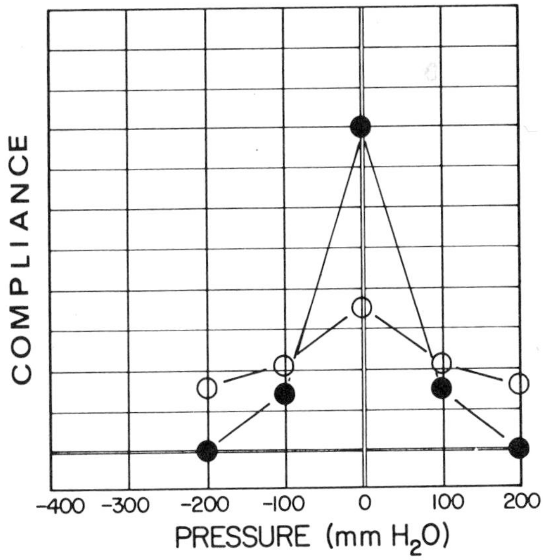

Fig. 7.5. Contours of tympanograms obtained on the same ear with two different impedance instruments.

these two measures in hand, the static compliance of the middle ear is determined by subtracting C_1 from C_2: C (static compliance) = $C_2 - C_1$.

Acoustic Reflex Threshold

The compliance of the middle ear is decreased when the two small muscles associated with the middle ear, the stapedius and the tensor tympani, contract. The mechanism becomes stiffer. This change in compliance is readily observable on the impedance meter. Activity of the tensor tympani can be elicited by nonacoustic stimuli. However, when the individual experiences a sufficiently loud sound, apparently only the stapedius muscle contributes importantly to the acoustic reflex. Thus, the acoustic reflex is sometimes called the stapedial reflex.

The acoustic reflex is a bilateral phenomenon. The muscles in both ears contract on the presentation of an adequate stimulus to one ear. Therefore, it is common to stimulate one ear while observing compliance change in the other. This contralateral measure is accomplished by utilizing an impedance headset which has a conventional earphone-cushion combination (attached to a pure tone audiometer) on one side and the impedance probe tube on the other. For special testing purposes, many impedance meters also provide for ipsilateral measures of the acoustic reflex, measuring the reflex in the ear to which the stimulus is delivered. For diagnostic use of ipsilateral reflex measures, see Jerger and Jerger (1977).

Acoustic reflex measures are usually expressed as the minimum decibel HL required to elicit the reflex. Acoustic reflex thresholds are obtained in much the same manner as behavioral thresholds of sensitivity. The major difference, of course, is that the clinician watches the impedance meter for a consistent change in compliance rather than requiring a voluntary response from the patient.

Since both ears are involved in the contralateral reflex measurement, both ears contribute to the result. As a result there has been some question regarding which ear should be considered the test ear. Forms on which reflex thresholds are recorded should clearly indicate the fashion in which results are reported. For example, our forms state, "probe in left ear, sound in right ear," leaving no room for confusion. As a generalization, the stimulated ear is considered the test ear even though the reflex generated by stimulation of that ear is actually measured on the other side. Important information is also gained from the ear in which the probe is located. You will learn about that later in this chapter.

In contralateral reflex testing it is common to test with pure tones at octave intervals between 500 and 4000 Hz. Broad bands of noise or filtered noise are also used for special purposes. Ipsilateral reflex testing is usually done at 1000 and 2000 Hz.

MEASUREMENT

Preparation for Testing

A procedure similar to the audiometer listening check described in Chapter 2 is advisable each day before using the impedance meter. Details will differ according to the model in use, and you must refer to the manufacturer's manual. Regardless of the type, you should check certain physical and acoustic properties for correct operation.

Be sure the probe assembly is clean and the openings are not plugged with ear wax. Follow the manufacturer's instructions and use the cleaning wire supplied to open the holes. Damage to the instrument is possible in some cases if instructions given in the manual are not followed. Be sure that there are no defective controls, and that the earphone cord and cushion are in good condition.

Check to ensure that an adequate supply of clean tips is available. Tips should be cleaned in some solution such as Zepharin, rinsed, and dried before use.

Check for air leaks in the pumping system by inserting the tip into a closed cavity and obtaining an air-tight seal. Your ear canal will work well. Be sure you can maintain a positive or negative pressure, with no change in the pressure meter over time. Leaks in the system commonly occur when tubes that transmit air or sound energy become loose at some connection, usually where the tubes attach to the probe tip assembly which fits into the ear. Do not check for leaks by holding your finger over the end of the probe tube. If the leak is in the microphone or earphone tube, your finger occluding the air tube will suggest that the system is all right, but an air pressure leak will persist via the transducer tube when the tip is in the ear canal.

Most impedance meters provide for probe tone calibration via appropriate cavities on the instrument into which the probe tone can be directed, measured, and adjusted. Follow the manufacturer's directions and utilize this procedure daily.

Listen to the pure tones which will be used as the stimulus for reflex testing. They should be of appropriate loudness and the circuit should be free of clicks or other noises. This daily check is not a substitute for the periodic calibration procedure described in Chapter 2.

Finally, obtain a tympanogram on your own ear. Having become familiar with your ear's characteristics, you can assess the impedance meter's function in this fashion, assuming of course that on a given day you do not have a cold or some other malady which affects the functioning of your ear. Along with the tympanogram, obtain acoustic reflexes. Having completed this brief pretest check, you are ready to meet your first patient of the day.

Otoscopic Observation

The use of an otoscope was discussed in Chapter 3. Perhaps you should review that section before reading further. In preparing for impedance testing, the purposes of otoscopic observation are (1) to look for wax in the ear canal and (2) to determine the size and shape of the external opening of the canal preparatory to selecting an adequate tip to insert over the probe tube.

If the canal is entirely occluded by wax, a valid measure of the middle ear system through tympanometry is not possible. We will discuss later the expected results of an occluded canal. It is possible to get a valid tympanogram when there is wax in the ear canal, providing the canal is not entirely blocked. Therefore, the observation of wax should not stop you from attempting a tympanogram. However, when wax is present, the probability of the probe tube becoming plugged is increased. This obstruction of the tube may happen as the tube is inserted in the canal or later during tympanometry as pressure changes in the canal force wax against the openings of the tube. In either case an invalid tympanogram will result. We will discuss the signs of this problem later.

You may observe eardrum perforation or a ventilating tube through the eardrum. Parents or patients may not always inform you of the presence of either. Fresh perforations of the drum are usually easy to see because of the discoloration of tissue surrounding the perforation. However, old healed perforations may be difficult to detect. Ventilating tubes are usually easy to see because they are in an easily observable area of the drum and are often brightly colored. Figure 7.6 shows a ventilating tube in place. The type shown in this figure is in common use. However, types with quite different appearance are used also. The interested reader is referred to Warder and Hughes (1977) for additional details. A characteristic tympanogram accompanies an eardrum perforation or ventilating tube. Details are presented later in this chapter.

As mentioned above, the other purpose of otoscopic observation is to discern the size and shape of the ear canal to help select an appropriate tip. You will also learn to make, based on the observation, an estimate of the difficulty to be expected in obtaining an air-tight seal for tympanometry. Canals which are elliptical in shape and which have a tendency toward collapsing are likely to give the most trouble.

Instructing the Patient

Minimum instructions are necessary for impedance testing. Under conventional conditions it is only necessary to tell the patient that no response is necessary during the test and to ask the patient to sit quietly, not talk, and avoid swallowing if possible. Later, prior to reflex testing,

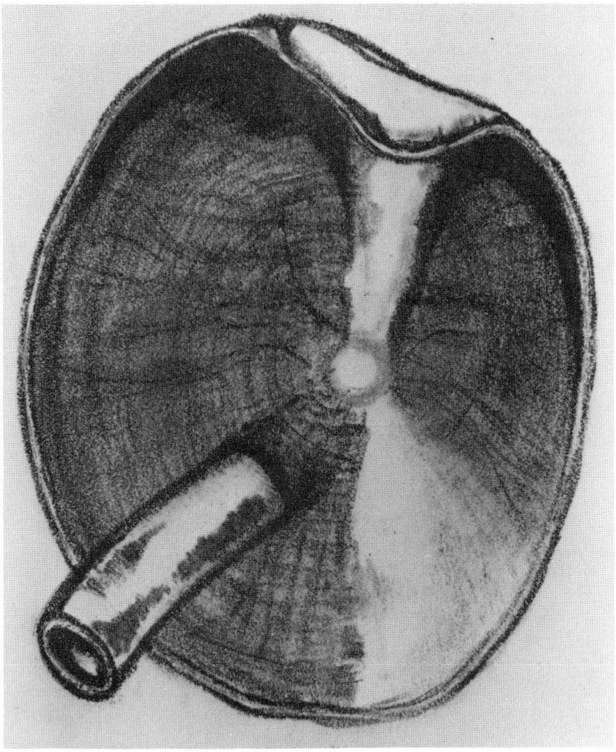

Fig. 7.6. Ventilating tube in place through the eardrum.

you may avoid startling the patient by indicating that loud sounds are about to be introduced.

Children are occasionally apprehensive about the idea of the probe tip being inserted into the ear canal. It sometimes helps to involve the child in the test by requesting assistance in picking out an appropriate tip to be placed over the probe tube. You should be sure that the probe tube cleaning wire, which looks like a hypodermic needle, is not visible before you introduce the child to the impedance meter.

Positioning the Headset

Be sure the impedance meter is ready for testing before you put the headset on the patient. If there is a manual air pump control, set it to the middle of its range before inserting the probe tube into the canal. Especially if a graphic recorder is in use to plot the tympanogram, a specific meter setting is necessary at the start of the test. Follow the instructions in the manual in this regard.

Select an appropriate tip and place it on the probe tube. Refer again to Figure 7.3, which shows tips of various styles. Those with the smoothly rounded tops are the most comfortable and are usually adequate for obtaining a seal. They have some tendency to be extruded when positive air pressure is pumped into the ear canal. Because of the comfort factor, I usually start with these tips and then go to others if I have difficulty obtaining or maintaining a seal. If you need to change the tip after the headset is on the patient, you may remove it and put on another without removing the headset. However, considerable force is necessary to replace the tip on some impedance meters. Be careful, therefore, that your hand does not slip, in which case you may sock the patient in the jaw.

Consistent with good audiometric practice, position the earphone cushion directly over one ear, with the earphone diaphragm right over the ear canal. Adjust the headset securely. The standard headset is too big for small heads. You should have an appropriately shaped piece of foam rubber available to place between the patient's head and the headset to improve the fit if necessary. When testing infants it may not be possible to keep the headset on the patient's head. It may be preferable to remove the earphone from the headset and hand hold the apparatus while inserting the probe tip in the ear and obtaining the tympanogram. For reflex testing, the earphone may be held against the other ear. This somewhat tedious procedure is illustrated in Figure 7.7.

Initially you will probably find problems with obtaining a seal the most frustrating part of impedance measurement. The difficulty will diminish with experience. The tip needs to be seated a little deeper and more firmly than most beginning clinicians expect. A little practice with a cooperative friend will reduce your anxiety and promote competence. During the insertion process, always watch the patient's facial expression for signs of discomfort.

Before inserting the tip, grasp the pinna gently and pull it upward and backward to straighten the canal. Adequate insertion may be promoted by asking the patient to open the mouth until insertion is completed. The resultant lowering of the mandible may help to get a seal in difficult cases but is usually not necessary.

Next, put positive pressure into the ear canal and ascertain by watching the manometer that the pressure is maintained. It is possible to obtain some tympanometric measures if a very slow leak is present but in almost all cases it is not necessary if adequate attention is given to achieving a seal.

In the uncommon instance when adequate insertion of an appropriate tip does not result in a seal the probe can be held by hand after insertion. Maintaining some inward pressure by hand may help keep the seal. However, holding the probe increases the possibility of occluding the opening of the tip by forcing it against the wall of the ear canal and

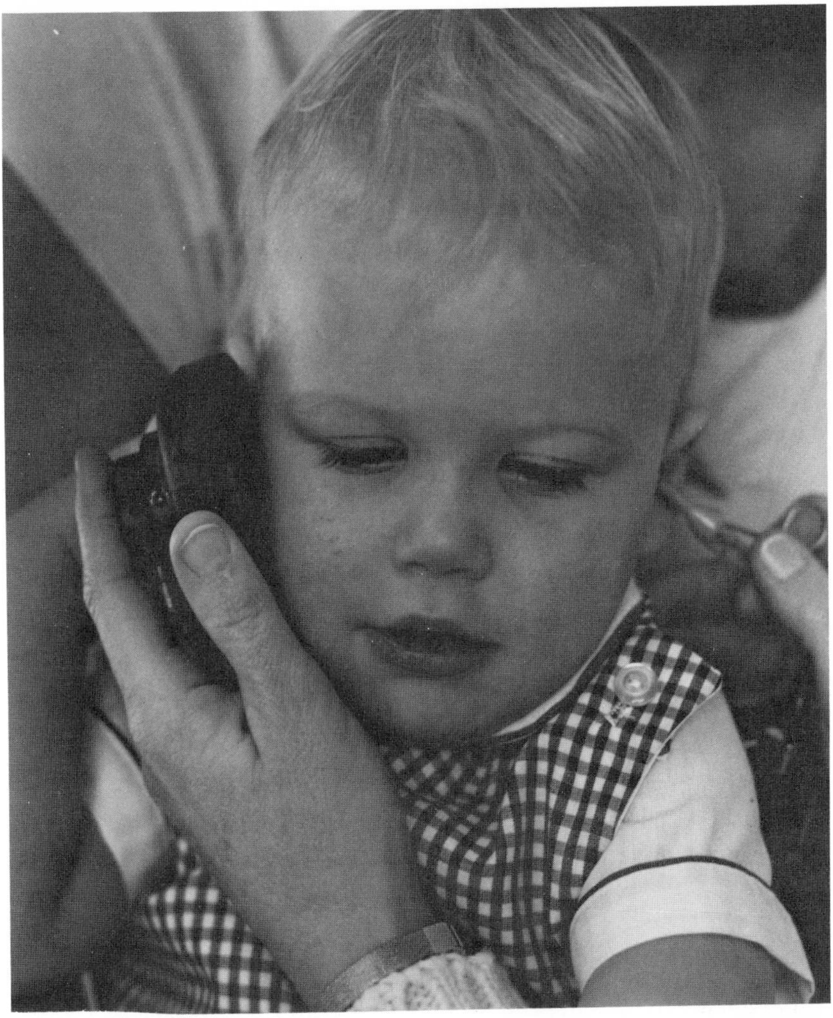

Fig. 7.7. Impedance measurement with an infant, illustrating how the probe tube and earphone can be hand held if the small size of the infant's head precludes standard positioning of the headset.

invalidating the tympanogram. Therefore, if you must hold the probe, accept the results only if they are consistent with an open probe tip. We will discuss how to make this judgment in a following section.

Obtaining the Tympanogram

Having obtained a seal, increase air pressure in the ear canal to +200 mm H_2O and begin obtaining the tympanogram. Details will vary according to the instrument you are using, clinic philosophy, and whether you are obtaining point-by-point information manually or a continuous measure recorded automatically. Follow the appropriate instructions in your manual. Regardless of details, the salient features are these: You will obtain compliance measures at different ear canal air pressure across a range from +200 to −200 (or −300 or −400) mm H_2O. Point-by-point measures are usually made at 100 mm H_2O pressure intervals. Increase the air pressure to +200 mm H_2O and read from the impedance meter the compliance which results at that setting. Record the value on the tympanogram as C_1. Change the canal pressure to +100 mm H_2O and so forth, reading and recording the compliance for each setting. Include −300 and −400 mm H_2O if the tympanogram is abnormal and it seems likely that the point of maximum compliance (C_2) may be forthcoming from these measures. These very negative values may be necessary to determine the peak of compliance in some ears. Record the peak compliance (in cm^3) and the canal pressure (in mm H_2O) at which it occurred. The canal air pressure which results in highest compliance is equivalent to the middle ear air pressure.

In summary, the tympanogram is quickly obtained following these steps: (1) obtain an air-tight seal; (2) take compliance measures while changing ear canal air pressure across a range ±200 mm H_2O, or to a more negative value if indicated; and (3) note the ear canal air pressure which resulted in the greatest compliance.

Determining Static Compliance

The static compliance can be computed from values derived from the tympanogram. The formula is $C_2 - C_1$. C_1 is the compliance obtained with +200 mm H_2O of pressure in the ear canal. C_2 is the peak compliance value. Record the results on the tympanogram form.

Obtaining Acoustic Reflex Thresholds

Most impedance instruments currently on the market incorporate a pure tone audiometer to supply the signals for acoustic reflex threshold testing. If yours does not you must, of course, supply one by attaching one earphone of an audiometer to the headset of the impedance unit.

Reflexes should be measured with the canal air pressure set to obtain maximum compliance. Small spontaneous compliance changes are usually present, causing some meter fluctuation. Usually the reflex can be detected in spite of this variability. However, if there are rapid and large random changes in compliance (as may occur if the eardrum is flaccid), compliance may be stablized with the canal pressure about −50 mm H_2O away from the compliance peak. This procedure will probably make reflex thresholds somewhat poorer. Rizzo and Greenberg (1979) reported that reflex thresholds of normals averaged about 6 dB poorer when ear canal pressure was changed from 0 to 80 mm H_2O. Obviously it is preferable to obtain reflex measures with canal air pressure adjusted to obtain maximum compliance.

A standard method for determining reflex threshold has not been established. One efficient procedure is to begin presentations just below the estimated reflex threshold. For example, when stimulating a normal ear, the best estimate for reflex threshold is 85 dB, so you might begin at 80 dB HL. Ascend in 5 dB steps, presenting a tone at each level, until a response occurs. Reduce the level 10 dB and ascend again to confirm the response. The lowest level at which an adequate compliance change can be reliably observed is the acoustic reflex threshold. The actual magnitude of change which constitutes a response will depend on the impedance instrument you are using and will be specified in the manual.

The magnitude of the reflex grows as signal level is increased above threshold. To confirm the reflex response in doubtful cases, present a signal 5 dB above the apparent threshold. An appreciable larger compliance change will result if the signal is actually above threshold. Another way to preclude acceptance of false positive responses is to look for a return to the prior compliance value when the stimulus terminates as well as for the compliance decrease after the onset of the stimulus.

CLASSIFYING TEST RESULTS

The purpose of basic impedance measurement is to confirm and extend information gained via conventional audiometry. Test results, therefore, are to be interpreted in conjunction with the information gained from the rest of the basic test battery. Integration of tympanometric and audiometric results is covered in Chapter 8. Classification of tympanograms and acoustic reflex thresholds is considered below.

Tympanograms

Jerger (1970) and Jerger and associates (1972) divided tympanograms into several types based on middle ear air pressure and static compliance. Feldman (1976b) developed a classification system based on a descriptive analysis of tympanogram pressure, amplitude, and shape. Jerger and his co-workers classified tympanograms into types A, B, and C.

Type A (Fig. 7.8) tympanograms are associated with normal middle ear function except for the two subtype A tympanograms described below. In all cases, type A tympanograms are consistent with normal Eustachian tube function. Type A tympanograms show a compliance maximum, or peak, with ear canal air pressure around 0 mm H_2O, or in any case less than −100 mm H_2O. Marked positive middle ear pressure is not common, although it might occur in early stages of suppurative

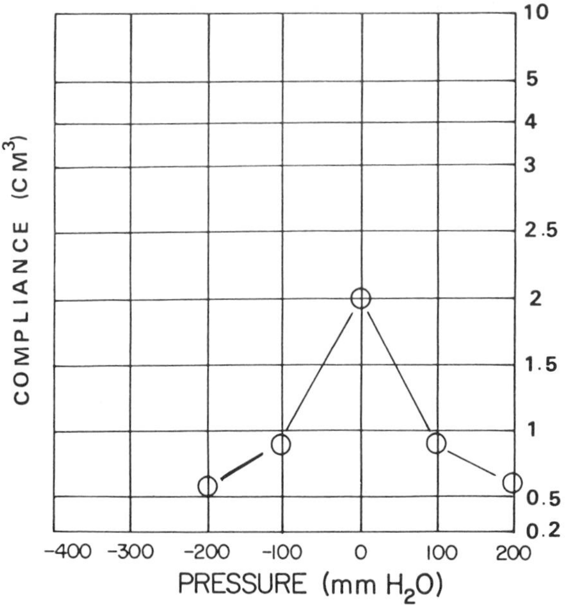

Fig. 7.8. Type A tympanogram, consistent with normal middle ear. Normal Eustachian tube function is indicated by the peak of compliance at 0 mm H_2O. Static compliance (C_2, 2.0 cm^3 − C_1, 0.6 cm^3) = 1.4 cm^3, within normal limits.

otitis media, an acute ear infection. More commonly marked positive middle ear pressure may be observed in an individual after forceful blowing of the nose. The pressure may exceed +200 mm H_2O in these cases, moving the compliance peak entirely off the tympanogram to the right. In such cases, the problem may be alleviated by asking the patient to swallow forcefully a few times and then repeating the preceeding measure.

Type B tympanograms (Fig. 7.9) show no peak of compliance at any measurable canal pressure. They are flat or rise slightly as air pressure in the ear canal is made more negative. This type results from an immobile eardrum, with little compliance change as canal pressure changes. Type B tympanograms are associated with fluid matter in the middle ear or other abnormalities which preclude mobility of the eardrum.

Type B tympanograms are commonly associated with serous otitis media. The terms serous otitis media, secretory otitis media, and middle ear effusion are used to describe the condition in which fluid is present in the middle ear cavity in association with Eustachian tube dysfunction. This problem is the most common cause of conductive hearing loss in children (Ginsberg and White, 1978). When the Eustachian tube does not open periodically to supply air to the middle ear space, negative

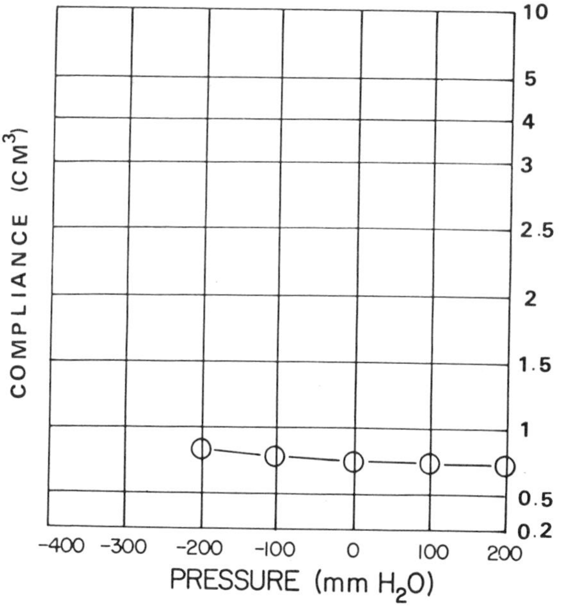

Fig. 7.9. Type B tympanogram, showing no peak of compliance.

middle ear pressure develops. Subsequently, fluid may also develop in the middle ear cavity.

Type C tympanograms (Fig. 7.10) show a peak of compliance equal to or more negative than −100 mm H_2O (Jerger, 1970). This indication of negative middle ear pressure suggests Eustachian tube dysfunction. As discussed below, there is some disagreement about the actual negative value which should differentiate normal and abnormal ears and the adequacy of tympanometry to assess Eustachian tube function.

Two additional tympanograms, types D and E, have been reported by Liden *et al.* (1974a). The type D shows a double peak, or notch, in the area where compliance is greatest. Liden *et al.* (1974b) reported a high incidence of type D tympanograms in otherwise normal individuals with scars on the eardrum or with flaccid drums and normal hearing. Otherwise, diagnostic significance has not been attached to the type D tympanogram. The type E tympanogram was described by the authors just cited as "undulating" in the region of maximum compliance. The rolling up-and-down compliance occurred in patients with ossicular discontinuity, disruption of the ossicular chain. The authors attributed this particular pattern to the fact that they used an 800-Hz rather than 220-Hz probe tone. The expected pattern in discontinuity associated with use of a 220-Hz probe tone is described below.

Jerger and associates (1974c) described two A subtypes. In these,

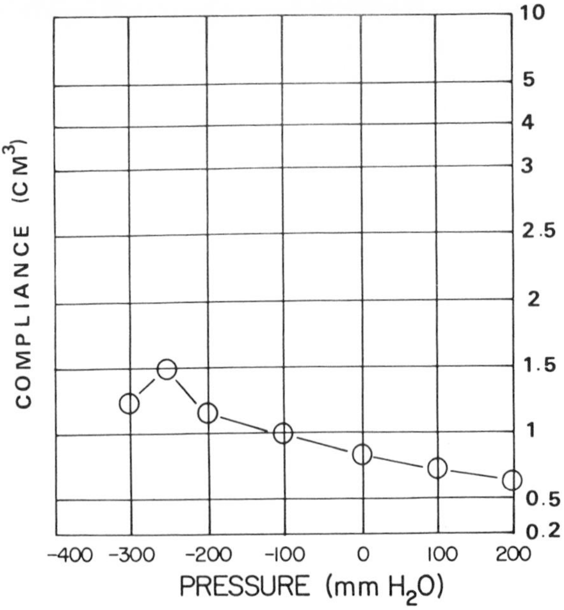

Fig. 7.10. Type C tympanogram. The negative pressure is consistent with Eustachian tube dysfunction.

middle ear air pressure was within normal limits, consistent with normal Eustachian tube function. However, static compliance was outside the range considered normal by these authors. They found a range of static compliance from 0.3 to 1.65 cm^3 in 825 subjects with presumably normal middle ears. There is not universal agreement regarding the normal range of static compliance. Northern and Grimes (1978) suggested 0.28–2.5 cm^3. They indicated that values which are clearly outside this range should be considered diagnostically significant.

The designation of abnormally stiff middle ear systems is A_s (Fig. 7.11). This type is commonly associated with otosclerosis. The A_d tympanogram type (Fig. 7.12) is reserved for abnormally compliant middle ear systems. This configuration is seen in ossicular discontinuity, accompanied by conductive hearing loss. It is also in patients who may have normal hearing sensitivity and flaccid eardrums. Diagnostic information based solely on static compliance is limited by the considerable overlap which exists among diagnostic categories. For example, while otosclerosis tends to stiffen the middle ear system, some otosclerotics exhibit static compliance within the normal range, and many individuals without otosclerosis exhibit reduced static compliance. Similar overlap exists among other diagnostic categories.

As mentioned above, Feldman (1976a) advocated interpretation of tympanometric information on the basis of tympanogram pressure,

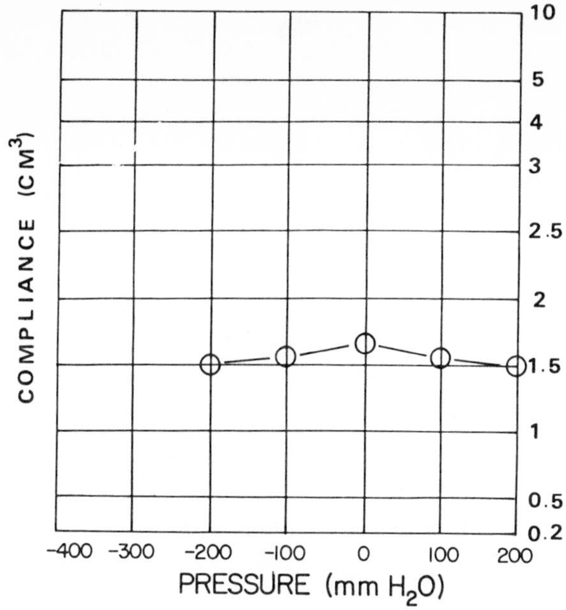

Fig. 7.11. Type A_s tympanogram, showing abnormally increased stiffness. Static compliance (C_2, 1.7 cm^3 − C_1, 1.5 cm^3) = 0.2 cm^3. Normal Eustachian tube function is indicated by the peak of compliance at 0 mm H_2O.

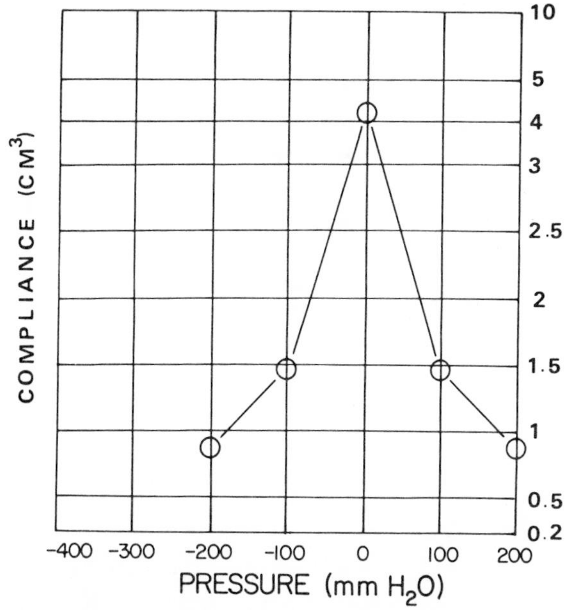

Fig. 7.12. Type A_d tympanogram, showing abnormal decrease in stiffness. Normal Eustachian tube function is indicated by the peak of compliance at 0 mm H_2O. Static compliance (C_2, 4.2 cm^3 − C_1, 0.8 cm^3) = 3.4 cm^3, above the normal range.

amplitude, and shape. In this system, pressure is divided into normal, negative, positive, and absent categories. The "absent" category indicates a fluid-filled middle ear. Amplitude consists of normal, flaccid, and stiff categories. Shape includes normal, peaked, flat, and notched classifications. The interaction of these factors indicates various disorders. A summary of Feldman's classifications, comparison with Jerger's typing system, and tympanometric interpretation are shown in Figure 7.13.

As discussed more extensively in Chapter 8, type A tympanograms are expected in those individuals with normal hearing or with sensorineural losses. These individuals should have normal middle ear mechanisms and therefore normal tympanograms. Individuals with conductive loss are expected to have type A_s, A_d, B, or C tympanograms. However, it is possible to observe any of these tympanograms with only a minimal reduction in hearing sensitivity or with only a small air-bone gap. Conversely, the conductive component may be large. This variability increases the importance of looking at all of the results of the basic test battery during interpretation.

Tympanometry has other applications. Whether a ventilating tube in the eardrum is open or obstructed can be established or the presence of an eardrum perforation can be confirmed. Similar tympanograms occur in these two situations. Compliance will not change across the pressure changes in the ear canal and the equivalent volume reading will be large, since the middle ear space will at all times be included in the measurement. Northern and Grimes (1978) indicate that the normal C_1 compliance (measured with +200 mm H_2O pressure in the canal) is 0.6–0.8 cm^3 in a child and 1.0–1.5 cm^3 in an adult, but the C_1 value for an adult may be 4 or 5 cm^3 or even more if a drum perforation or patent ventilating tube is present. Additionally, there may be a loss of all or part of the ear canal pressure when the patient swallows if the Eustachian tube is functioning properly. This pressure loss is due to pressure escaping through the middle ear and Eustachian tube. Conversely, if the ventilating tube is not open, the equivalent volume (C_1) should be within the expected range. The shape of the tympanogram in such a case will be determined by conditions prevailing in the middle ear.

Flat tympanograms may also be expected when the canal is securely plugged with earwax. In this case the equivalent volume is often smaller than usual, because wax has reduced cavity size. When wax is observed, the tympanogram may be useful to determine if the canal is entirely occluded. If not, compliance should change along with ear canal air pressure unless, of course, a middle ear pathology prevents the change. One precautionary note: a flat tympanogram with extremely small equivalent volume (plotted right along the bottom of the tympanogram) suggests that the probe tube itself is occluded, either by wax or by its

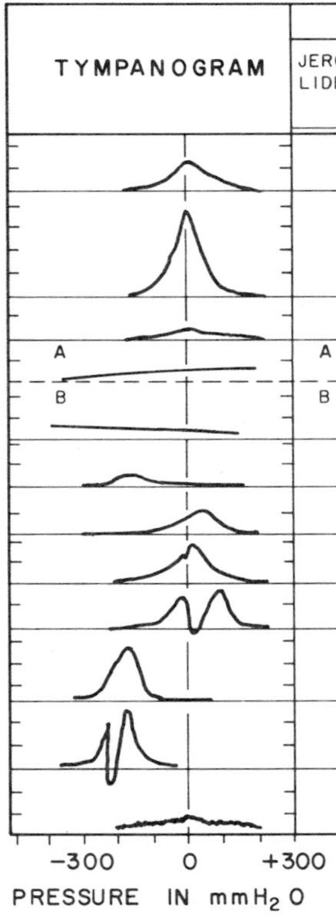

CLASSIFICATION: JERGER (1970) LIDEN et al (1974) TYPE	FELDMAN (1975) PRESSURE	FELDMAN (1975) AMPLITUDE	FELDMAN (1975) SHAPE	INTERPRETATION
A	NORMAL	NORMAL	NORMAL	NORMAL MIDDLE EAR
A_D	NORMAL	FLACCID	PEAKED	EAR DRUM ABNORMALITY OR, WITH HEARING LOSS, OSSICULAR DISCONTINUITY
A_S	NORMAL	STIFF	NORMAL	OTOSCLEROSIS
A ? B	ABSENT–NEG.	STIFF	FLAT	(A=HIGH FREQUENCY, B=LOW FREQUENCY PROBE TONE) FLUID–FILLED MIDDLE EAR
B ? B	ABSENT–NEG.	STIFF	FLAT A+B CONVERGE	
C	-125 mm	STIFF	NORMAL	LOW COMPLIANT MIDDLE EAR SYSTEM SEEN IN SEROUS OTITIS MEDIA
?	+ 90 mm	NORMAL	NORMAL	OVER–INFLATED BY VALSALVA MANEUVER OR ACUTE OTITIS MEDIA
D	NORMAL	FLACCID	NOTCHED	SCARRED EARDRUM
E	NORMAL	FLACCID	DEEP, BROAD NOTCHING	(HIGH FREQUENCY PROBE TONE) OSSICULAR DISCONTINUITY
C	-200 mm	FLACCID	NORMAL	OSSICULAR DISCONTINUITY AND POOR EUSTACHIAN TUBE FUNCTION
? C/E	-200 mm	FLACCID	DEEP, BROAD NOTCHING	(HIGH FREQUENCY PROBE TONE) OSSICULAR DISCONTINUITY AND POOR EUSTACHIAN TUBE FUNCTION
A_S	NORMAL	STIFF	VASCULAR PERTURBATION	GLOMUS TUMOR

Fig. 7.13. Classification and interpretation of tympanograms. (Modified and reprinted with permission from: Feldman, A.: *Ann. Otol. Rhinol. Laryngol., 85 (Suppl. 25)*: 202–208, 1976.)

opening being pressed against the canal wall. In this instance, remove the probe tube, clean it, and reobtain the tympanogram.

Acoustic Reflex Thresholds

Acoustic reflex threshold measurements add information about the type of hearing loss: conductive, sensory, or neural. Jerger (1970) found the modal value for the acoustic reflex threshold in normal ears to be 85 dB HL, regardless of subject age (across a range from 2 to 59 years). However, in about ⅓ of the subjects in the age range from 2 to 5 years, reflexes could not be elicited at 110 dB HL. Jerger could not determine whether this high incidence of absent reflexes was associated with a maturational factor or if there was a higher incidence of undetected middle ear problems in the young age group which obscured or otherwise prevented measurement of the reflex. Jerger, assessing normal ears, found a distribution of reflex thresholds about 40 dB wide, ranging from 70 to 110 dB HL.

Jerger (1970) reported that the sensation level necessary to elicit the acoustic reflex was progressively reduced in ears with sensorineural (presumably cochlear) hearing loss. He concluded that reflexes occurring at sensation levels less than 60 dB indicated the presence of loudness recruitment. As mentioned earlier, loudness recruitment has been reported in sensory rather than neural losses (Jerger and Harford, 1960), and its measurement contributes to the differential diagnosis of cochlear versus retrocochlear disorder. Jerger and co-workers (1972) reported reflex thresholds in cochlear losses as low as 25 dB SL. On the other hand, retrocochlear problems are expected to result in an increase in threshold, absence of the reflex, or abnormal decay of the acoustic reflex (Jerger *et al.*, 1974b).

If the inner ear is normal, the acoustic reflex requires a signal about 85 dB above the air conduction threshold. Therefore, reflex thresholds will be elevated when the stimulated ear has a conductive loss. Elicitation of the acoustic reflex becomes unlikely in conductive losses when the air conduction thresholds reach about 25 dB, since maximum output levels of the conventional audiometer then prevent a presentation level sufficient to overcome the conductive component. The measure provides useful corroborative information to the pure tone audiogram. If air-bone gaps suggest a larger conductive component but acoustic reflexes are present, retesting is in order.

Even if the stimulated ear is normal, slight middle ear pathology in the ear to which the probe tone is directed may prevent measurement of the reflex. It is even possible for the reflex to be obscured although the probe tone ear does not show an appreciable air-bone gap. Children may have bone conduction sensitivity of −10 to −20 dB, lower than can be measured with the conventional audiometer, which has a minimum output of 0 dB HL. Thus, small conductive components may exist without a measurable air-bone gap. In any case, an air-bone gap of 5–10 dB or larger is expected to obscure the reflex. Jerger and associates (1974c) reported 50% presence of reflex with a 5 dB air-bone gap in the ear with the probe tone, and less than 25% presence when the air-bone gap was 10 dB. Uncommon exceptions include some conductive disorders which do not inhibit measurement of the reflex. Middle ear cholesteatoma (cyst) may not inhibit reflexes if it does not involve the eardrum or ossicular chain. In rare cases reflexes may persist with ossicular discontinuity if fibers associated with the chain remain attached or if the disruption is medial (inward) to the attachment of the stapedius muscle to the stapes (Wilber, 1976).

IMPEDANCE MEASUREMENTS AND SCREENING

The purpose of screening is to differentiate normal and abnormal individuals within a given population. I have postponed discussion of impedance measures for screening until the end of the chapter so that you can approach this complex issue with some knowledge of impedance testing.

Most of the discussion of impedance measurement in screening has centered around children—primarily school age children. Eagles *et al.* (1967) established that pure tone audiometric screening can be quite efficient for detecting children who have handicapping losses of auditory sensitivity and problems of sufficient magnitude to cause major difficulty in classroom communication. However, the same study established that pure tone audiometric screening is inefficient to detect ear pathologies manifested by otologic abnormalities. In fact, 50% of the children with otologic abnormalities (inflamed eardrums, drum perforations, chronic otitis media) retained hearing sensitivity good enough to pass routine pure tone screening tests.

The advent of impedance measurement brought hope for a more sensitive method of detecting auditory disorders in children on a screening basis. Problems developed in experimental programs. The most common was over-referral. That is, some children referred for medical examinations after failing impedance screening were reported to be otologically normal. There was difficulty in setting failure criteria which would detect serious and continuing problems without an unacceptable number of children who had no apparent problems also being referred.

The number of false positives can be high in any screening program. For example, Melnick and associates (1964) found that 50% of the children who failed an initial pure tone screening passed on being rescreened. The stringency which can be assigned to criteria for failure depends on the intended followup. If additional audiologic testing is to be the next step, criteria can be more stringent. In this instance, false positive cases can be weeded out and those with problems can be referred on for medical examination with additional information useful to the physician making the examination. However, in some programs medical examination may be the next step after screening failure. This procedure is risky under any circumstances because of the limited information available to the parent and the physician. If this procedure is followed the criteria need to be less stringent to reduce the number of apparent false positives. Walton (1975) commented that the problem of apparent over-referral is complicated by the inability of otoscopic examination to detect small middle ear disorders to which tympanometry is sensitive. Additionally, some middle ear disorders fluctuate and may be present during tympanometric screening but absent at the time of medical examination.

McCandless and Thomas (1974) suggested a combination of tympanometric and acoustic reflex screening. They used criteria for failure of middle ear pressure more negative than −100 mm H_2O and absence of acoustic reflex for a 1000 Hz tone at 100 dB HL. They reported a false negative rate of only 4–6% and commented that most children whose ears appeared near normal otoscopically but who failed the screening procedure were found to have beginning or resolving otitis media.

To detect children with middle ear problems but avoid a large number of false positives, Brooks (1977) recommended a screening procedure based on two tests separated by an optimum interval. He reported that a 6-week interval between tests was adequate to reduce referral of children with transient problems which resolved spontaneously while children with continuing middle ear problems still obtained the necessary medical attention.

Here are some procedures which may permit the efficient use of tympanometric screening without undue problems associated with false positive referrals. As a preliminary, I should remind you that tympanometric screening is only useful for detecting conductive hearing disorders. Usually programs which use tympanometric screening incorporate conventional screening with a 4000 Hz pure tone at an appropriate level (for example, 25 dB HL) to search for individuals with sensorineural loss. Sensorineural loss, when present, commonly involves this frequency.

One procedure based on a tympanometric screening model is to refer for further testing children who have type B tympanograms or those with negative middle ear pressure of −160 mm H_2O or greater. Recall that the type B tympanogram is one which shows no peak of compliance and is commonly seen in cases of middle ear effusion. The value −160 mm H_2O was selected because of an initial recommendation of Walton (1975). Children who fail according to these criteria are then given additional audiologic evaluation. They are referred for medical examination if any two of the following three conditions are present: (1) a consistent air-bone gap of 10 dB or more at adjacent octave intervals, (2) generally absent acoustic reflexes, or (3) persistence of negative middle ear pressures of −160 mm H_2O or greater.

The American Speech and Hearing Association (1978b) has proposed guidelines for screening of middle ear function. Children are to be divided into three classes on the basis of tympanometric and reflex screening. Class 1 children pass the screening by showing essentially normal middle ear pressures and reflex responses to a 1000 Hz tone at 100 dB HL. Class 2 (at risk) children have abnormal middle ear pressure more negative than −200 mm H_2O *or* absent reflex. They are rescreened in 3–5 weeks. Class 3 children (fail) have abnormal middle ear pressure *and* an absent reflex. They are referred for audiologic and medical examination.

Research regarding the best procedures for incorporating tympanometry into screening programs is continuing. For detecting medical ear disorders, it holds promise as a sensitive screening device. Paradise and Smith (1979) studied the literature on tympanometric screening. In view of unsolved problems they concluded that rather than large-scale screening programs we need extensive research on both tympanometric screening and secretory otitis media, the major disorder contributing to tympanometric failures. For programs whose aim in screening is detection of presently handicapping hearing losses, pure tone screening appears to be adequate. For those programs which also intend to detect ear disorders and prevent the development of handicapping hearing problems, tympanometric screening may be useful. Research to date indicates, however, that tympanometric screening is not a shortcut to cheaper or easier identification programs and that effective programs will require adequate audiologic and otologic input.

SUMMARY

Conventional audiometry delineates types of hearing loss—conductive, sensorineural, or mixed. In some cases, masking problems or other procedural difficulties make validity of conventional test results questionable. The purpose of impedance measurement is to confirm and extend information gained via conventional procedures.

The tympanogram is a measure of middle ear function. Specifically it measures compliance as a function of changing ear canal air pressures. The tympanogram permits specification of middle ear pressure. If Eustachian tube function is normal, middle ear pressure should approximate the ambient pressure, that is, the pressure of the atmosphere surrounding the individual. Thus, tympanometry permits measurement of Eustachian tube function. Absence of a compliance peak as ear canal pressure changes suggests the presence of fluid in the middle ear space or other conditions precluding mobility of the eardrum. Reduced compliance measured at the eardrum may suggest additional pathologies.

Because compliance changes in conjunction with the acoustic (stapedial) reflex, the threshold of that reflex can be established. In normal ears a hearing level approximating 85 dB is needed, with considerable variability, to elicit the reflex. Occurrence of the reflex at sensation levels less than 60 dB is consistent with loudness recruitment and a cochlear rather than retrocochlear disorder in cases of sensorineural losses. A conductive component of about 25 dB in the stimulated ear or 5–10 dB in the ear with the probe tone is expected to prevent measurement of the reflex. Therefore, the presence of the reflex is incompatible with significant conductive loss in the ear which contains the probe tube.

Experimental use of tympanometric screening has shown that the procedure can be useful for detecting middle ear disorders which would be missed in conventional pure tone screening. There have been some problems with over-referral. In the preceding pages, some procedures for reducing over-referral are suggested. If the goal of a screening program is to detect currently handicapping hearing loss, pure tone screening is adequate. If the goal is to detect ear disorders and prevent the development of handicapping problems, tympanometric screening is a promising tool which requires further investigation.

STUDY QUESTIONS

1. Review the following characteristics of the Impedance Record: What are the units on (a) the abscissa? (b) the ordinate? Which ear is considered the test ear in acoustic reflex testing?
2. How do you identify each of the following tympanogram types? What is the interpretation of each type: (a) type A? (b) type B? (c) type C? (d) type A_s? (e) type A_d?
3. How is static compliance computed? What is the expected range of static compliance in normal ears?
4. What are the expected range and modal value of acoustic reflex thresholds in normal ears? What is the relationship between loudness recruitment and acoustic reflex thresholds? How is this relationship recorded on the Impedance Record?
5. Review the procedures for impedance testing. What are some methods which may help if you are having difficulty (a) keeping the headset on the patient because of small head size? (b) maintaining an acoustic seal? (c) observing reflex responses because of meter fluctuation?
6. What are the potential advantages and disadvantages of impedance screening in a hearing conservation program?

CHAPTER 8

Interpreting Test Results

In the previous chapters we have discussed the basic audiologic battery. The battery includes pure tone air and bone conduction thresholds, speech thresholds, speech discrimination testing, and impedance measurements. We will now look more closely at interpretation of the test battery and discuss the meaning and utility of the results. We will also consider interaction of the tests: how they support each other and extend information gained from individual tests. You should realize, however, that this book cannot tell you all you need to know about interpreting audiometric test results. You must improve your skill through experience and continued study, as more is learned about the relationship between test results and auditory disorders.

A review of audiometric standards may be in order at this point. Audiometers are currently calibrated to ISO 1964 or ANSI 1969 norms. However, if you look at old audiograms for comparison with a patient's present hearing, you must consider the possibility that test results were obtained with an audiometer calibrated to the 1951 ASA norms, which are considerably different from those of the present. Audiograms obtained with ISO or ANSI calibrated audiometers will contain a printed statement to that effect. However, ASA audiograms commonly contained no statement relative to calibration standards. You can identify them by this omission, the date, or by the fact that it was conventional on ASA audiograms for the decibel scale to include the range from -10 to 100 dB HL, while ISO or ANSI audiograms usually range from 0 to 110 dB HL. The ISO and ANSI standards are more stringent than the ASA standard. Therefore, at any given decibel HL, the ISO or ANSI output is weaker. As a result, thresholds obtained via an ISO or ANSI calibrated audiometer will look poorer than when obtained with an ASA audiometer. To convert thresholds from ASA to ISO or ANSI standards "make the thresholds poorer"—*add* the differences between

Table 8.1
Difference in Decibels Between ASA and ISO-ANSI Threshold Norms, Rounded to the Nearest 5 dB[a,b]

Frequency in Hz									
125	250	500	1000	1500	2000	3000	4000	6000	8000
10	15	15	10	10	10	10	5	10[c]	10

[a] To convert ASA audiograms to ISO-ANSI, add these values to the ASA thresholds.
[b] To convert ISO-ANSI thresholds to ASA, subtract these values from the ISO or ANSI thresholds.
[c] ISO value is 10 dB; ANSI value is 5 dB.

the norms. Conversely, to convert from ISO or ANSI to ASA "make the thresholds better"—*subtract* the values which represent the differences between the two norms. A conversion chart is given in Table 8.1.

PURPOSES OF THE BASIC TEST BATTERY

The specific goals of an audiologic evaluation will vary, depending on the patient. However, the main purposes of the basic evaluation are listed below:

1. Pure tone air conduction and speech threshold testing measures auditory sensitivity, revealing magnitude of hearing loss.
2. Bone conduction thresholds, when compared with air conduction results, differentiate conductive, sensorineural, and mixed loss. Impedance measures provide additional information about the nature of the conductive or sensorineural loss.
3. Discrimination testing, in conjunction with sensitivity measures, permits an estimate of the communication handicap to be expected from the hearing loss.
4. Interpretation of the battery and observation of patient behavior may indicate need for additional testing, such as hearing aid evaluation, site-of-lesion tests, medical examination, or evaluation by other professionals.

SOME NONAUDITORY FACTORS WHICH INFLUENCE MAGNITUDE OF HANDICAP

Many factors influence the amount of handicap in hearing loss. I have called some "nonauditory" because they are not a part of the hearing loss itself. Other factors, designated "auditory," are an integral part of the hearing loss. The factors discussed below are important in determining how handicapping a given hearing loss will be. Some are easy to measure, others are difficult. It is important to consider these factors in the overall analysis of the hearing disorder.

Age at Onset

Congenital hearing loss (present at birth), or a loss which develops before the acquisition of language, produces a greater handicap than an equal loss acquired later in life. Learning language and speech in the presence of hearing loss is a difficult task. Speech disorders are often the most noticeable result of congenital hearing loss. However, language deficits are a more important problem. Reading, writing, and speaking skills are dependent on language ability.

There is evidence that hearing affects vocal behavior from an early age. Weir (1966) reported that normal hearing infants of various nationalities develop patterns of vocalization characteristic of their native language by the age of 5 months. McNeill (1965) estimated that the basic components of a normal hearing child's native language are acquired by age 3–4½ years. Congruent with this estimate, Goetzinger (1978) reported that 3 years of age is the critical time for onset of hearing loss. Losses acquired before this age should be considered prelinguistic, and the children involved will in later years behave in a fashion similar to those with congenital loss as far as language development is concerned.

Goetzinger (1962) estimated that congenital sensorineural hearing loss of 30–45 dB can cause language and speech retardation of about 12–18 months at a chronological age of 3 years. Evidence that the language deficit does not disappear as the child grows older was accumulated by Goetzinger *et al.* (1964). They found that 9–16 year old school children with small congenital hearing losses had poorer reading scores than normal hearing children of the same age in the school system.

With greater hearing loss, the problem is more severe. A survey from Gallaudet College (Ries, 1972) showed that the typical adult deaf person (18 years and older) was reading at the level of the typical hearing student in the fourth grade. The median Verbal Aptitude scores from the Graduate Record Examination of seniors graduating from Galluadet College (a college for deaf students) during the period 1957 to 1964 ranged from 240 to 330, while the median for the normative group of hearing college students for that period was 490 (Babbidge, 1965).

The general conclusion of these studies is that congenital or prelinguistic hearing loss will result in greater handicap than similar loss developed later in life. Language level is likely to be below normal and the development of normal speech is extremely difficult.

Hearing losses acquired in adulthood may bring special problems associated with age at onset. Losses acquired during the working years may be a threat to job security. Hearing loss acquired in old age may be complicated by other accumulating physical disorders as well as social and economic problems.

Manner of Onset

Different behavior results from sudden bilateral loss than from loss with gradual onset. Depending on magnitude, sudden hearing loss can have catastrophic effects. Life style is often disrupted. In adults, loss of job is possible. Depending on the circumstances, there may be questions in the patient's mind about the cause of the loss and anxiety about auditory recovery or further deterioration of hearing. On the whole, sudden loss is likely to be associated with medical, psychological, social, and occupational problems of great magnitude. A prompt multidisciplinary rehabilitative program is indicated.

Hearing loss with gradual onset often spares the individual the trauma of sudden loss. The problems are no less real, however, and may be just as great. In the early stages of slowly progressive loss, the person may not identify the problem as hearing loss because of the gradual deterioration. This likelihood is increased if the loss begins in the higher frequencies which contribute less to the perceived loudness of speech, although important for intelligibility. It may be a long while before the individual identifies the problem and seeks professional help. Because the problem develops so slowly the individual has time to adapt to changes in hearing as they occur. There may be real difficulty understanding and accepting the magnitude of the problem. These are prerequisites to doing something about it. Finally, the magnitude of the handicap will be affected by whether the loss continues to progress, or stabilizes at some level. For example, presbycusis (loss associated with aging) typically continues to progress at a slow rate and may be accompanied by other physical and mental deterioration. On the other hand, the progression of noise induced loss is expected to stop if the individual is no longer exposed to the noise or takes effective measures to protect the ears.

Intelligence

A highly intelligent hearing impaired person has the potential to minimize the handicap associated with hearing loss better than does a less intelligent person. Particularly in congenital loss, the demands on intelligence of learning language and speech and of the entire educational process are great. Some causes of hearing loss are associated with multiple handicaps, including mental retardation (Vernon, 1966 and 1967a-c).

Motivation

Problems associated with hearing loss may be poorly understood and very difficult to solve. Professional help may not be readily available or affordable. Therefore, individuals may not be motivated to work actively to overcome their problems. They may give up, making unsatisfactory adjustments as necessary to exist without effective communication. These may include withdrawing from social events, changing jobs, or reducing competitiveness in society. In addition to understanding the problem and what can be done, most hearing impaired persons need counseling and support to maintain the motivation needed to combat the many problems of hearing loss.

Training

An effective training program facilitates use of residual hearing. Children born with severe or profound loss may not learn the utility of sound and may not use their residual hearing consistently unless trained to do so. Many adults with acquired hearing loss who try a hearing aid do not learn to use it effectively. Therefore, they may reject the aid or use it with less than optimum results. Thus, training in many areas relating to hearing impairment is an important determinant of the extent of handicap associated with a given hearing loss.

Other Handicapping Conditions

Hearing loss, both congenital and acquired, may be associated with other physical and mental problems. Visual problems, neuromotor disorders, and mental retardation are examples. These disorders may mask symptoms of hearing loss and delay its identification. The multiple handicap makes habilitation more difficult. For example, visual impairment removes the modality which may otherwise be heavily relied upon in training hearing impaired individuals.

Demands on Hearing

The role which hearing plays in our lives fluctuates from time to time and from person to person. Hearing is obviously important in early childhood for language and speech development and later for education. While hearing is important in most occupations, the demands placed on hearing by various occupations vary considerably. Some jobs require the person to hear everything that is said. Other jobs require communication under difficult conditions, such as listening in noise or hearing faint or distant speech. While the personal and social demands on hearing are retained by retired individuals, occupational demands are reduced. Thus, demands placed on the person's hearing are an important contributor to magnitude of handicap and to determination of rehabilitative needs.

Family Support

Assistance and encouragement from family are important both to children with congenital hearing loss and adults with acquired loss. The attitude of family members and the understanding they display are important though complex factors which contribute heavily to the manner in which the hearing impaired person copes with hearing loss. Kapteyn (1977) reported family support to be an important factor in successful orientation to hearing aid use.

Socioeconomic Status

Socioeconomic factors play a role in obtaining adequate medical treatment of reversible hearing loss. Training or rehabilitation programs are beyond the economic reach of many hearing impaired persons. The cost of hearing aids is a particular problem for many elderly hearing impaired individuals.

SOME AUDITORY FACTORS WHICH INFLUENCE AMOUNT OF HANDICAP

The nonauditory factors discussed above will obviously influence the amount of handicap resulting from a given hearing loss. Therefore, people with the same audiometric characteristics will not exhibit the same handicaps. It is necessary to assess each hearing impaired person on the basis of nonauditory as well as auditory factors. Such assessment enables us to estimate the effect of hearing loss on social, educational, and vocational life. We can also predict the need for and the expected effectiveness of rehabilitation.

From the auditory tests of the basic battery, information is gained about (1) type of loss, (2) magnitude of loss, (3) configuration of loss, and (4) auditory discrimination ability. These auditory factors influence the amount of handicap. You should remember that they are interrelated and influence each other even though discussed separately below.

Type of Loss

You are by now familiar with the concept that hearing losses are classified as conductive, sensorineural, or mixed. Conductive losses result from disorders in the outer or middle ear which reduce the effective intensity of sound reaching the inner ear. Sensorineural losses are associated with disorders in the inner ear or auditory nerve. Mixed losses consist of both a conductive and a sensorineural component present in the same ear. Audiometric and behavioral characteristics of each type of loss are discussed below.

Conductive Loss. Conductive loss is (1) potentially correctible and (2) involves only loss of sensitivity with no accompanying loss of auditory discrimination ability. As with all generalizations, there are exceptions. Some congenital conductive disorders and some chronic middle ear infections are difficult cases which may not be resolved by surgical or medical treatment. Because of these reasons and because some people do not elect surgical correction, permanent conductive problems will be encountered. People with acquired conductive loss, provided with effective amplification, show no reduction in discrimination scores. However, you may see reduction in these scores in children with large bilateral conductive loss because of the effect of the hearing loss on language ability.

People with conductive loss are expected to speak at a reduced intensity level because they can hear themselves well by bone conduction and do not react with the Lombard reflex (an increase in the voice level to compensate for background noise) to the same extent as normals. Persons with conductive loss are also supposed to hear better in noise than in quiet, a phenomenon called Paracusis of Willis. This improvement may occur when the person with conductive loss benefits from increase of the speaker's voice due to background noise level but, because of the loss, fails to hear much of the noise. For this phenomenon to operate, the magnitude of the loss and the level of the noise must be just right. There are many exceptions to both of the generalizations mentioned above, depending on the individual personality, speaking habits, and communication situation.

The audiometric Weber is expected to lateralize to the involved ear in unilateral conductive loss. In bilateral losses, as a rule, the Weber should lateralize to the ear with the greater conductive component. Refer to audiograms in this chapter for illustrations of Weber test results.

Recall that the audiometric indicators of conductive loss are air-bone gap and abnormal tympanograms. Acoustic reflexes are generally absent or have elevated thresholds. Figures 8.1–8.3 show audiometric test results in conductive disorders.

Sensorineural Loss. Sensorineural loss is expected to be permanent and irreversible, and may be progressive. Some sensorineural losses have a temporary component. For example, noise exposure may result in a temporary threshold shift although the long term effect of noise exposure can be irreversible loss. Surgery may improve hearing in a limited number of sensorineural losses with specific etiologies, such as Meniere's disease and VIIIth nerve tumor, if performed at the right

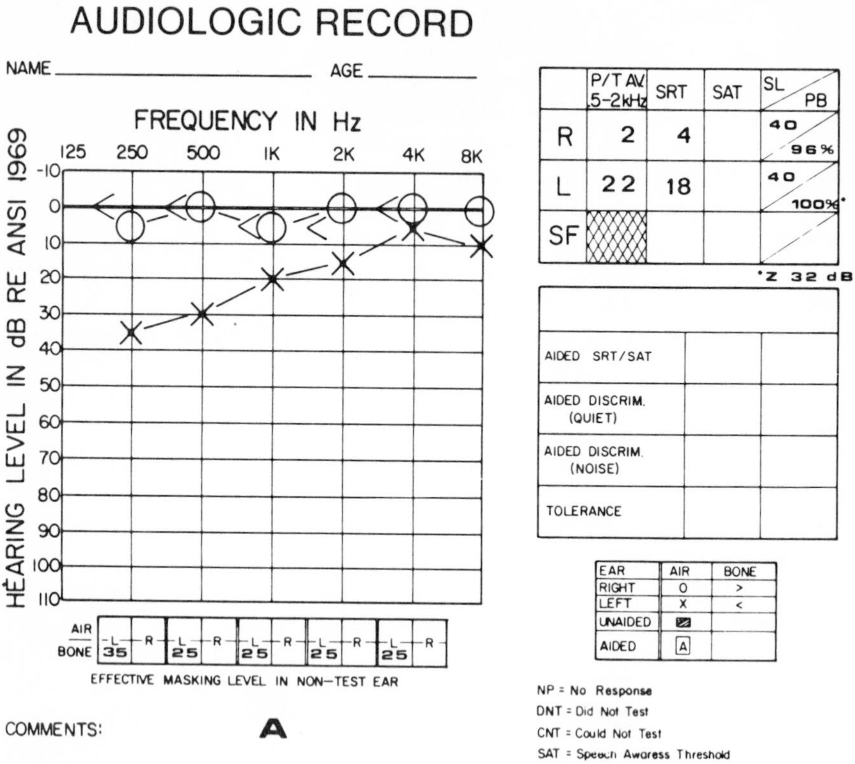

Fig. 8.1. Conductive disorder associated with serous otitis media on the left ear. Note that masking was necessary during bone conduction testing of the left ear, and effective masking levels are recorded below the audiogram. In our clinic we record the amount of effective masking at the bottom of the audiogram under the *test* ear. In this example the right ear was masked while obtaining left ear bone conduction thresholds. The reduction in pure tone air conduction thresholds (*A*) is small and reflects the increased stiffness of the middle ear system and resultant decrease in low frequency sensitivity. Bone conduction thresholds and discrimination scores are normal. The type B tympanogram (*B*, see page 213) is consistent with fluid in the middle ear space. Absent acoustic reflexes with the probe in the impaired ear is consistent with the conductive nature of the disorder. Reflexes are present with the probe in the normal ear, although at elevated thresholds in the lower frequencies, reflecting the increased intensity needed to overcome the effect of the conductive blockage.

time. However, the great majority of sensorineural losses once acquired are permanent. Because the disorder ordinarily is associated with loss in discrimination ability as well as in sensitivity, a more handicapping problem results than from a conductive loss of equal magnitude. Sensorineural disorders may result in complete deafness, while the maximum conductive loss is 60–70 dB (Goetzinger, 1978).

Loudness recruitment is usually associated with sensory loss (hearing loss of cochlear origin), which constitutes the majority of sensorineural

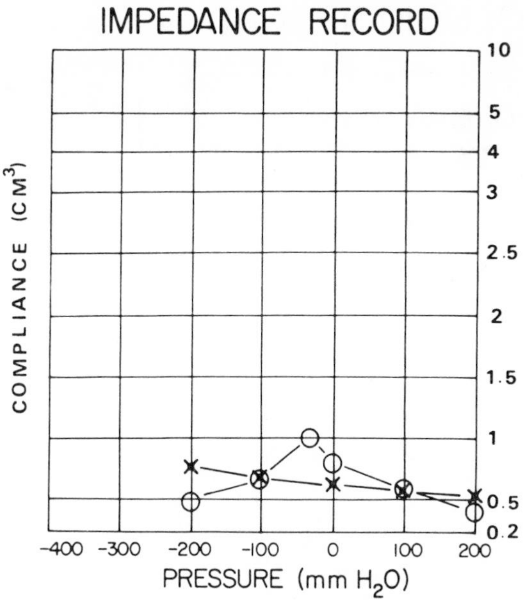

		PROBE IN LEFT EAR SOUND IN RIGHT EAR				PROBE IN RIGHT EAR SOUND IN LEFT EAR			
	HZ	500	1000	2000	4000	500	1000	2000	4000
REFLEX	HL	NR	NR	NR	NR	110	110	95	95
	SL								

	RE	LE
MIDDLE EAR PRESSURE	-30	-

	RE	LE
C_2	1.00	
C_1	.42	
COMPLIANCE IN CM^3	8	-

B

losses. The recruiting patient with sensory loss will not hear low intensity sounds at all, may just barely hear sounds of moderate intensity, but the recruitment of loudness may cause intense sounds to be perceived as loudly as by a normal ear. This disruption of the normal loudness function may be annoying to the individual and may be associated with tolerance problems when hearing aid use is attempted.

Sensorineural loss causes disproportionately increased difficulty in noise (Olsen and Tillman, 1968). Many people with mild sensorineural loss report no difficulty in communicating in quiet but almost always complain of problems with hearing in noisy places, such as in groups of people.

In sensorineural loss, the audiometric Weber test is expected to lateralize to the better ear.

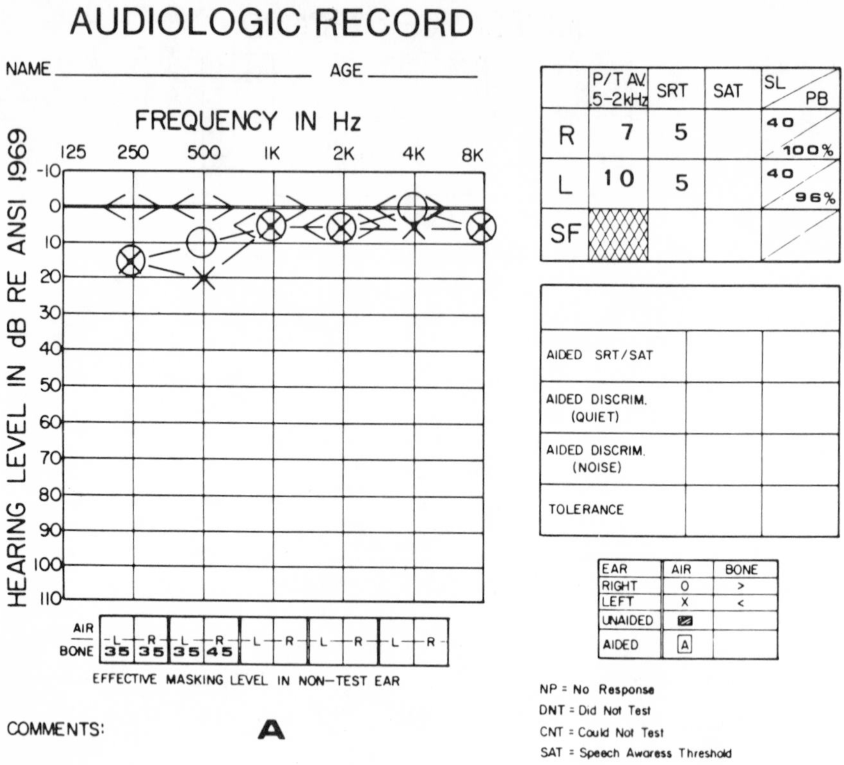

Fig. 8.2. Slight conductive disorder associated with Eustachian tube dysfunction. The change in air conduction thresholds (*A*) is small. Bone conduction thresholds and discrimination scores are normal. Type C tympanograms (*B*, see page 215) indicate abnormal negative middle ear air pressure resulting from failure of the Eustachian tubes to equalize air pressure. Absent acoustic reflexes support the conductive component. This disorder may be transitory and is often associated with the common cold, other upper respiratory problems, or allergenic reactions. Recurrent fluctuating hearing loss may occur in children with chronic problems of this sort.

Audiometrically, sensorineural loss is characterized by interweaving air and bone conduction thresholds and normal tympanograms. Acoustic reflexes are expected if the loss is sensory in nature and the magnitude of the loss is not too great to permit elicitation of the reflex. As reported earlier, reflex thresholds are expected at reduced sensation levels, indicating loudness recruitment. Jerger (1970) reported that reflex thresholds at SLs less than 60 dB indicate the presence of recruitment. He reported the occurrence of reflexes in sensory losses at SLs as low as 25 dB. You may expect to see reflexes in some sensory losses as great as 85 dB and perhaps, in some cases, even greater. In neural (retrocochlear) disorders, on the other hand, acoustic reflexes tend to have elevated

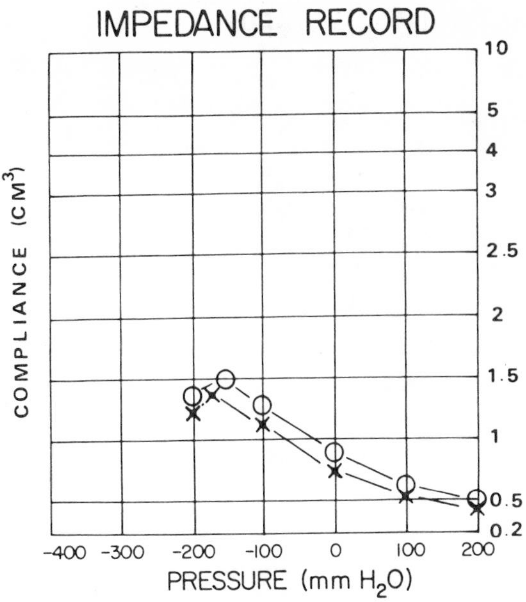

		PROBE IN LEFT EAR SOUND IN RIGHT EAR				PROBE IN RIGHT EAR SOUND IN LEFT EAR			
	HZ	500	1000	2000	4000	500	1000	2000	4000
REFLEX	HL	NR	NR	NR	NR	NR	NR	NR	NR
	SL								

	RE	LE
MIDDLE EAR PRESSURE	-155	-185

	RE	LE
C_2	1.5	1.3
C_1	.5	.4
COMPLIANCE IN CM^3	1.0	.9

B

thresholds, be absent, or show reflex decay (Jerger *et al.* 1974b). Figures 8.4–8.8 show audiometric results in sensorineural losses of various origins.

Mixed Loss. A mixed loss consists of a conductive and a sensorineural component in the same ear. Added together, the components constitute the total hearing loss. Behavior of the patient will reflect attributes of both a conductive and a sensorineural disorder. Discrimination scores are expected to be reduced consistent with the magnitude of the sensorineural component. Recruitment may be present but may not manifest itself with the usual tolerance reactions, since the conductive component acts as a buffer, reducing the intensity of sound reaching the inner ear. The conductive component of the disorder may be correctible. The feasibility of correction is related to the relative size of

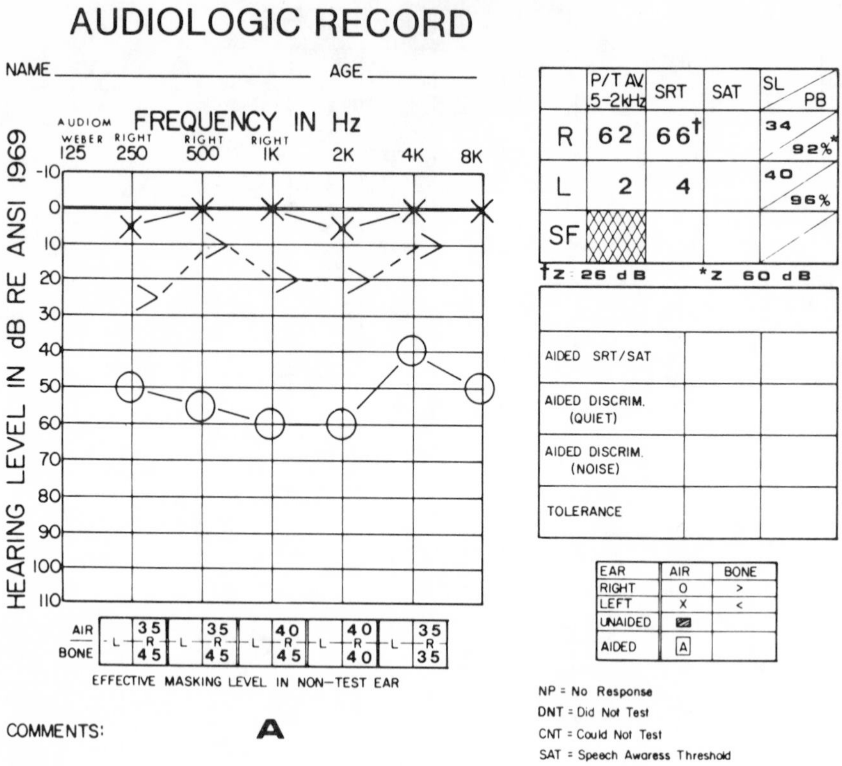

Fig. 8.3. Unilateral conductive loss associated with ossicular discontinuity. There is a large air-bone gap on the affected ear (*A*). Bone conduction thresholds and discrimination scores are normal. The A_d tympanogram (*B*, see page 217) reflects the decreased stiffness. Acoustic reflexes are absent bilaterally. Reflexes are absent with the probe in the affected ear because of the discontinuity and with the probe in the normal ear because sufficient effective intensity cannot be generated in the affected ear due to the large conductive loss.

the two components. The patient with a small conductive and a large sensorineural component may not elect correction if the procedure involves complex and expensive surgery due to the small improvement which would be possible and the fact that amplification would be necessary even after successful surgery because of the sensorineural component. On the other hand, if the sensorineural component is small enough to permit hearing function without amplification once the conductive component is corrected, surgery is more feasible.

The many causes of conductive and sensorineural loss can combine to form a mixed loss. Both components may begin at the same time, as with a mixed loss resulting from acoustic trauma that causes damage to both conductive and sensorineural mechanisms. Or, one component may be present for some time before the other is added. It is important

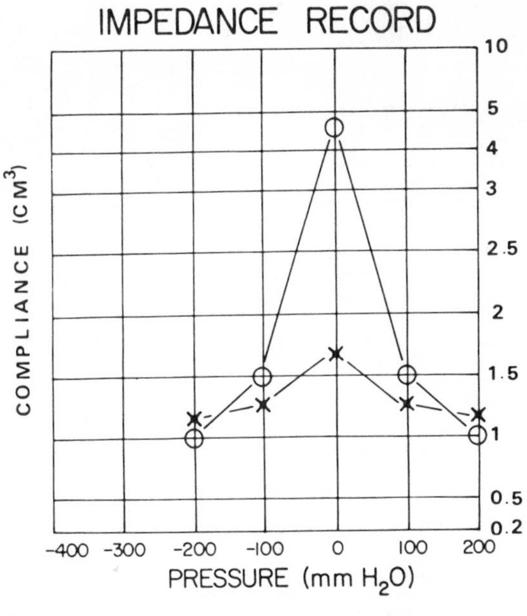

		PROBE IN LEFT EAR SOUND IN RIGHT EAR				PROBE IN RIGHT EAR SOUND IN LEFT EAR			
	HZ	500	1000	2000	4000	500	1000	2000	4000
REFLEX	HL	NR	NR	NR	NR	NR	NR	NR	NR
	SL								

	RE	LE
MIDDLE EAR PRESSURE	0	0

	RE	LE
C_2	4.60	1.7
C_1	1.04	1.2
COMPLIANCE IN CM^3	3.56	.5

B

to remember that individuals with sensorineural loss are susceptible to the same influences which cause conductive loss in normal individuals. A cold or a buildup of wax in the ear canal can add a small conductive component to any ear. While this small change in sensitivity may not be noticed in a normal hearing individual, it may be sufficient to severely reduce the communication ability of the person with existing sensorineural loss. It is particularly important to be alert for this complication in children with sensorineural loss. Children are more liable to small conductive disorders than are adults and may not report their onset. The addition of a small conductive component may prevent the child, who otherwise functions acceptably, from hearing in the classroom; or it may make the child's hearing aid inadequate for the duration of the conductive complication.

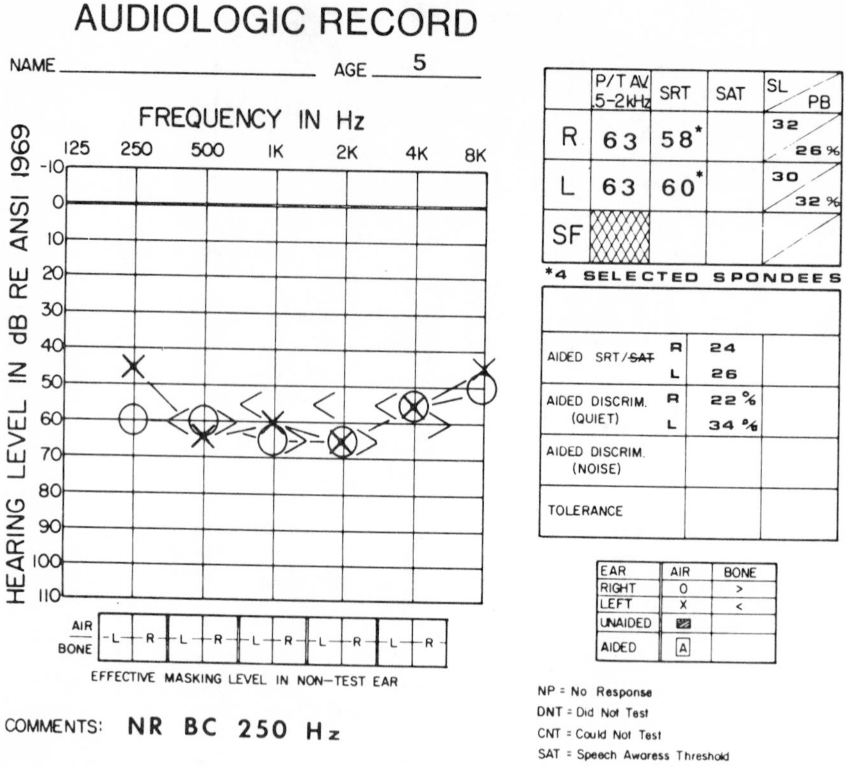

Fig. 8.4. Sensorineural loss resulting from postmaternal rubella. The mother had rubella (German measles) early in pregnancy. This "cookie-bite" configuration is typical of rubella induced loss, although there is great variability in both magnitude and configuration. Tympanograms were normal and acoustic reflexes were absent.

Test results in a patient with mixed loss are shown in Figure 8.9. Remembering that bone conduction testing measures inner ear function, it should be clear that reduction in bone conduction thresholds constitutes a measure of the size of the sensorineural loss. Since the air-bone gap is the audiometric indicator of conductive loss, you can see how the size of the air-bone gap is an indicator of the magnitude of the conductive component in a mixed loss.

Magnitude of Hearing Loss

It is necessary to have some method for selecting one number from the audiogram to represent the overall magnitude of the hearing loss. The usual procedure is to average thresholds for certain pure tone frequencies. Because of the large amount of information lost in this abstraction process, it becomes difficult to generalize with high accuracy about the effect of hearing loss of particular magnitudes. In addition, certain losses, such as the unilateral and the high frequency losses discussed below, constitute exceptions which do not fit well into classification schemes.

Additional problems with handicap scales that are based on sensitivity alone relate to three factors. First, they do not consider the effect of auditory discrimination ability. If the loss is sensorineural, rather than conductive, discrimination ability will be reduced, with a greater handicap in every listening condition. Furthermore, sensorineural losses of different origins result in a wide range of discrimination scores. Phonemic regression, inordinately poor discrimination ability, makes some sensorineural losses more handicapping than others of the same magnitude.

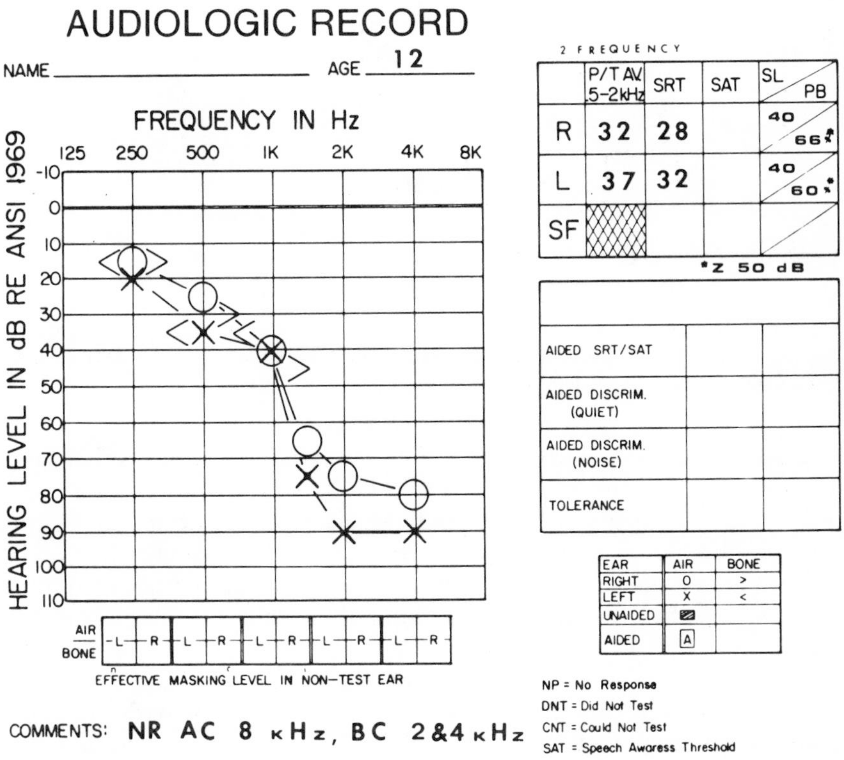

Fig. 8.5. High frequency sensorineural loss associated with complications arising from Rh incompatibility. Losses of this sort may be undetected, particulary if other disorders are present to mask the behavioral effect of the loss. Athetoid type cerebral palsy is another disorder associated with Rh incompatibility problems. The resulting motor impairment may make testing difficult.

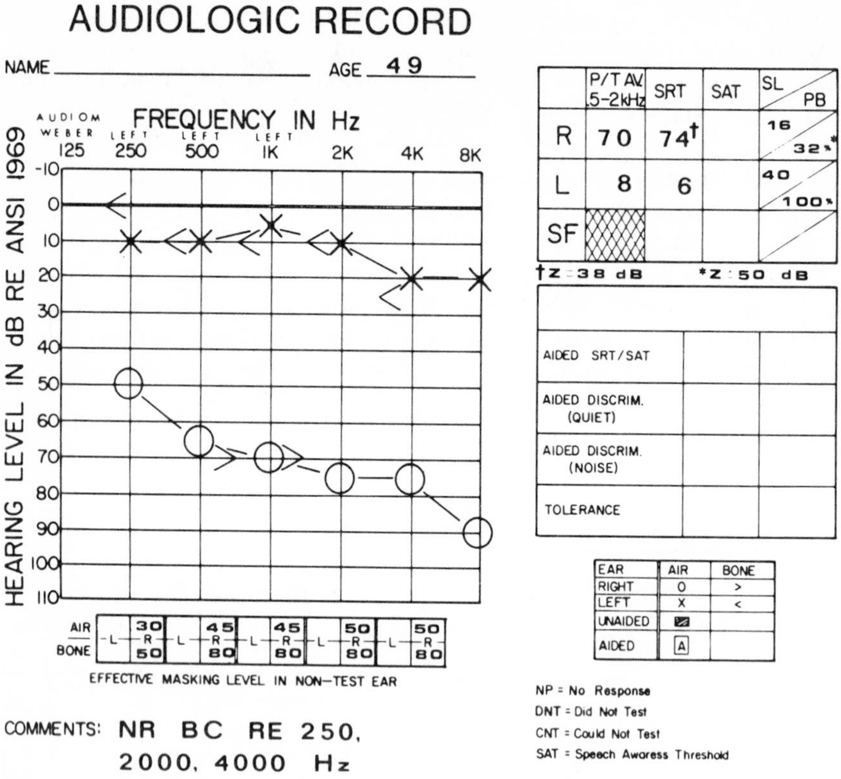

Fig. 8.6. Meniere's disease. This disorder is usually unilateral and results in a progressive hearing loss, as shown in the audiogram. Tympanograms are normal and acoustic reflexes are present at reduced sensation levels.

A second problem with sensitivity-based handicap scales is that they do not consider the effect of different listening conditions on the individual's performance. Many individuals with sensorineural loss do fairly well when listening in quiet places but suffer a great reduction in performance when listening in noise or in other unfavorable circumstances. Sensitivity scales have traditionally been based on the person's ability to perform in quiet, inasmuch as the average used for classification has been thresholds at 500, 1000, and 2000 Hz. The result has often been underestimation of handicap for individuals with predominately high frequency loss. As indicated below, some attention has recently been paid to reducing this problem.

The third problem with sensitivity-based handicap scales is that they do not take into consideration the configuration of the audiogram. Thus, they are more applicable to fairly flat audiograms than to those which show unequal sensitivity across frequency. The most common example of the latter is provided by people with high frequency loss. Often a significant handicap can exist because of high frequency loss, while the handicap, as measured by the sensitivity scale, will be zero. Sensitivity-based scales tend to underestimate handicap in cases of high frequency loss.

Keeping these limitations in mind, we will now consider two methods of classifying hearing loss according to sensitivity. The first divides hearing losses into groups, gives each group a name, and generalizes about the amount of handicap to be expected in each group. The second estimates percentage of hearing impairment.

Classification of Hearing Loss. Use of this procedure permits classification of the magnitude of loss in either ear and the overall magnitude, based on sensitivity in the better ear. Several scales exist, each originating from the experience and perceptions of different clinicians. A commonly used one is shown in Table 8.2.

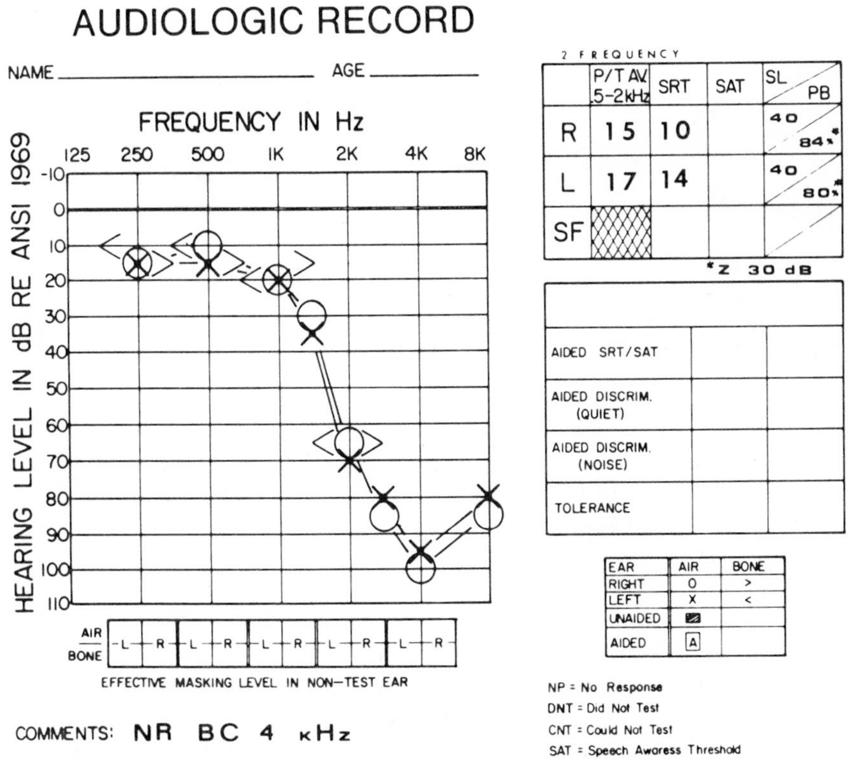

Fig. 8.7. Noise induced loss. This slowly progressive loss results from long-term noise exposure, usually associated with occupational noise. However, recreational activities, such as the shooting of guns, may be responsible. The greatest loss is usually in the region of 3000–6000 Hz.

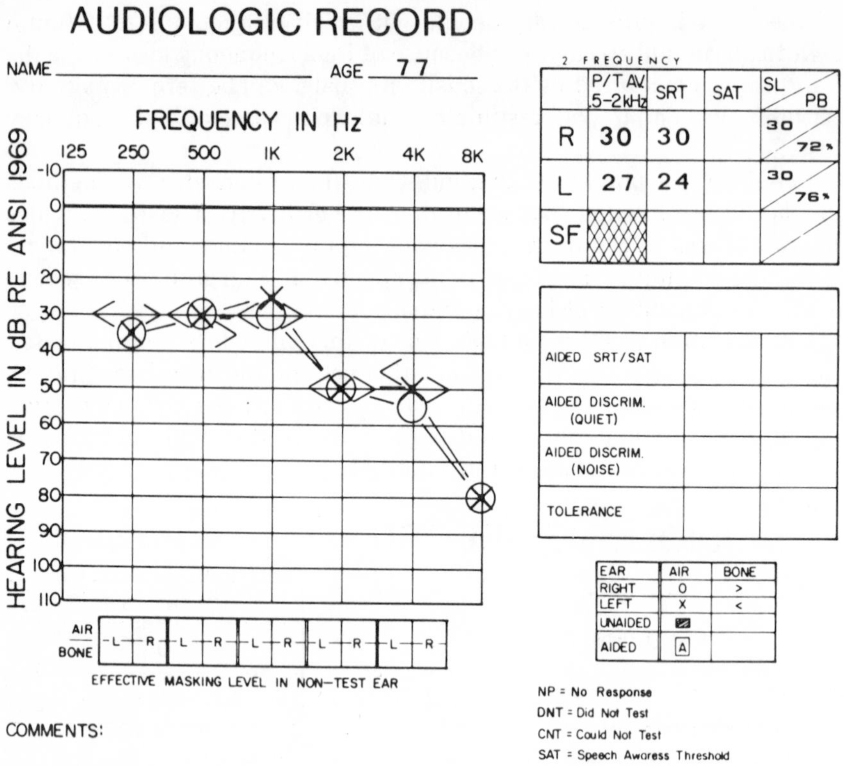

Fig. 8.8. Presbycusis. This sensorineural disorder associated with aging typically presents a mild bilaterally equal loss that slopes gently downward for successively higher frequencies. Discrimination scores are variable and may, as in this case, be reduced more than would be expected from the magnitude of the loss.

The names of the various classifications are generally descriptive of difficulty to be expected. There is no universal agreement for the names or decibel ranges. As you study Table 8.2, remember all of the nonauditory factors discussed earlier in this chapter which affect how a given hearing loss relates to behavior. Finally, remember that when we classify hearing loss, we are treating as discrete a disorder which really exists as a continuum, from the best possible hearing to the worst. Therefore, in addition to the other variables besides hearing loss which affect the performance of the hearing impaired, it also follows that those whose hearing falls into the upper part of a particular category will tend to do better than those in the lower area of the category.

Percentage of Impairment. It is an appealing, though problematic, concept to express hearing loss in terms of the percentage of impairment. Laws often utilize percentage impairment in their terminology, and the use of percentage impairment is common in medicolegal cases. Formulas to compute percentage impairment are based entirely on sensitivity. They do not consider auditory discrimination ability and take no direct account of the configuration of the audiogram. They do not consider the effect of adverse listening conditions or the variation in impairment caused by more or less critical demands on hearing experienced by different individuals. Therefore, individuals with quite different auditory handicaps may have the same percentage of impairment, as derived from the formulas discussed below.

An early formula was known as the A.M.A. (American Medical Association) Percentage of Hearing Loss formula (Carter, 1947). This procedure gave weights to four pure tone frequencies according to their presumed importance: 500 Hz, 15%, 1000 Hz, 30%; 2000 Hz, 40%; and 4000 Hz, 15%.

A procedure which became widely used was adopted by the American Academy of Opthalmology and Otolaryngology (AAOO), using only the frequencies 500, 1000, and 2000 Hz (Lierle, 1959). These three frequencies were weighted equally, and the number used to obtain percentage of impairment was derived from the average of the thresholds at these three frequencies. After the average was obtained, 26 dB were subtracted. This value, 26 dB, represented the "low fence," beyond which impairment was presumed to start. The value, 26 dB, came from the value of 15 dB re: the 1951 ASA norms, the low fence in effect when the AAOO method was developed. Rounded to the nearest decibel, 15 dB re: the ASA norms is the same SPL as 26 dB re: the ISO norms. For each decibel of hearing loss beyond 26, 1½% of impairment was attributed. As a result, 100% impairment occurred if the average loss was 93 dB. Overall, or binaural, percentage of impairment was computed by multiplying the percentage of impairment in the better ear by five, adding the result to the percentage of impairment of the poorer ear and dividing the sum by six. The rationale for this procedure was that the better ear contributed more importantly to hearing ability and should be weighted more heavily when estimating impairment. An example of percentage of impairment calculated by use of the AAOO method is shown in Figure 8.10.

As discussed above, there were problems with the AAOO method which are inherent to any procedure that estimates impairment on the basis of sensitivity alone. There was an additional difficulty. The procedure used only the frequencies 500, 1000, and 2000 Hz and weighted them equally. It attributed no impairment to average losses less than 26 dB. The result was essentially a procedure which estimated handicap for an individual listening in quiet under good conditions. An individual can have a substantial high frequency loss and still be rated

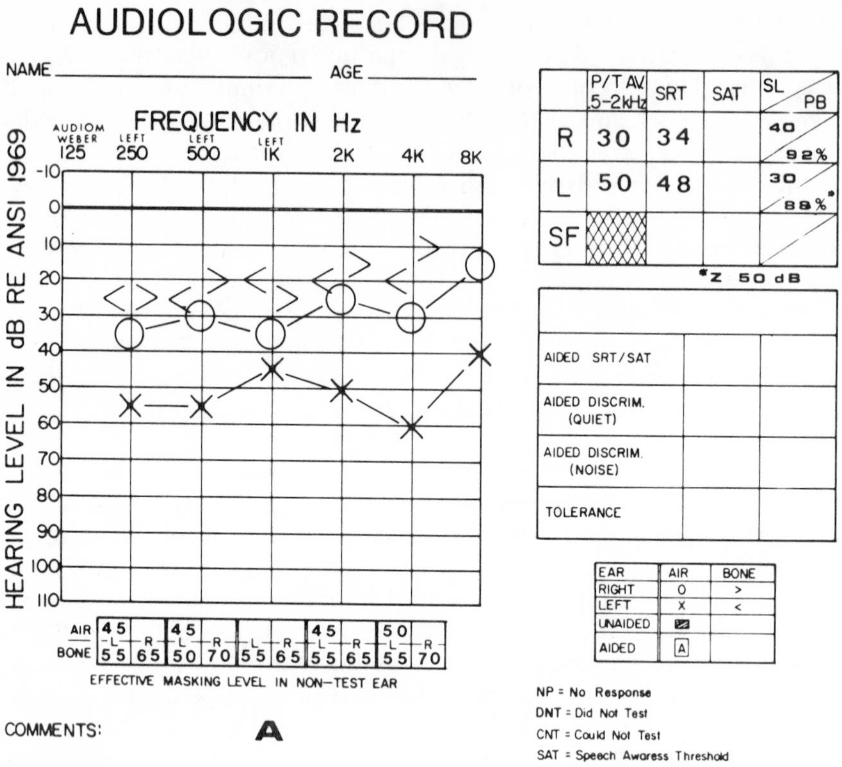

Fig. 8.9. Mixed loss associated with otosclerosis, showing both a sensorineural and conductive component. (*A*), Audiologic Record; (*B*, see page 225), Impedance Record.

0% impairment using the AAOO procedure. Such a person may get along well in quiet under good listening conditions but experience substantial difficulty when listening in noisy circumstances or in other unfavorable listening circumstances.

Recently the AAOO formula was revised (American Academy of Otolaryngology Committee on Hearing and Equilibrium, and the American Council of Otolaryngology Committee on the Medical Aspects of Noise, 1979). The new formula utilizes the thresholds at 500, 1000, 2000, *and 3000* Hz. Impairment begins after 25 rather than 26 dB. Otherwise, the procedure remains the same. The new formula is intended to reflect more realistically the ability to understand speech in the presence of some background noise. The difference in percentage of impairment between the two formulas is shown in Figure 8.10.

Other formulas have been developed which place even more emphasis on hearing sensitivity for higher frequencies. To obtain more detail regarding these formulas see Scott (1977). For a detailed study of the

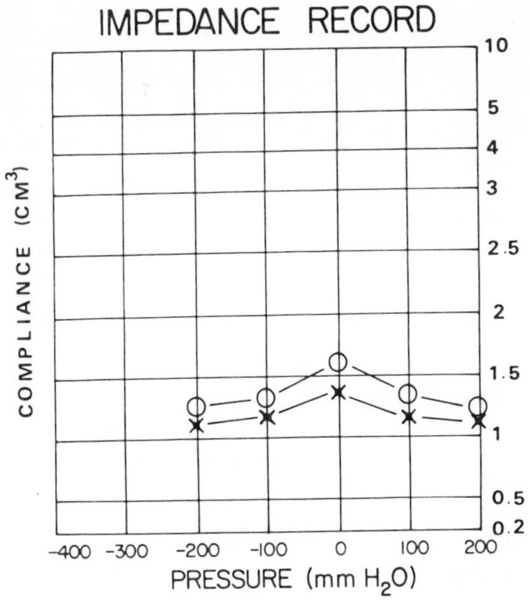

		PROBE IN LEFT EAR SOUND IN RIGHT EAR				PROBE IN RIGHT EAR SOUND IN LEFT EAR			
	HZ	500	1000	2000	4000	500	1000	2000	4000
REFLEX	HL	NR	NR	NR	NR	NR	NR	NR	NR
	SL								

	RE	LE
MIDDLE EAR PRESSURE	O	O

	RE	LE
C_2	1.60	1.4
C_1	1.26	1.2
COMPLIANCE IN CM^3	.34	.2

B

problems of hearing conservation in industry, you should look at Olishifski and Harford (1975).

Configuration of Hearing Loss

Audiograms are divisible into the following types based on configuration or curve—the levels at which thresholds fall across the audiogram. Not all audiograms fit neatly into these categories and some have characteristics of more than one type. Based on behavioral characteristics, it is useful to consider the following configurations: (1) flat loss, (2) high frequency loss, (3) low frequency loss, (4) trough-shaped loss, and (5) irregular loss (Carhart, 1945). An additional category considers behavior in unilateral loss. A description of each class appears in Table 8.3.

Table 8.2
Classification of Magnitude of Hearing Loss (Based on Appropriate Two or Three Frequency Pure Tone Threshold Average)

Classification	Threshold in dB (PTA)
Normal	0–10
Borderline normal	11–25
Mild loss	26–45
Moderate loss	46–65
Severe loss	66–85
Profound loss	86 +

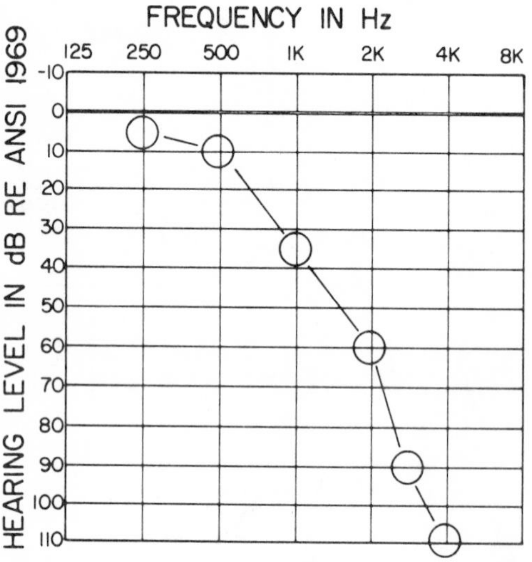

Fig. 8.10. Audiogram showing percentage impairment using the AAOO and the AAO methods. AAOO percentage impairment is (35 [PTA] −26 [low gate] ×1.5) 13.5%. AAO impairment is (49 [PTA] −25 [low gate] ×1.5) 36%.

Flat Configuration. Audiograms with fairly flat configuration may result from either conductive or sensorineural causes, although most sensorineural losses tend toward greater loss for higher frequencies. Usually we think of flat configurations in sensorineural loss as less handicapping than other types and recommend the ear with the flatter configuration for amplification (Hodgson, 1977). There are exceptions to this generalization. In a given case, auditory discrimination ability, tolerance for intense sounds, or magnitude of hearing loss may play a more important role than configuration in determining feasibility of amplification.

High Frequency Configuration. While high frequency configurations usually are associated with sensorineural disorders, conductive com-

Table 8.3
Audiometric configurations[a]

Configuration	Description
Flat	No more than 5–10 dB change per octave
High frequency	Progressively greater loss for higher frequencies, slope 15 dB/octave or steeper
Low frequency	Progressively less loss for higher frequencies
Trough	Twenty decibels or more loss in the mid frequencies than at extremes
Irregular	Loss which does not fit above categories
Unilateral	Normal hearing in one ear with a significant loss in the other ear.

[a] Modified from Carhart (1945).

ponents of this nature have been reported in ossicular discontinuity (Anderson and Barr, 1971). Additionally, some conductive disorders may result in mass tilt—a high frequency loss with near normal sensitivity below 1000 Hz. However, if you obtain an air-bone gap limited to the higher frequencies you should suspect the possibility of a collapsing ear canal causing invalid results. This artifact tends to be greater for the higher frequencies.

Individuals with normal hearing sensitivity across part of the range important for hearing and understanding speech, but with a high frequency loss, may show behavior atypical of that we expect in hearing loss. Because of the good low frequency sensitivity, they hear and respond to most environmental sounds and are ordinarily aware when people are talking to them. Depending on the severity of the loss, they may have little or no difficulty in one-to-one speaking situations under good listening conditions. Their ability to follow speech, however, may deteriorate when listening in unfavorable conditions, such as in noise. A school child with high frequency loss may show no difficulty when talking directly to the teacher in a quiet classroom before school but may have great trouble understanding the teacher in the noisy classroom during school hours. Because of the atypical behavior, high frequency loss tends to be detected later in children than other types of loss. The apparent response inconsistencies associated with difficult listening situations and the language delay usually resulting from longstanding hearing loss may cause the child to be misdiagnosed as mentally retarded, emotionally disturbed, or aphasic. These problems are illustrated in Figure 8.11. The child, in a school which had no hearing conservation program, had a history of school problems. Some time was spent in special classes, first for retarded children, then for the emotionally disturbed. Only when the child moved to a school which had a hearing screening program was the hearing loss detected. The mag-

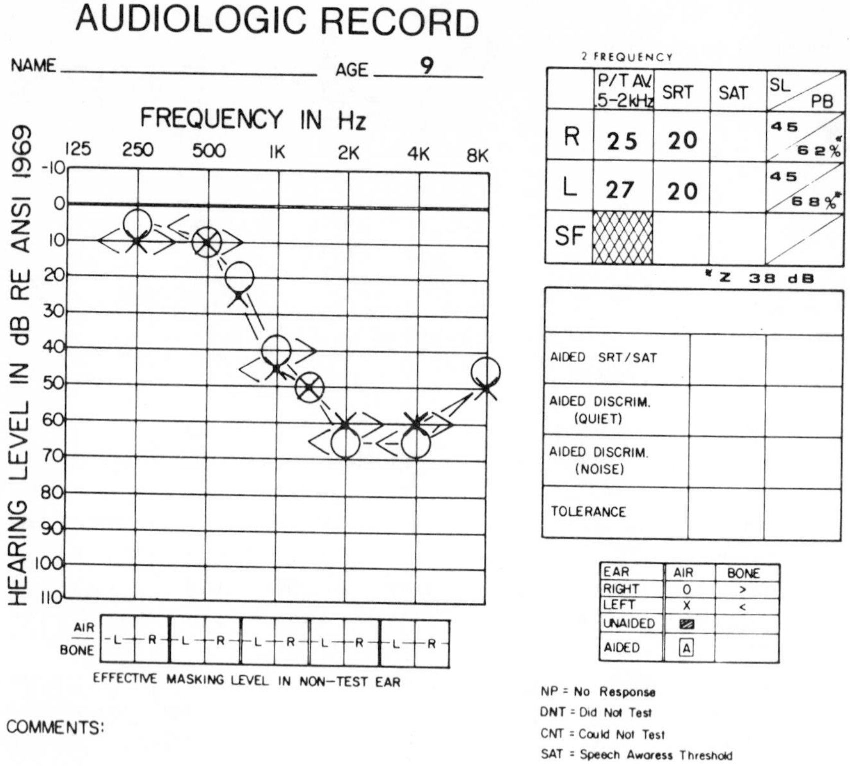

Fig. 8.11. Child with high frequency loss identified late. The loss was not identified and evaluated until the child was 9 years old although there was a long history of school problems and suspected mental retardation.

nitude of this loss seems entirely adequate to account for the child's behavior and school problems.

Merklein and Briskey (1962) found that 10 of 25 students enrolled in a program for aphasic children had handicapping hearing loss. Elliott and Armbruster (1967) reported additional learning problems and a higher incidence of aphasic labels in children whose hearing loss had been identified later than in another group of hearing impaired children identified earlier in life. These findings emphasize the importance of early and correct identification of hearing loss, of informing other professionals who deal with children of the problem, and of careful hearing evaluation in diagnosing the problems of children.

Adults also have problems with undetected high frequency loss, particularly if acquired loss comes on slowly over a period of months or years. Adults may be aware of the nature of the problem, explaining that they hear but do not always understand. However, they may, with a slowly acquired hearing loss, attribute their problem to the belief that people do not talk as clearly as they used to.

A great deal of progress has occurred in the use of amplification for those with high frequency loss. These amplification procedures are reviewed by Hodsgon (1977a).

Low Frequency Configuration. Losses with greater reduction of sensitivity in the lower audiometric frequencies are usually associated with conductive disorders (stiffness tilt). However, sensorineural configurations of this sort do exist and may present special problems of identification, based on the individual's behavior. Ross and Matkin (1967) described children with low frequency loss who presented problems in identification, confusing behavior, and delayed language. They typically had good articulation ability and could respond to faint (even whispered) speech, probably because of their ability to hear high frequency consonant sounds. They were often misdiagnosed as having normal hearing.

Trough Configuration. Trough, or "cookie bite," configurations exhibit better sensitivity at both frequency extremes than across the middle frequencies. This configuration is usually associated with sensorineural loss. With great variability it has been associated with the postmaternal rubella syndrome (Hodgson, 1969). In extreme cases, low and high frequency sensitivity may be normal with a reduction of sensitivity in the mid frequencies most important for the audibility of speech. In these instances, detection of the loss may be delayed because the good low and high frequency sensitivity permits the individual to respond to many environmental sounds.

Irregular Configuration. Those configurations which do not fall into one of the categories discussed above may be classified as "irregular," and therefore may be a heterogeneous group. They may be either conductive or sensorineural. There are sometimes extreme irregularities in audiograms, with one audiometric frequency much better or poorer than the others. These extreme irregularities may cause unusual auditory behavior. In cases of less extreme irregularity, the result may be more reminiscent of a flat audiometric configuration.

A Special Case—Unilateral Hearing Loss. The person with normal hearing in one ear and a significant loss in the other has problems which have not always been recognized. Perhaps because the ordinary hearing evaluation is not designed to measure the problems of the person with unilateral loss, these problems have sometimes been minimized. Nevertheless, unilaterals usually complain of the following: (1) problems understanding when the speaker is located on the side of the poor ear, especially in unfavorable listening conditions; (2) difficulty understanding in noise or other poor listening conditions, and (3) some difficulty in locating the source of sounds in space.

Twenty persons with unilateral loss reported that extraneous noise was the factor which contributed most to listening difficulty (Giolas and Wark 1967). In quiet places, they reported listening to a speaker at a distance as the greatest problem. Especially in noise, they reported that the difficulty of listening was increased when speakers were positioned on the side of the impaired ear.

Kasten and associates (1967–1968) reported the head shadow to be about 6 dB for spondee words. That is, when a person with unilateral loss listens to spondees with the head between the good ear and the speech source, speech threshold is about 6 dB poorer than if the good ear is directed toward the speech source. The head shadow is greater than 6 dB for higher frequencies, probably causing an additional effect on auditory discrimination ability. Considering the PI functions discussed in Chapter 6, it is easy to understand the effect the head shadow can have on the unilateral who must listen to faint or distant speech or speech at an unfavorable signal-to-noise ratio.

The school child with unilateral loss presents a special problem. In quiet when the teacher speaks from nearby no particular problem is evident. However, a much different situation results if the child sits near the back of a noisy classroom. For this reason, preferential seating near the front of the classroom, with seating that permits the good ear to be directed toward the area where the teacher is usually located, is of great importance to the child with unilateral loss. Preferential seating is not always easy to establish or maintain, and children should be monitored carefully.

Harford and Musket (1964) and Harford and Barry (1965) made early reports on the successful use of amplification with patients who had unilateral loss. Considerable progress has since been made in the application of hearing aids for unilateral losses, and Hodgson (1977b) reviews the concepts and hearing aids that are involved.

Auditory Discrimination Ability

The handicap resulting from auditory discrimination deficit is difficult to predict because of variability in discrimination scores and because of the other factors we have discussed which influence the performance of a hearing impaired person. Nevertheless, auditory discrimination ability is one of the most important determinants of hearing handicap. The following remarks about the relationship between discrimination scores and auditory handicap are based on the expected results from a discrimination test such as the recorded W-22 test administered to an individual with an acquired loss and normal language ability.

Carhart (1960) estimated that discrimination scores better than 80%

indicate discrimination ability adequate for everyday listening, scores between 80% and 68% indicate mild handicaps, scores between 68% and 56% result in moderate handicap, and scores poorer than 56% represent a severe discrimination impairment associated with major disability. An expanded general guide to interpreting discrimination test results is shown in Table 8.4. You must remember, as always, when using guides of this sort that people near the extremes of a category tend to be less representative of that class that those nearer the middle. Also keep in mind the many other variables which influence behavior in the hearing impaired.

The guide applies to performance when listening without visual clues. Many people with poor discrimination ability perform much better than the guide suggests when both looking at and listening to the speaker. Others do not take advantage of visual clues. The importance of measuring the contribution of lip reading to auditory performance is discussed by Dodds and Harford (1968). They advocate administration of lip reading tests with and without a hearing aid in those cases where poor discrimination ability may otherwise suggest that amplification would not be useful. The aided improvement may be sufficient to justify use of amplification. Steele and co-workers (1978) reported the success-

Table 8.4
Expected Relationship Between Auditory Discrimination Score and Communication Difficulty. Estimate is Based on Score in the Better Ear Obtained From the Recorded W-22 or Other Comparable Test

Discrimination Score %	Classification of Discrimination Ability	Magnitude of Problem
92–100	Excellent	None
82–90	Good	Little or no difficulty in good listening conditions. Some trouble in poor listening conditions, especially with unfamiliar or technical words
72–80	Fair	Some trouble in good listening conditions. Significant difficulty in poor listening conditions without supplemental visual input.
52–70	Poor	Constant difficulty. Without lip reading can just follow familiar conversation under good listening conditions.
22–50	Very poor	Cannot get along with hearing alone. Hearing becomes an aid to lip reading.
0–20	Extremely poor	Hearing alone is not useful for understanding speech. Can be an aid to lip reading ability.

ful use of the NU 6 PB lists in a combined auditory and visual presentation. Cooper and Langley (1978) reported the experimental use of the Modified Rhyme Test to obtain measures of auditory, lip reading, and combined auditory and lip reading performance. They feel their procedure will be useful for both diagnostic and rehabilitative evaluations.

Figure 8.12 provides an example of an individual who performed poorly when looking only or when listening only. You can see that significant improvement occurred when visual and auditory inputs were combined.

OTHER HANDICAP SCALES

Some procedures have attempted to base prediction of handicap on more than one of the auditory measures discussed above, or on entirely different measures.

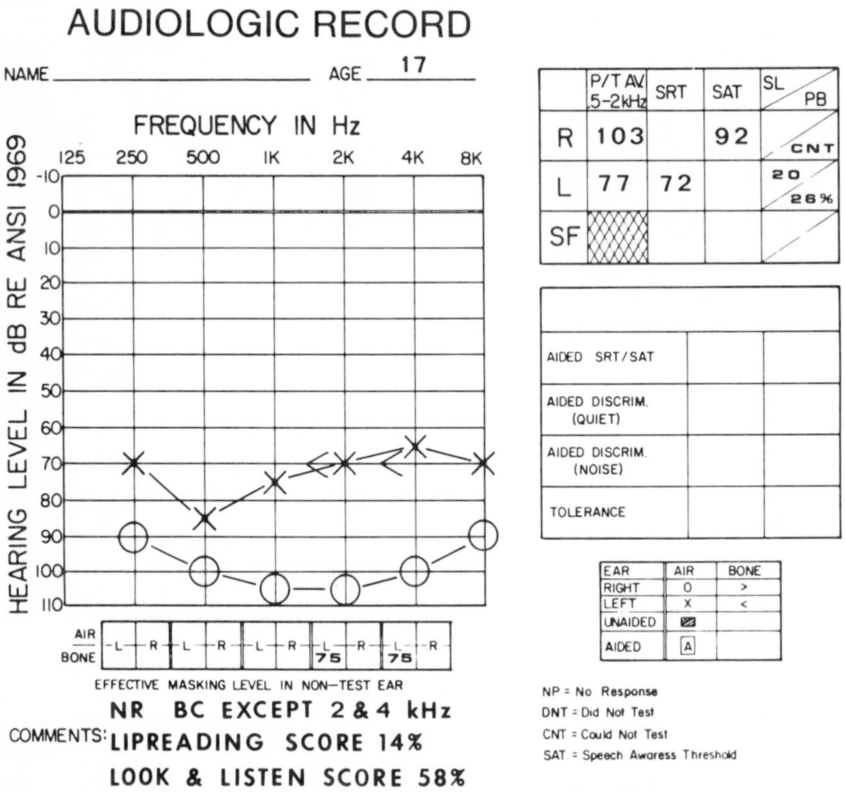

Fig. 8.12. Example of improvement in performance when listening and lip reading are combined. Score when listening only is 26%. Score when lip reading only is 14%. Score when both looking and listening is 58%. In each case, the test consisted of a list of PB-K words.

The Social Adequacy Index was developed by Walsh and Silverman (1946) and used by Davis (1948) in an attempt to predict social handicap by using two measures, the speech reception threshold and the auditory discrimination score. Predictive ability was not very good. The normative data were collected using the Rush Hughes recording for discrimination testing, a test which did not remain in widespread clinical use.

High and associates (1964) developed a subjective scale for the self assessment of hearing handicap. Their research, as well as the later study of Speaks *et al.* (1970), did not establish the general clinical utility of the Hearing Handicap Scale. Dirks and Carhart (1962) developed a questionnaire to assess the difficulty hearing impaired listeners feel they have in different listening conditions. More recently, Rupp *et al.* (1977) reported a scale designed to predict probability of successful hearing aid use. This scale is based on such factors as age, auditory sensitivity, auditory discrimination ability, visual acuity, and several others.

The Hearing Performance Inventory (Giolas *et al.* 1979) was developed to assess handicap in everyday listening situations. The scale considers problems in these areas: (1) understanding speech, (2) intensity, (3) response to auditory failures, (4) social, (5) personal, and (6) occupational. The inventory is intended as a tool to help organize and plan rehabilitation services.

Jerger and Jerger (1979) reported development of a procedure for Quantification of Auditory Handicap (QUAH). Subjects listen to sentences in the presence of a competing signal consisting of a single voice at a message-to-competition ratio of 0 dB. The test consists of 25 questions or commands which require a specific motor response, such as the drawing of a circle. The authors reported the test to be quickly and easily administered, and it awaits further validation. Because of the problems we have discussed regarding the prognostic value of conventional discrimination tests, I am happy to see innovative experiments with new techniques to evaluate auditory handicap.

THE AUDIOLOGIC REPORT

The purpose of the audiologic report is the interpretation, not the mere repetition, of auditory test results. Specifically, the goals of a good report are to interpret to the referring source the auditory test results, to make recommendations based on the test results, and to provide a clear and accurate record in the patient's file. The exact form and nature of the report will vary according to circumstances and whether the audiologist is serving as consultant in a given case or has assumed responsibility for management of the patient. Regardless of form, there are these requisites of a good report: results should be interpreted accurately, clearly, and briefly. Terminology must be on a level which will be meaningful to the referring source. Appropriate recommendations must be included.

Typically the audiologic report should contain the following:

1. Identifying information. There should be a clear record of the patient's name, address, age and phone number; the date of the evaluation; and the name of the evaluator. This information should be clear and complete. Occasionally I see an old report with the day and month given but the year of the evaluation omitted, effectively preventing any assessment of change in hearing over time.
2. Source of referral and reason for referral. The referring source and the names of others who receive a copy of the report should be included. The reason for referral and the patient's chief complaint, or primary concern, should be noted.
3. Pertinent history. History, as related to you, should be briefly recorded: cause of loss, age at onset, prior evaluations and training.
4. Behavior during testing and test reliability. Behavior which may effect test results should be noted, along with any special procedures necessitated. Include only pertinent information which will help the reader interpret the report or be useful if the patient is evaluated again. Include a statement about reliability of the patient's responses and the confidence you have in the validity of test results.
5. Description of hearing based on the routine test battery. Interpret the pure tone air and bone conduction results. Indicate if speech thresholds support pure tone test findings or, if not, the probable reason for the discrepancy. Interpret impedance measures, explaining the findings in terms of middle ear and sensorineural status. Interpret discrimination test results. Make a unifying statement about the implications of the overall results.
6. Description of special tests. Describe and interpret any nonstandard or special test results which were obtained. Conditioned Orientation Reflex (COR) audiometry may have been necessary to test a very young child, or the Peabody Picture Vocabulary Test (PPVT) may have been used as a screening measure with a child who has a congenital loss and a possible receptive language deficiency.
7. Recommendations. The patient may need additional auditory testing (a hearing aid evaluation, for example) or referral to other professionals. The appearance of a medical problem indicates the need for examination by a physician. Particularly in children, observation of behavior or interpretation of test results may suggest the need for neurological, psychological, or visual examination. Auditory test findings may contribute to recommendations regard-

ing educational needs: preferential classroom seating, educational placement, or the need for language training.

Sample reports are shown below. The first is the report of a child with congenital loss. The Audiologic Record is shown in Figure 8.13. The report of an adult with acquired loss follows. The Audiologic Record of the adult is shown in Figure 8.14. The form of the Audiologic Report may vary from clinic to clinic. To illustrate, the child's report is written in the form of a report to be filed in the clinic folder, with a carbon copy sent to the referring source. The adult's report is in the form of a letter to the referring physician, a copy of which is filed in the clinic folder. In either case, an accompanying sheet in the clinic folder will detail identifying information.

Audiologic Report of a Hearing Impaired Child

Ann, accompanied by her father, came to the clinic on referral of Dr. Jones for a complete audiologic evaluation to determine current hearing

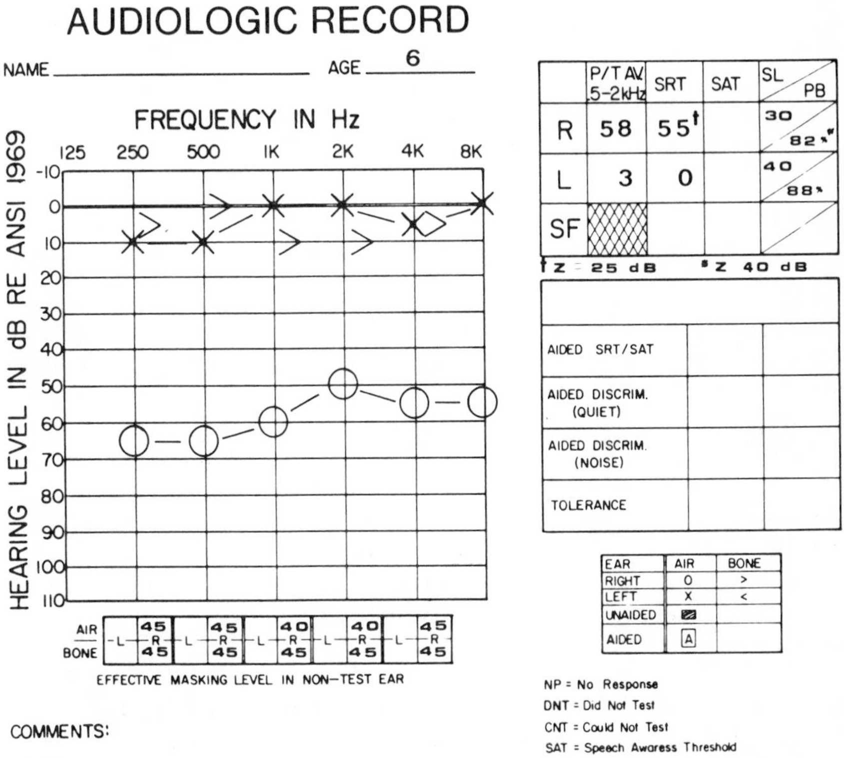

Fig. 8.13. Test results for a child with a congenital hearing loss. See text for Audiologic report.

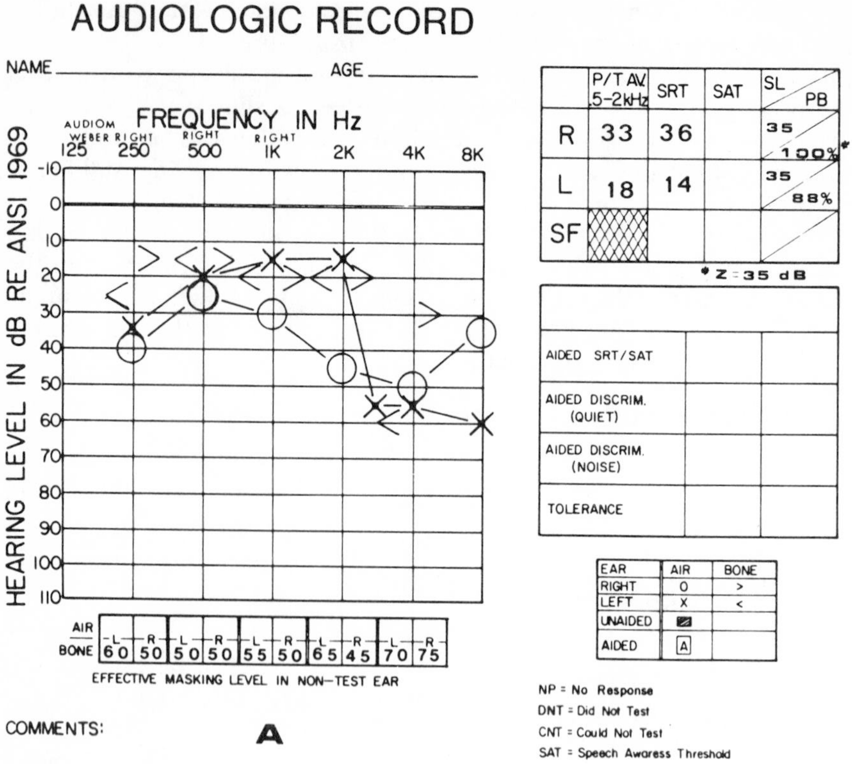

Fig. 8.14. Test results for an adult with acquired loss. (*A*), Audiologic Record; (*B*, see page 237), Impedance Record. See text for audiologic report.

status prior to plastic surgery on the right pinna for cosmetic purposes. Medical history, according to the father, revealed congenital unilateral atresia accompanied by microtia of the right ear. A similar condition was reported in a paternal second cousin.

Modified conditioned play audiometry revealed a moderate unilateral, conductive hearing loss in the right ear with a rising configuration in the lower test frequencies. In sharp contrast there was normal hearing sensitivity in the left ear. Speech reception thresholds were in good agreement with the pure tone averages, suggesting that the measurements are reliable. Tympanometry was not attempted due to the atretic canal.

Speech discrimination was tested under earphones while using PB-K-50 word lists with the scores indicating good discrimination ability for both ears. These scores may be depressed somewhat because of scoring problems associated with Ann's articulation, which included distortions

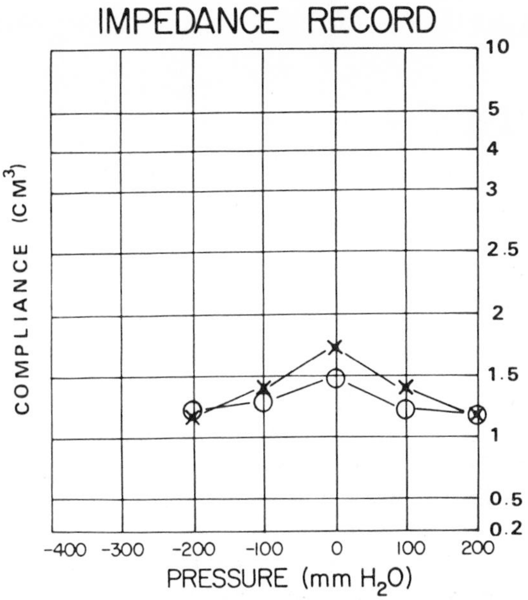

		PROBE IN LEFT EAR SOUND IN RIGHT EAR				PROBE IN RIGHT EAR SOUND IN LEFT EAR			
	HZ	500	1000	2000	4000	500	1000	2000	4000
REFLEX	HL	100	105	NR	NR	NR	NR	NR	NR
	SL								

	RE	LE
MIDDLE EAR PRESSURE	0	0

	RE	LE
C_2	1.4	1.7
C_1	1.2	1.2
COMPLIANCE IN CM^3	.2	.5

B

and omissions. The audiologic results and their implications were discussed with the father. It was explained that (1) Ann may have difficulty localizing sound, the relevance of this problem relating to warning signals while crossing busy streets or bike riding was stressed; (2) Ann may experience difficulty understanding speech in noisy situations, especially if the competition is directed towards the good (left) ear and the speech signal toward the poor (right) ear; and (3) preferential seating in an educational setting should be arranged toward the front and right of the classroom so she can favor her better (left) ear. Finally, an annual hearing evaluation was recommended to monitor Ann's hearing status since maintenance of normal hearing sensitivity in the left ear is critical.

If questions or concerns arise regarding this report, please feel free to contact me.

(signed) Noel D. Matkin, Ph.D.

cc: Joe Jones, M.D.

Audiologic Report of a Hearing Impaired Adult

John Smith, M.D.
ENT Associates
000 Main Street
Tucson, AZ 85718

Re: Mary A.
DOB: 12-9-45

Dear Dr. Smith:

On your referral, I saw Mrs. A. for an audiologic evaluation on January 9, 1980. As you know, she reports a slowly progressive hearing loss of several months duration. She was cooperative during the evaluation and responded reliably.

Pure tone test results are shown on the enclosed audiogram and indicate a high frequency loss of sensitivity on the left ear with no consistent air-bone gap. On the right ear there is a mild loss with a more gradually sloping configuration and a substantial air-bone gap. Speech thresholds support pure tone results. Discrimination for comfortably loud speech is excellent on the right ear and good on the left ear.

Audiometric Weber, elevated acoustic reflex thresholds on stimulating the right ear, and absent reflexes with the probe in the right ear support the pure tone findings of a conductive component on the right ear. Tympanograms indicate normal Eustachian tube function bilaterally. Decreased static compliance on the right ear indicates abnormal stiffness of the right middle ear mechanism.

Mrs. A. was advised to return to you for further otologic recommendations. Mrs. A. works in an office where she must listen to faint speech under quiet conditions. She reports some difficulty. Part time amplification may be helpful, and a hearing aid evaluation is recommended if medical resolution of the problem is not feasible.

Thank you for referring this patient. If you have any questions, please call me at 626-1266.

Sincerely yours,
(signed) William R. Hodgson, Ph.D.

SUMMARY

Interpretation of the basic audiometric test battery requires understanding the purposes of the tests involved, how they are administered, and what they mean. You must learn the many factors, nonauditory and auditory, which combine to determine the amount of handicap resulting from hearing loss and the avenues which are available to reduce the handicap.

You must know how to classify hearing loss according to type, magnitude, and configuration. Estimation of the problems and rehabilitation potential associated with discrimination deficit must be learned. You must be familiar with how test results inter-relate in order to assess the overall validity of the evaluation and what all of the information means in terms of the patient's needs and potentials. You must learn to detect and resolve incongruous test results.

You must know how to explain the test results, implications, and recommendations to the patient, referring sources, and other interested parties. Your explanation must be correct, clear, concise, and convincing.

STUDY QUESTIONS

1. Refer to Table 8.1 to answer the following questions. Would a person's hearing appear to be *better* or *poorer* when testing with an ANSI calibrated versus an ASA calibrated audiometer? Change the following ASA audiogram to ANSI thresholds:

	Frequency in Hz					
	250	500	1000	2000	4000	8000
dB re: 1951 ASA norms	20	30	45	60	70	80
dB re: 1969 ANSI norms	___	___	___	___	___	___

2. Review the purposes of the basic test battery. What does each test of the basic battery contribute to realizing the purposes?
3. How do the nonauditory factors discussed in Chapter 8 influence the amount of handicap associated with a given hearing loss?
4. How do the auditory factors discussed in Chapter 8 influence auditory behavior?
5. What are the advantages and limitations of plans which classify hearing loss, such as those shown in Table 8.2 and Figure 8.10?
6. What are the general relationships between auditory discrimination scores and magnitude of handicap?
7. What are the special auditory problems of those with (a) unilateral hearing loss? (b) high frequency hearing loss?
8. Review the information which should be included in the audiologic report. Can you find all of this information in the audiologic reports included in Chapter 8?
9. What factors contribute to effective interpretation of test results to the patient?

BIBLIOGRAPHY

Allen, G., and Fernandez, C.: The mechanism of bone conduction. *Ann. Otol., Rhinol., Laryngol., 69*:5–28, 1960.

AMA Council on Physical Medicine and Rehabilitation: Minimum requirements for acceptable pure tone audiometers for diagnostic purposes. *JAMA 146*:255–257, 1951.

American National Standards Institute: *Volume Measurements of Electrical Speech and Program Waves.* ANSI C16.5-1954 (R1961). New York: American National Standards Institute, 1961.

American National Standards Institute: *Standard Specifications for Audiometers.* ANSI S3.6-1969 (R1973). New York: American National Standards Institute, 1969.

American National Standards Institute: *Specifications for an Artificial Head Bone.* ANSI S3.13-1972. New York: American National Standards Institute, 1972.

American National Standards Institute: *Standard Criteria for Permissible Ambient Noise During Audiometric Testing.* ANSI S3.1-1977. New York: American National Standards Institute, 1977.

American National Standards Institute: *Methods for Manual Pure-Tone Threshold Audiometry.* S3.21-1978. New York: American National Standards Institute (1978).

American Speech and Hearing Association: Guidelines for audiometric symbols. *Asha, 16*:260–264, 1974.

American Speech and Hearing Association: Guidelines for determining threshold level for speech. *Asha, 19*:241–243, 1977.

American Speech and Hearing Association: Guidelines for manual pure-tone threshold audiometry. *Asha, 20*:297–301, 1978*a*.

American Speech and Hearing Association: Guidelines for acoustic immittance screening of middle ear function. *Asha, 20*:550–555, 1978*b*.

American Speech and Hearing Association: *PSB Accreditation Manual.* Rockville, MD: American Speech and Hearing Association, 1978*c*.

American Standards Association: *American Standard Specification for Audiometers for General Diagnostic Purposes.* Z24.5-151. New York: American National Standards Institute, 1951.

Anderson, H., and Barr, B.: Conductive high-tone hearing loss. *Arch. Otolaryngol., 93*:599–605, 1971.

Arlinger, S., Kylen, P., and Hellqvist, H.: Skull distortion of bone conducted signals. *Acta Otolaryngol., 85*:318–323, 1978.

Babbidge, H.: *Education of the Deaf.* Washington, DC: U.S. Dept. of Health, Education, and Welfare, 1965.

Barry, S., and Resnick, S.: Absolute thresholds for frequency-modulated signals: Effects of rate, pattern, and percentage of modulation. *J. Speech Hear. Disord., 43*:192–199, 1978.

Beasley, W.: *The National Health Survey; Hearing Studies Series.* Bulletin #2, Washington, DC: U.S. Public Health Service, 1938.

Beasley, D., and Rintelmann, A.: Central auditory processing. In *Hearing Assessment,* edited by W. Rintelmann, Ch. 10 Baltimore: University Park Press, 1979.

Beattie, R., Edgerton, B., and Svihovec, D.: A comparison of the Auditec of St. Louis cassette recordings of NU-6 and CID W-22 on a normal-hearing population. *J. Speech Hear. Disord., 42*:60–64, 1977*a*.

Beattie, R., Forrester, P., and Ruby, B.: Reliability of the Tillman-Olsen procedure for determination of spondee threshold using recorded and live voice presentations. *J. Am. Aud. Soc., 2*:159–162, 1977*b*.

Beattie, R., Svihovec, D., and Edgerton, B.: Relative intelligibility of the CID spondees as presented via monitored live voice. *J. Speech Hear. Disord., 40*:84–91, 1975.

Beattie, R., Svihovec, D., and Edgerton, B.: Comparison of speech detection and spondee thresholds and half-list versus full-list intelligibility scores with MLV and taped presentations of NU-6. *J. Am. Aud. Soc., 3*:267–272, 1978.

Bekesy, G.: *Experiments in Hearing.* New York: McGraw-Hill, 1960.

Berlin, C., and Cullen, J.: The physical basis of impedance measurement. In *Handbook of Clinical Impedance Audiometry*, edited by J. Jerger, Ch. 1, Dobbs Ferry, NY: American Electromedics Corp., 1975.

Bienvenue, G., and Michael, P.: Noise attenuation characteristics of the MX-41/AR and the Telephonics circumaural audiometric headsets. *J. Am. Aud. Soc., 4*:1–5, 1978.

Bluestone, C.: Assessment of Eustachian tube function. In *Handbook of Clinical Impedance Audiometry*, edited by J. Jerger, Ch. 6, Dobbs Ferry, NY: American Electromedics Corp., 1975.

Brooks, D.: Middle-ear impedance measurements in screening. *Audiology, 16*:288–293, 1977.

Campbell, R.: An index of pseudo-discrimination loss. *J. Speech Hear. Res., 8*:77–84, 1965.

Carhart, R.: An improved method for classifying audiograms. *Laryngoscope, 55*: 640–662, 1945.

Carhart, R.: Monitored live-voice as a test of auditory acuity. *J. Acoust. Soc. Am., 17*:339–349, 1946.

Carhart, R.: Clinical application of bone conduction audiometry. *Arch. Otolaryngol., 51*: 798–807, 1950.

Carhart, R.: Basic principles of speech audiometry. *Acta Otolaryngol., 40*:62–71, 1951.

Carhart, R.: Speech audiometry in clinical evaluation. *Arch. Otolaryngol., 41*:18–22, 1952.

Carhart, R.: The determination of hearing loss. *DM&S Bulletin* IB 10-115, Veterans Administration, 1960.

Carhart, R.: Problems in the measurement of speech discrimination. *Arch. Otolaryngol., 82*:253–260, 1965.

Carhart, R., and Hayes, C.: Clinical reliability of bone conduction audiometry. *Laryngoscope, 59*:1084–1101, 1949.

Carhart, R., and Jerger, J.: Preferred method for clinical determination of pure-tone thresholds. *J. Speech Hear. Disord., 24*:330–345, 1959.

Carter, H.: Tentative standard procedure for evaluating the percentage loss of hearing in medicolegal cases. *JAMA, 133*:396–397, 1947.

Chaiklin, J., and Ventry, I.: Spondee threshold measurement: A comparison of 2- and 5-dB methods. *J. Speech Hear. Disord., 29*:47–59, 1964.

Chandler, J.: Partial occlusion of the external auditory meatus: Its effect upon air and bone conduction hearing acuity. *Laryngoscope, 74*:22–54, 1964.

Cooper, J., and Langley, L.: Multiple choice discrimination tests for both diagnostic and rehabilitative evaluation: English and Spanish. *J. Acad. Rehabilitative Audiol., 11*:132–141, 1978.

Cox, J., and Bilger, R.: Suggestion relative to the standardization of loudness balance data for the Telephonics TDH-39 earphone. *J. Acoust. Soc. Am., 32*:1081, 1960.

Cozad, R.: A survey of hearing conservation programs conducted by public health and school nurses. *J. Sch. Health, 36*:454–461, 1966.

Danaloff, R., Schuckers, G., and Feth, L.: *The Physiology of Speech and Hearing*. Englewood Cliffs, NJ: Prentice-Hall, Inc., 1980.

Davis, H.: The articulation area and the social adequacy index for hearing. *Laryngoscope, 58*:761–778, 1948.

Davis, H.: Audiometry: Pure-tone and simple speech tests. In *Hearing and Deafness*, edited by H. Davis and S. Silverman, Ed. 4, Ch. 7, New York: Holt, Rinehart and Winston, 1978.

Davis, H., and Kranz, F.: The international standard reference zero for pure-tone audiometers and its relation to the evaluation of the impairment of hearing. *J. Speech Hear. Res., 7*:7–16, 1964.

Dirks, D.: Factors related to bone conduction reliability. *Arch. Otolaryngol., 79*:551–558, 1964.

Dirks, D.: Bone-conduction testing. *Handbook of Clinical Audiology* (Rev. Ed.), edited by J. Katz, Ch. 10, Baltimore: Williams & Wilkins, 1978.

Dirks, D., and Carhart, R.: A survey of reactions from users of binaural and monaural hearing aids. *J. Speech Hear. Disord., 27*:311–322, 1962.

Dirks, D., and Kamm, C.: Bone-vibrator measurements: Physical characteristics and behavioral thresholds. *J. Speech Hear. Res., 18*:242–260, 1975.

Dirks, D., and Malmquist, C.: Comparison of frontal and mastoid bone-conduction thresholds in various conductive lesions. *J. Speech Hear. Res., 12*:725–746, 1969.

Dirks, D., and Swindeman, J.: The variability of occluded and unoccluded bone conduction thresholds. *J. Speech Hear. Res., 10*:232–249, 1967.

Dirks, D., Lybarger, S., Olsen, W., and Billings, B.: Bone conduction calibration: Current status. *J. Speech Hear. Disord., 44*:143–155, 1979.

Dodds, E., and Harford, E.: Application of a lipreading test in a hearing aid evaluation. *J. Speech Hear. Disord., 33*:167–173, 1968.

Eagles, E., Wishik, S., and Doerfler, L.: Hearing sensitivity and ear disease in children: A prospective study. *Laryngoscope, Suppl.*, 1–274, 1967.

Egan, J.: Articulation testing methods. *Laryngoscope, 58*:955–991, 1948.

Eldert, E., and Davis, H.: The articulation function of patients with conductive deafness. *Laryngoscope, 61*:891–909, 1951.

Elliott, L., and Armbruster, V.: Some possible effects of the delay of early treatment of deafness. *J. Speech Hear. Res., 10*:209–224, 1967.

Elliott, L., Connors, S., Kille, E., Levin, S., Ball, K., and Katz, D.: Children's understanding of monosyllabic nouns in quiet and in noise. *J. Acoust. Soc. Am., 66*:12–21, 1979.

Fairbanks, G.: Test of phonemic differentiation: The rhyme test. *J. Acoust. Soc. Am., 30*: 596–601, 1958.

Feldman, A.: Tympanometry. In *Acoustic Impedance and Admittance—The Measurement of Middle Ear Function*, edited by A. Feldman and L. Wilber, Ch. 6, Baltimore: Williams & Wilkins, 1976a.

Feldman, A.: Tympanometry: Application and interpretation. *Ann. Otol. Rhinol., Laryngol., 85, Suppl. 25*:202–208, 1976b.

Feldman, A., and Wilber, L. (Eds.): *Acoustic Impedance and Admittance—The Measurement of Middle Ear Function*, Baltimore: Williams & Wilkins, 1976.

Finitzo-Hieber, T., Gerling, I., Cherow-Skalka, E., and Matkin, N.: A sound effects recognition test for the pediatric audiological evaluation. *Ear and Hearing* (in press).

Fletcher, H.: *Speech and Hearing*, New York: D. Van Nostrand, 1929.

Fletcher, H.: Auditory patterns. *Rev. Mod. Physics, 12*:47–65, 1940.

Fletcher, H., A Method of calculating hearing loss for speech from an audiogram. *Acta Otolaryngol., Suppl. 90*:26–37, 1950.

Fletcher, H. *Speech and Hearing in Communication*, New York: D. Van Nostrand, 1953.

French, N., and Steinberg, J.: Factors governing the intelligibility of speech sounds. *J. Acoust. Soc. Am., 19*:90–119, 1947.

Frisina, D.: Audiometric evaluation and its relation to habilitation and rehabilitation of the deaf. *Am. Ann. Deaf, 107*:478–481, 1962.

Gaeth, J.: A study in phonemic regression in relation to hearing loss. Unpublished doctoral dissertation, Northwestern University, 1948.

Gang, R.: The effects of age on the diagnostic utility of the rollover phenomenon. *J. Speech Hear. Disord., 41*:63–69, 1976.

Gengel, R.: On the reliability of discrimination-performance in persons with sensorineural hearing-impairment using a closed-set test. *J. Aud. Res., 13*:97–100, 1973.

Ginsberg, I., and White, T.: Otological considerations in audiology. In *Handbook of Clinical Audiology* (Rev. Ed.), edited by J. Katz, Ch. 2, Baltimore: Williams & Wilkins, 1978.

Giolas, T., and Epstein, A.: Comparative intelligibility of word lists and continuous discourse. *J. Speech Hear. Res., 6*:349–358, 1963.

Giolas, T., and Randolph, K.: *Basic Audiometry,* Lincoln, NE: Cliffs Notes, 1977.

Giolas, T., and Wark, D.: Communication problems associated with unilateral hearing loss. *J. Speech Hear. Disord., 32*:336–343, 1967.

Giolas, T., Owens, E., Lamb, S., and Schubert, E.: Hearing performance inventory. *J. Speech Hear. Disord., 44*:169–195, 1979.

Glorig, A.: *Audiometry: Principles and Practices,* Baltimore: Williams & Wilkins, 1965.

Glattke, T.: Anatomy and physiology of the auditory system. In *Audiological Assessment* (Rev. Ed.), edited by D. Rose, Ch. 2, Englewood Cliffs, NJ: Prentice-Hall, 1978.

Goetzinger, C.: Effects of small perceptive losses on language and on speech discrimination. *Volta Rev., 64*:408–414, 1962.

Goetzinger, C.: The psychology of hearing impairment. In *Handbook of Clinical Audiology* (Rev. Ed.), edited by J. Katz, Ch. 37, Baltimore: Williams & Wilkins, 1978.

Goetzinger, C., and Angell, S.: Audiological assessment in acoustic tumors and cortical lesions. *EENT Monthly, 44*:39–49, 1965.

Goetzinger, C., Harrison, C., and Baer, C.: Small perceptive hearing loss: Its effect in school-age children. *Volta Rev., 65*:124–131, 1964.

Goodhill, V., Dirks, D., and Malmquist, C.: Bone-conduction thresholds; relationships of frontal and mastoid measurements in conductive hypacusis. *Arch. Otolaryngol., 91*:250–256, 1970.

Goodhill, V., and Holcomb, A.: Cochlear potentials in the evaluation of bone conduction. *Ann. Otol. Rhinol. Laryngol., 64*:1213–1233, 1955.

Green, D.: Pure tone air-conduction testing. In *Handbook of Clinical Audiology* (Rev. Ed.), edited by J. Katz, Ch. 9, Baltimore: Williams & Wilkins, 1978.

Hallpike, C., and Hood, J.: Some recent work on auditory adaptation and its relationship to the loudness recruitment phenomenon. *J. Acoust. Soc. Am. 23*: 270–274, 1951.

Harford, E., and Barry, J.: A rehabilitative approach to the problem of unilateral hearing impairment: The contralateral routing of signals (CROS). *J. Speech Hear. Disord., 30*: 121–138, 1965.

Harford, E., and Musket, C.: Binaural hearing with one hearing aid. *J. Speech Hear. Disord., 29*:133–146, 1964.

Harris, J., Haines, H., and Myers, C.: A helmet-held bone conduction vibrator. *Laryngoscope, 63*:998–1007, 1953.

Haskins, H.: A phonetically balanced test of speech discrimination for children. Unpublished master's thesis, Northwestern University, 1949.

High, W., Fairbanks, G., and Glorig, A.: Scale for self-assessment of hearing handicap. *J. Speech Hear. Disord., 29*:215–230, 1964.

Hirsh, I., Davis, H., Silverman, S., Reynolds, E., Eldert, E., and Benson, R.: Development of materials for speech audiometry. *J. Speech Hear. Disord., 17*:321–337, 1952.

Hirsh, I., Reynolds, E., and Joseph, M.: Intelligibility of different speech materials. *J. Acoust. Soc. Am., 26*:530–538, 1954.

Hodgson, W.: Audiological report of a patient with left hemispherectomy. *J. Speech Hear. Disord., 32*:39–45, 1967.

Hodgson, W.: Auditory characteristics of post-rubella impairment. *Volta Rev., 71*:97–103, 1969.

Hodgson, W.: A comparison of WIPI and PB-K discrimination test scores. Paper presented at the meeting of the American Speech and Hearing Association, Detroit, October, 1973.

Hodgson, W.: Clinical measures of hearing aid performance. In *Hearing Aid Assessment and Use in Audiologic Habilitation,* edited by W. Hodgson and P. Skinner, Ch. 8, Baltimore: Williams & Wilkins, 1977a.

Hodgson, W.: Special cases of hearing aid assessment: CROS aids. In *Hearing Aid*

Assessment and Use in Audiologic Habilitation, edited by W. Hodgson and P. Skinner, Ch. 10, Baltimore, Williams & Wilkins, 1977b.

Hodgson, W.: Testing infants and young children. In *Handbook of Clinical Audiology* (Rev. Ed.), edited by J. Katz, Ch. 33, Baltimore: Williams & Wilkins, 1978.

Hodgson, W., and Skinner, P. (Eds.): *Hearing Aid Assessment and Use in Audiologic Habilitation,* Baltimore: Williams & Wilkins, 1977.

Hodgson, W., and Tillman, T.: Reliability of bone conduction occlusion effects in normals. *J. Aud. Res., 6*:141–151, 1966.

Hood, J.: Principles and practices of bone conduction audiometry. *Laryngoscope, 70*:1211–1228, 1960.

Hopkinson, N.: Speech reception threshold. In *Handbook of Clinical Audiology* (Rev. Ed.), edited by J. Katz, Ch. 12, Baltimore: Williams & Wilkins, 1978.

House, A., Williams, C., Hecker, M., and Kryter, K.: Articulation-testing methods: Consonantal differentiation with a closed-response set. *J. Acoust. Soc. Am., 37*:158–166, 1965.

Hudgins, C., Hawkins, J., Karlin, J., and Stevens, S.: The development of recorded auditory tests for measuring hearing loss for speech. *Laryngoscope, 57*:57–89, 1947.

Hughson, W., and Thompson, E.: Correlation of hearing acuity for speech with discrete frequency audiograms. *Arch. Otolaryngol., 36*:526–540, 1942.

International Electrotechnical Commission: *An IEC Mechanical Coupler for the Calibration of Bone Vibrators Having a Specified Contact Area and Being Applied with a Specific Static Force,* IEC-373, 1971.

International Standards Organization: *Standard Reference Zero for the Calibration of Pure-Tone Audiometers.* ISO Recommendation R 389. New York: American National Standards Institute, 1964.

Jerger, J.: Clinical experience with impedance audiometry. *Arch. Otolaryngol., 92*:311–324, 1970.

Jerger, J.: Forum: The future of Audiology. *Asha, 16*:249–250, 1974.

Jerger, J.: Impedance terminology. *Arch. Otolaryngol., 101*:589–590, 1975.

Jerger, J., Anthony, L., Jerger, S., and Mauldin, L.: Studies in impedance audiometry III: Middle ear disorders. *Arch. Otolaryngol., 99*:165–171, 1974c.

Jerger, J., Burney, P., Mauldin, L., and Crump, B.: Predicting hearing loss from the acoustic reflex. *J. Speech Hear. Disord., 39*:11–22, 1974a.

Jerger, J., and Harford, E.: Alternate and simultaneous binaural balancing of pure tones. *J. Speech Hear. Res., 3*:15–30, 1960.

Jerger, H., Harford, E., Clemis, J., and Alford, B.: The acoustic reflex in eighth nerve disorders. *Arch. Otolaryngol., 99*:409–413, 1974b.

Jerger, J., and Hayes, D.: Hearing aid evaluation: Clinical experience with a new philosophy. *Arch. Otolaryngol., 102*:214–225, 1976.

Jerger, J., and Jerger, S.: Psychoacoustic comparison of cochlear and VIII nerve disorders. *J. Speech Hear. Res., 10*:659–688, 1967.

Jerger, J., and Jerger, S.: Audiological comparison of cochlear and eighth nerve disorders. *Ann. Otol. Rhinol. Laryngol., 83*:275–285, 1974.

Jerger, S., and Jerger, J.: Extra- and intra-axial brain stem auditory disorders. *Audiology, 14*:93–117, 1975.

Jerger, S., and Jerger, J.: Diagnostic value of crossed vs. uncrossed acoustic reflexes. *Arch. Otolaryngol., 103*:445–453, 1977.

Jerger, S., and Jerger, J.: Quantifying auditory handicap. A new approach. *Audiology, 18*: 225–237, 1979.

Jerger, J., Jerger, S., and Mauldin, L.: Studies in impedance audiometry I: Normal and sensorineural ears. *Arch. Otolaryngol., 96*: 513–523, 1972.

Jerger, S., Jerger, J., Mauldin, L., and Segal, P.: Studies in impedance audiometry II: Children less than 6 years old. *Arch. Otolaryngol., 99*:1–9, 1974d.

Jerger, J., Speaks, C., and Trammell, J.: A new approach to speech audiometry. *J. Speech*

Hear. Disord., *33*:318–328, 1968.

Jerger, J., and Tillman, T.: A new method for the clinical determination of sensorineural acuity level (SAL). *Arch. Otolaryngol.*, *71*:948–953, 1960.

Jirsa, R., and Hodgson, W.: Effects of harmonic distortion in hearing aids on speech intelligibility for normals and hypacusics. *J. Aud. Res.*, *10*:213–217, 1970.

Kapteyn, T.: Satisfaction with fitted hearing aids. II. An investigation into the influence of psycho-social factors. *Scand. Audiol.*, *6*:171–177, 1977.

Karlin, J., Abram, M., Stanford, F., and Curtis, J.: Auditory tests of the ability to hear speech in noise. OSRD, Report #3516, 1944.

Kasten, R., Lotterman, S., and Hinchman, S.: Head shadow and head baffle effects in ear level aids. *Acustica*, *17*:154–160, 1967–1968.

Katz, D., and Elliott, L.: Development of a new children's speech discrimination test. Paper presented at the meeting of the American Speech and Hearing Association, San Francisco, November, 1978.

Katz, J (Ed.), *Handbook of Clinical Audiology* (Rev. Ed.), Baltimore: Williams & Wilkins, 1978.

Keaster, J.: A quantitative method of testing the hearing of young children. *J. Speech Disord.*, *12*:159–160, 1947.

Kirikae, I.: An experimental study on the fundamental mechanism of bone conduction. *Acta Otolaryngol.*, *Suppl. 145:* 1959.

Konig, E.: Variations in bone conduction as related to the force of pressure exerted on the vibrator. *Beltone Institute for Hearing Research*, No. 6, 1957.

Kreul, E., Bell, D., and Nixon, J.: Factors affecting speech discrimination test difficulty. *J. Speech Hear. Res.*, *12*:281–287, 1969.

Kreul, E., Nixon, J., Kryter, K., Bell, D., Lang, J., and Schubert, E.: A proposed clinical test of speech discrimination. *J. Speech Hear. Res.*, *11*: 536–552, 1968.

Lehiste, I., and Peterson, G.: Linguistic considerations in the study of speech intelligibility. *J. Acoust. Soc. Am.*, *31*:280–286, 1959.

Lezak, R.: Determination of an intensity level to obtain PB max. *Laryngoscope*, *73*:267–274, 1963.

Graham, A. (Ed.). *Sensorineural Processes and Disorders*, Boston: Little, Brown & Co., 1967.

Liden, G., Harford, E., and Hallen, O.: Tympanometry for the diagnosis of ossicular disruption. *Arch. Otolaryngol.*, *99*:23–29, 1974a.

Liden, G., Harford, E., and Hallen, O.: Automatic tympanometry in clinical practice. *Audiology*, *13*:126–139, 1974b.

Liden, G., Nilsson, G., and Anderson, H.: Masking in clinical audiometry. *Acta Otolaryngol.*, *50*:125–136, 1959.

Lierle, D.: Guide for the evaluation of hearing impairment. *Am. Acad. Ophthal. Otolaryngol. Trans.*, *63*:236–238, 1959.

Lybarger, S.: Interim bone conduction thresholds for audiometry. *J. Speech Hear. Res.*, *9*: 483–487, 1966.

Martin, F.: Speech audiometry and clinical masking. *J. Aud. Res.*, *6*:199–203, 1966.

Martin, F., and Pennington, C.: Current trends in audiometric practices. *Asha*, *13*:671–677, 1971.

Matkin, N.: Hearing aids for children. In *Hearing Aid Assessment and Use in Audiologic Habilitation*, edited by W. Hodgson and P. Skinner, Ch. 9, Baltimore: Williams & Wilkins, 1977.

McCandless, G., and Thomas, G.: Impedance audiometry as a screening procedure for middle ear disease. *Am. Acad. Ophthal. Otolaryngol. Trans.*, *78*:98–102, 1974.

McNeill, D.: The capacity for language acquisition. In U.S. Dept. of Health, Education, and Welfare, *Research on Behavioral Aspects of Deafness*, Washington, DC: Vocational Rehabilitation Administration, 1965.

Melnick, W., Eagles, E., and Levine, H.: Evaluation of a recommended program of identification audiometry with school-age children. *J. Speech Hear. Disord., 29*:3–13, 1964.

Merklein, R., and Briskey, T.: Audiometric findings in children referred to a program for language disorders. *Volta Rev., 64*:295–298, 1962.

Merrell, H., and Atkinson, C.: The effect of selected variables upon discrimination scores. *J. Aud. Res., 5*:285–292, 1965.

Naunton, R., and Elpern, B.: Interaural phase and intensity relationships: The Weber test. *Laryngoscope, 74*:55–63, 1964.

Niemeyer, W., and Sesterhenn, G.: Calculating the hearing threshold from the stapedius reflex threshold for different sound stimuli. *Audiology, 13*:421–427, 1974.

Northern, J., and Downs, M.: *Hearing in Children* (Rev. Ed.), Baltimore: Williams & Wilkins, 1978.

Northern, J., and Grimes, A., Introduction to acoustic impedance. In *Handbook of Clinical Audiology* (Rev. Ed.), edited by J. Katz, Ch. 29, Baltimore: Williams & Wilkins, 1978.

Norton, D., and Hodgson, W.: Intelligibility of black and white speakers for black and white listeners. *Language and Speech, 16*:207–210, 1973.

Olishifski, J., and Harford, E. (Eds.): *Industrial Noise and Hearing Conservation*. Chicago: National Safety Council, 1975.

Olsen, W., and Matkin, N.: Speech audiometry. In *Hearing Assessment*, edited by W. Rintelmann, Ch. 5, Baltimore: University Park Press, 1979.

Olsen, W., and Tillman, T.: Hearing aids and sensorineural hearing loss. *Ann. Otol. Rhinol. Laryngol., 77*:717–726, 1968.

O'Neill, J., and Oyer, H.: *Applied Audiometry*, New York: Dodd, Mead & Co., 1966.

Orchik, D., Krygier, K., and Cutts, B.: A comparison of the NU-6 and W-22 speech discrimination tests for assessing sensorineural loss. *J. Speech Hear. Disord., 44*:522–527, 1979.

Paradise, J., and Smith, C.: Impedance screening for preschool children. *Ann. Otol. Rhinol. Laryngol., 88*:56–65, 1979.

Peterson, G., and Lehiste, I.: Revised CNC lists for auditory tests. *J. Speech Hear. Disord., 27*:62–70, 1962.

Pollack, I., Rubenstein, H., and Decker, L.: Intelligibility of known and unknown message sets. *J. Acoust. Soc. Am., 31*:273–279, 1959.

Posner, J., and Ventry, I.: Relationships between comfortable loudness levels for speech and speech discrimination in sensorineural loss. *J. Speech Hear. Disord., 42*:370–375, 1977.

Price, L.: Pure tone audiometry. In *Audiological Assessment* (Rev. Ed.), edited by D. Rose, Ch. 6, Englewood Cliffs, NJ: Prentice-Hall, Inc., 1978.

Ries, P.: *Academic Achievement Test Results of a National Testing Program for Hearing Impaired Students*. Washington, DC: Office of Demographic Studies, Gallaudet College, 1972.

Rintelmann, W., and Schumaier, D.: Factors affecting speech discrimination in a clinical setting: List equivalence, hearing loss, and phonemic regression. *J. Aud. Res., Suppl. 2*: 12–15, 1974.

Rintelmann, W., Schumaier, D., and Burchfield, S.: Influence of test form on speech discrimination scores of normal listeners on N.U. auditory test no. 6. *J. Aud. Res., Suppl. 2*:8–11, 1974b.

Rintelmann, W., Schumaier, D., and Jetty, A.: List equivalency and reliability for normal listeners on N.U. auditory test no. 6: Comparison with data from original talker. *J. Aud. Res., Suppl. 2*: 3–7, 1974a.

Rintelmann, W., *et al.*: Six experiments on speech discrimination utilizing CNC monosyllables (Northwestern University test no. 6). *J. Aud. Res., Suppl. 2*: 1974.

Rizzo, S., and Greenberg, H.: Influence of ear canal air pressure on acoustic reflex threshold. *J. Am. Aud. Soc., 5:*21–24, 1979.
Roach, R., and Carhart, R.: A clinical method for calibrating the bone-conduction audiometer. *Arch. Otolaryngol., 63:*270–278, 1956.
Rose, D.: A 10-word speech discrimination screening test. Paper presented at the meeting of the American Speech and Hearing Association, Las Vegas, November, 1974.
Ross, M., and Lerman, J.: A picture identification test for hearing-impaired children. *J. Speech Hear. Res., 13:*44–53, 1970.
Ross, M., and Matkin, N.: The rising audiometric configuration. *J. Speech Hear. Disord., 32:*377–382, 1967.
Rupp, R., Higgins, J., and Maurer, J.: A feasibility scale for predicting hearing aid use (FSPHAU) with older individuals. *J. Acad. Rehabilitative Audiol., 10:*81–104, 1977.
Sanders, J.: Masking. In *Handbook of Clinical Audiology,* edited by J. Katz, Ch. 11, Baltimore: Williams & Wilkins, 1978.
Sanders, J., and Rintelmann, W.: Masking in audiometry. *Arch. Otolaryngol., 80:*541–556, 1964.
Scott, B.: Noise induced hearing loss. *Hearing Instruments, 28:*14–15, 28, 1977.
Schuknecht, H.: Presbycusis. *Laryngoscope, 65:*402–419, 1955.
Shambaugh, G., Jr.: *Surgery of the Ear.* Philadelphia: W. B. Saunders, 1959.
Shaw, E.: Ear canal pressure generated by circumaural and supraaural earphones. *J. Acoust. Soc. Am., 39:*471–479, 1966.
Siegenthaler, B., and Smith, D.: Speech reception thresholds by different methods of test administration. *J. Acoust. Soc. Am., 33:*1802, 1961.
Sivian, L., and White, S.: On minimum audible sound fields. *J. Acoust. Soc. Am., 4:*288–321, 1933.
Small, A.: *Elements of Hearing Science; a Programmed Text.* New York: John Wiley & Sons, 1978.
Snow, J., Rintelmann, W., Miller, J., and Konkle, D.: Central auditory imperception. *Laryngoscope, 87:*1450–1471, 1977.
Speaks, C., and Jerger, J.: Method for measurement of speech identification. *J. Speech Hear. Res., 8:*185–194, 1965.
Speaks, C., Jerger, J., and Trammell, J.: Measurement of hearing handicap. *J. Speech Hear. Res., 13:*768–776, 1970.
Staab, W., and Rintelmann, W.: Status of warble-tone in audiometers. *Audiology, 11:*244–255, 1972.
Steele, J., Binnie, C., and Cooper, W.: Combining auditory and visual stimuli in the adaptive testing of speech discrimination. *J. Speech Hear. Disord., 43:*115–122, 1978.
Stisen, B., and Dahm, M.: Sensitivity and mechanical impedance of artificial mastoid type 4930. *Bruel & Kjaer Technical Information*, 1969.
Studebaker, G.: Placement of vibrator in bone conduction testing. *J. Speech Hear. Res., 5:* 321–331, 1962.
Studebaker, G.: Clinical masking of air- and bone-conduction stimuli. *J. Speech Hear. Disord., 29:*23–35, 1964.
Studebaker, G.: Clinical masking of the nontest ear. *J. Speech Hear. Disord., 32:*360–371, 1967.
Thurlow, W., Davis, H., Silverman, S., and Walsh, T.: Further statistical study of auditory tests in relation to the fenestration operation. *Laryngoscope, 59:*113–129, 1949.
Tillman, T.: Clinical applicability of the SAL test. *Arch. Otolaryngol., 78:*36–48, 1963.
Tillman, T., and Carhart, R.: An expanded test for speech discrimination utilizing CNC monosyllabic words: Northwestern University auditory test no. 6. SAM-TR-66-55, 1966.
Tillman, T., Carhart, R., and Wilber, L.: A test for speech discrimination composed of

CNC monosyllabic words (N.U. auditory test no. 4). SAM-TDR-62-135, 1963.

Tillman, T., and Jerger, J.: Some factors affecting the spondee threshold in normal-hearing subjects. *J. Speech Hear. Res.*, 2:141–146, 1959.

Tillman, T., and Olsen, W.: Speech audiometry. *Modern Developments in Audiology* (Rev. Ed.), edited by J. Jerger, Ch. 2, New York: Academic Press, 1973.

Tonndorf, J.: Bone conduction; studies in experimental animals. *Acta Otolaryngol., Suppl. 213,* 1966.

Tonndorf, J.: Bone conduction. In *Foundations of Modern Auditory Theory,* edited by J. Tobias, Ch. 5, New York: Academic Press, 1972.

Tyszka, F., and Goldstein, D.: Interaural phase and amplitude relationships of bone-conduction signals. *J. Acoust. Soc. Am.*, 57:200–206, 1975.

Ventry, I., and Chaiklin, J.: The efficiency of audiometric measures used to identify functional hearing loss. *J. Aud. Res.*, 5:196–211, 1965.

Vernon, M.: Prematurity and deafness: The magnitude and nature of the problem among deaf children. *Except. Child.*, 33:289–298, 1966.

Vernon, M.: Characteristics associated with post rubella deaf children: Psychological, educational, and physical. *Volta Rev.*, 69:176–185, 1967a.

Vernon, M.: Meningitis and deafness: The problem, its physical, audiological, psychological, and educational manifestations in deaf children. *Laryngoscope,* 77:1856–1874, 1967b.

Vernon, M.: Rh factor and deafness: The problem, its psychological, physical, and educational manifestations. *Except. Child.*, 34:5–12, 1967c.

Walsh, T., and Silverman, S.: Diagnosis and evaluation of fenestration. *Laryngoscope,* 56: 536–555, 1946.

Walton, W.: *A Tympanometry-ASHA Model for Identification of the Hearing Impaired.* Windsor, CT: Capitol Region Educational Council, 1975.

Ward, W.: "Sensitivity" versus "acuity." *J. Speech Hear. Res.*, 7:294–295, 1964.

Warder, F., and Hughes, L.: Tympanostomy tubes. *Hearing Loss in Children,* edited by B. Jaffe, Ch. 33, Baltimore: University Park Press, 1977.

Weir, R.: Some questions on the child's learning of phonology. In *The Genesis of Language,* edited by F. Smith and G. Miller, pp. 153–168, Cambridge: The MIT Press, 1966.

Weiss, E.: An air damped artificial mastoid. *J. Acoust. Soc. Am.*, 32: 1582–1588, 1960.

Wiener, F., and Ross, D.: The pressure distribution in the auditory canal in a progressive sound field. *J. Acoust. Soc. Am.*, 18:401–408, 1946.

Wilber, L.: Comparability of two commercially available artificial mastoids. *J. Acoust. Soc. Am.*, 52:1265–1266, 1972.

Wilber, L.: Acoustic reflex measurement—procedures, interpretations and variables. In *Acoustic Impedance and Admittance—The Measurement of Middle Ear Function,* edited by A. Feldman and L. Wilber, Ch. 9, Baltimore: Williams & Wilkins, 1976.

Wilber, L.: Calibration, pure tone, speech and noise signals. In *Handbook of Clinical Audiology* (Rev. Ed.), edited by J. Katz, Ch. 8, Baltimore: Williams & Wilkins, 1978.

Wilson, R., Coley, K., Haenel, J., and Browning, K.: Northwestern University auditory test no. 6: Normative and comparative intelligibility functions. *J. Am. Aud. Soc.*, 1:221–228, 1976.

Yost, W., and Nielsen, D.: *Fundamentals of Hearing,* New York: Holt, Rinehart and Winston, 1977.

Zwislocki, J.: Acoustic attenuation between the ears. *J. Acoust. Soc. Am.*, 25:752–759, 1953.

Author Index

Subject Index